THE
COMPENDIUM
COLLECTION

Exotic Animal Medicine in Practice

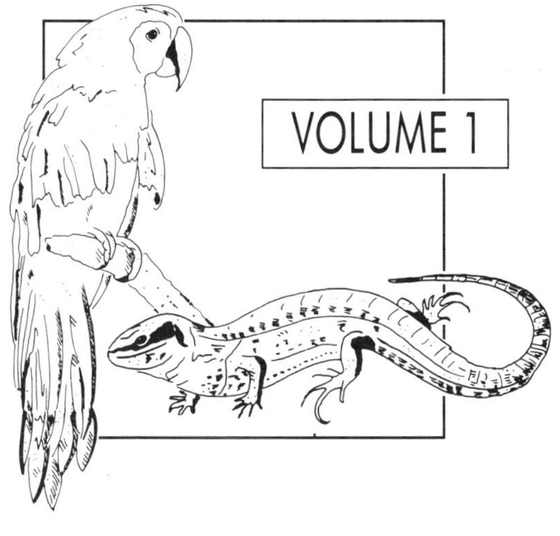

VOLUME 1

DUDLEY E. JOHNSTON, MVSc, EDITOR

Preface

The Compendium Collection gathers together the best, most practical information from the pages of *The Compendium on Continuing Education for the Practicing Veterinarian*. This edition, *Exotic Animal Medicine in Practice*, includes two volumes. Volume 1 is a republication of the articles that appeared in the fifth anniversary series. Because of its enthusiastic reception and repeated requests for copies of that text, we chose to make those same articles available once again under one convenient cover. In addition, we have expanded our coverage of this burgeoning area of veterinary practice by providing more recently published articles on exotic animal topics in Volume 2. In both volumes the articles have been updated, as necessary, by the authors to reflect new information and developments that have occurred since their original publication in the journal. Such new information has been appended to the article, following the references. Articles that do not include these updates were judged to have withstood the test of time in terms of the practicality and timeliness of their content without the need for any such material.

Editor

DUDLEY E. JOHNSTON, MVSc, Diplomate ACVS, is Head of Small Animal Surgery and Director of the small animal hospital at the University of Pennsylvania. He is also Professor of Surgery in the university's School of Veterinary Medicine.

Dr. Johnston, a graduate of the University of Sydney School of Veterinary Science in Australia, did his graduate studies in experimental surgery and radiology at the University of Toronto. Before coming to the University of Pennsylvania, he was in private mixed practice for eight years in Australia and was then Head of Surgery at the University of Melbourne School of Veterinary Science.

Published by Veterinary Learning Systems
Trenton, New Jersey

Contents

The Biology, Care, and Diseases of the Syrian Hamster*

August H. Battles, DVM
Department of Special Clinical Sciences
College of Veterinary Medicine
University of Florida
Gainesville, Florida

Hamsters are rodents with anatomic, physiologic, and clinical peculiarities that have made them useful as research animals. They are not native to the United States but were brought there for research purposes.[1] Although there are many species of hamsters, the Syrian (golden) hamster is the most common.[2]

The hamster is relatively resistant to diseases compared with other rodents. Proliferative ileitis, thought to be a bacterial disease, is the most frequently seen disease. Viral infections have been reported often, but most cause few clinical diseases. Protozoa, nematodes, cestodes, and mites are capable of parasitizing a hamster.[2] The incidence of neoplasms is low in hamsters, with lymphomas being the most common.[3] In aged hamsters, amyloidosis and atrial thrombosis are frequently seen and are responsible for the death of a large percentage of the aged.[3,4] Hamsters with dental disease, although not often reported, are seen by clinical veterinarians. Reproductive problems also occur and are frequently related to management, which plays an important part in disease prevention in hamsters.

This article reviews the biology and care of hamsters as well as the common problems presented to veterinary practitioners.

History

Hamsters were introduced into the United States in 1938. The Syrian hamster ranges in the wild from Rumania and Bulgaria southeastward through Asia Minor, Israel, and northwestern Iran. They were first used as laboratory research animals in 1930, at which time a litter of eight was brought to what is now Israel. All present domesticated strains of Syrian hamsters developed from this stock.[1]

Chinese hamsters were brought to the United States in 1948. From 1949 to 1952, they were domesticated and reproduction in captivity began. This species is useful in research because it offers a unique morphologic feature of having the lowest number of chromosomes of the common laboratory animal and is susceptible to diabetes mellitus and other diseases of public health significance. Chinese hamsters, however, are more difficult to breed in captivity than Syrian hamsters are.[5]

*This work was supported in part by the National Institute of Health Grant RR07001.

Characteristics

Hamsters are rodents in the family Cricetidae. Cricetidae are characterized by having large cheek pouches, short tails, and thick bodies.[6] The two most common genera of hamsters in the Cricetidae are the Syrian (*Mesocricetus auratus*) and the Chinese (*Cricetulus griseus*).[2] The Syrian hamster has 22 pairs of chromosomes and the Chinese hamster has 11.[5,7]

Varieties of Syrian hamsters include the wild type or reddish brown, cinnamon, cream, white piebald, and longhaired "teddy bear." Reddish golden brown is the most common. Chinese hamsters are smaller than Syrian hamsters and are dark brown.

Rodents are remarkably uniform in characteristics, especially in dentition. Like other rodents, hamsters have four incisors—two upper and two lower. The incisors grow throughout life, and there is no nerve in the incisor teeth except at the base. The outer surface of incisor teeth is to some extent self-sharpening. Rodents lack canine and premolar teeth.

The radius and ulna are distinct bones of the lower arm, and the elbow joint allows free rotation of the forearm. The hand has five fingers and the foot three to five toes. The penis of rodents has a baculum (os penis). The brain has a smooth cerebrum and large olfactory bulbs. The functions of the areas of the cerebrum are generalized rather than specialized.[6]

Adult Syrian hamsters weigh between 85 to 150 g, with the female being larger and maturing earlier. Newborn hamsters (pups) weigh approximately 2 to 4 g, with the male being slightly larger. The maximum weight is attained by six months of age.[8]

Hamsters have well-developed cheek pouches that are used to transport and store food and to conceal a newborn litter when danger is present (Figure 1). The cheek pouch, an evagination of the lateral buccal wall, is devoid of glands, highly distensible, lined with stratified squamous epithelium, and well vascularized.[7,8]

The stomach is divided into two distinct regions that are separated by a constriction and are described as the *squamous* and *glandular stomachs*.[8] The nonglandular forestomach is characteristic of ruminants in that it contains microorganisms and a high pH suggestive of a fermentation process.[9]

Adult male and female hamsters can be differentiated easily; the caudal area of a male is elongated because the testicles are carried caudally and well outside and behind the body. The vesicular gland and testes appear large in relation to the body size. The abdominal cavity of males may seem to be filled with the vesicular gland, which is an outpouching of the vas deferens with branching tubules. In addition to the vesicular gland, there are two additional accessory sex glands—the coagulating gland and the prostate. The sex of younger hamsters can be determined by measuring the distance between the anus and the genitals, which is greater in males. In the perineal area of females, there are three openings: the anus, the vulva, and the urethra. The uterus is bicornuate, with each uterine horn having a separate opening into the vagina. The female generally has 12 to 14 nipples.[7]

The anatomic and functional peculiarities of hamsters are noted in some of the glands. Sebaceous glands, referred to as *hip glands*, are located on either flank in both males and females (Figure 2) and are used as sex

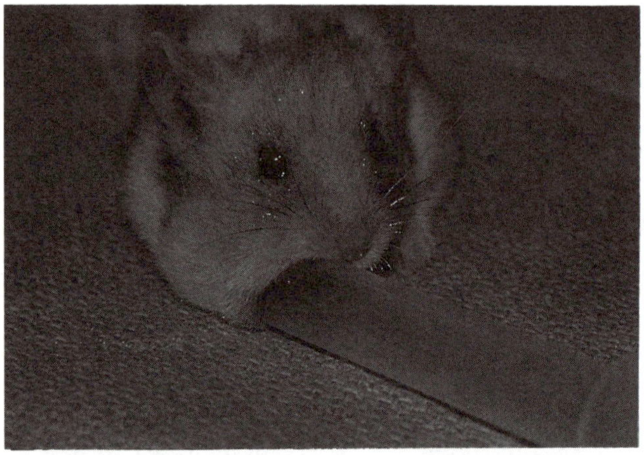

Figure 1—The cheek pouch of a mature Syrian hamster with a 3-cc syringe case inserted to demonstrate the size of the pouch.

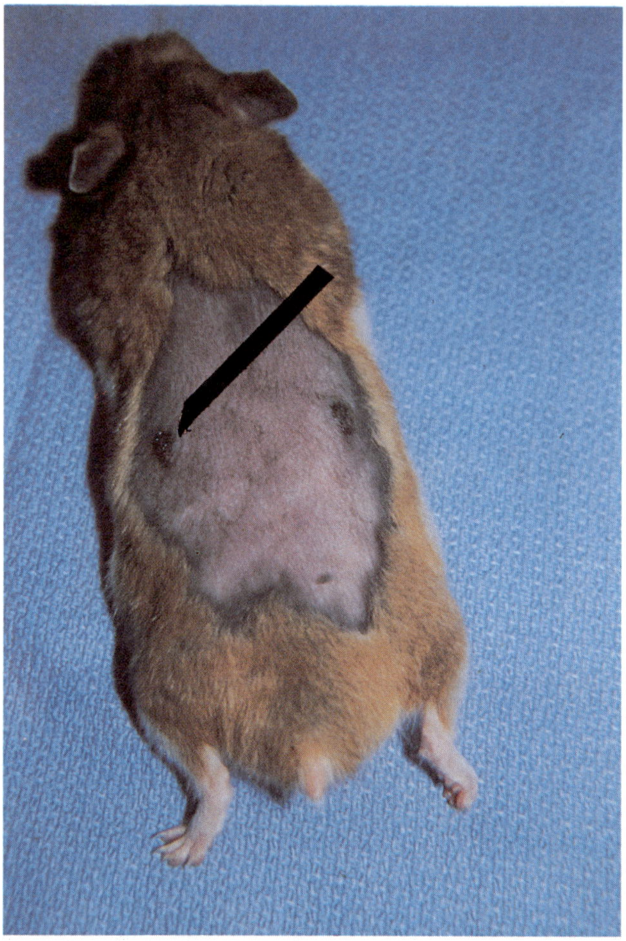

Figure 2—The black spots on the back of a hamster (one marked with an arrow) are called the *hip glands*.

glands and for olfactory marking of territory. They can be visualized if the hair is clipped over the flank. In sexually aroused males, these glands become matted from secretions and are readily visible.[8] Hamsters will scratch themselves, as if the area was pruritic. The harderian glands have also been shown to secrete sexually attractive substances.[10] The adrenal glands of male hamsters are larger than those of females. In other rodents, the size of the adrenal glands does not differ between the sexes.[11]

Syrian hamsters have a relatively short life span, usually 18 to 24 months; unlike many other mammals, females have a shorter life span than males. Old-age lesions, such as cardiac thrombosis and amyloidosis, that affect the life span occur earlier in the females.[12] Female Syrian hamsters have a reproductive life span of one year, while males have a reproductive life span of two years.[13]

Sexual maturity of Syrian hamsters occurs around two months and is two weeks earlier in females than in males. The estrous cycle is four days.[13] Estrus usually begins in the evening hours, with ovulation occurring between 12:00 midnight and 1:00 AM. Females demonstrate lordosis. On the morning after estrus, a characteristic thick, white, opaque, smelly discharge may be expressed from the vagina. On Day 3, a waxy discharge may be present. On Day 4, there is a translucent mucous discharge. If bred, sperm may be seen in the vaginal smear. A copulation plug may be found in the cage the morning after breeding. The plug is a white, waxy mass extruded in the form of a cast of the vaginal cavity and is composed of secretions from the male's accessory sex glands and secretions and cells from the female's vaginal wall.[14] Estrus occurs one to eight days after parturition.[13]

The average duration of pregnancy is 15½ days; it is characterized by a series of changes in the vaginal excretions. When correlated with weight changes, these excretions can be used to distinguish pregnant from nonpregnant individuals as early as 10 days of gestation. On Day 4 of pregnancy, the vagina contains a stringy transparent fluid that may appear to have many bubbles; and on Day 5 or 6 it may contain white flakes. The flocculent content continues to increase until Day 9 or 10, at which time the discharge becomes white and waxy, similar to the discharge after the evening of estrus.[14]

Pseudopregnancy can occur in a nonfertile mating and lasts from 8 to 12 days. A pseudopregnant female resembles a pregnant female until termination of the pseudopregnancy. During the final two days of pseudopregnancy, there is a decrease in body weight. At the end of pseudopregnancy, a normal estrous cycle is resumed.[14]

The average litter size is six to eight pups. Before parturition, a female is restless and exhibits excessive grooming and nest-building tasks. A bloody discharge may be present before the first fetus is born. Newborns are hairless, blind, and have closed ears and undeveloped limbs. Teeth are evident at birth. Hair growth begins at nine days of age.[15] Pups are capable of eating hard food at 7 to 10 days of age and open their eyes at 14 to 15 days of age. Weaning occurs at 21 to 25 days of age.[8]

Unlike seasonal hibernators, Syrian hamsters may hibernate in response to lowered environmental temperatures (below 40° F [4.4°C]). All will not hibernate spontaneously, but instead hibernation depends on such variables as food supply. The duration of hibernation is short, usually two to three days, but may be as long as five to seven days. Hibernation is not a continuous state, with arousal and return to hibernation occurring within a 12-hour period or less.[16]

Basic physiologic norms of hamsters are listed in Table I.[7,8,17]

Husbandry

Hamsters are nocturnal, burrow-dwelling animals with brief periods of diurnal activity. They may develop a pugnacious disposition if they are aroused during their rest period. Food and water consumption take place mainly during the evening hours. Females (when larger than the males) are the dominant individuals; a female can be very aggressive toward a smaller male, especially during anestrus, and has been known to inflict serious injury. Frequent, gentle handling of hamsters will keep them tame and easy to handle. Hamsters have a tendency to seek dark, protected areas.[6]

The nutritional requirements of omnivorous hamsters have not been determined specifically, but a pelleted rodent diet containing 15% to 20% protein is currently recommended.[18] Hamsters eat approximately 12 g of

TABLE I
Physiologic Data[7,8,17]

Body temperature	37° to 38°C (98° to 99°F)
Respiratory rate	35–135 breaths/min
Blood volume	0.078 ml/g body weight
Heart rate	250–500 beats/min
Packed cell volume	36% to 55%
Red blood cells	6 to 10 × 10^6/mm^3
White blood cells	3 to 11 × 10^3/mm^3
Neutrophils	10% to 42%
Lymphocytes	50% to 95%
Eosinophils	0% to 4.5%
Monocytes	0% to 3%
Basophils	0% to 10%
Platelets	200 to 500 × 10^3/mm^3
Urine	Crystalluria, cream-colored, turbid, pH 8.0
Serum protein	4.5–7.5 g/dl
Albumin	2.6–4.1 g/dl
Globulin	2.7–4.2 g/dl
Serum glucose	60–150 mg/dl
Blood urea nitrogen	12–25 mg/dl
Creatinine	0.91–0.99 mg/dl
Total bilirubin	0.25–0.60 mg/dl
Cholesterol	25–135 mg/dl
Serum calcium	5–12 mg/dl
Serum phosphorus	3.4–8.2 mg/dl

feed and drink 10 ml of water/100 g of body weight/day and, like rabbits and many other rodents, are coprophagic.[8] Lesions often develop around the nares when hamsters are fed from narrow, slotted food hoppers in a shoe-box-style cage often used for other rodents. Hoppers with slots 7/16 of an inch wide are recommended to allow easy removal of food pellets.[19] A pregnant hamster at 13 days of gestation should have a one-week supply of food (about 50% more feed than the normal adult diet) placed in the cage to minimize daily disturbance. A newborn hamster begins to eat at 7 to 10 days of age. Food for a lactating female should be placed on the cage floor; otherwise she will become preoccupied with removing feed from the hopper and neglect the pups. The food on the floor will also allow the young easy access.

Housing

Several types of cages are available for housing hamsters. Because hamsters chew plastic, wood, and soft metals, the cage should have only rounded corners with no areas available for the hamster to chew. A dark place to hide, such as a can, and sufficient litter material in which to burrow are desirable. The recommended temperature for hamsters is 65° to 70°F (18.3° to 21.1°C), but adult hamsters can tolerate lower environmental temperatures; a temperature of 71° to 75°F (21.6° to 23.8°C), however, is recommended for pups.[8] An adult hamster requires a floor space of at least 122.6 cm² (19 in.²) and a cage height of 15.2 cm (6 in.). A 12-hour light cycle is preferred.[20]

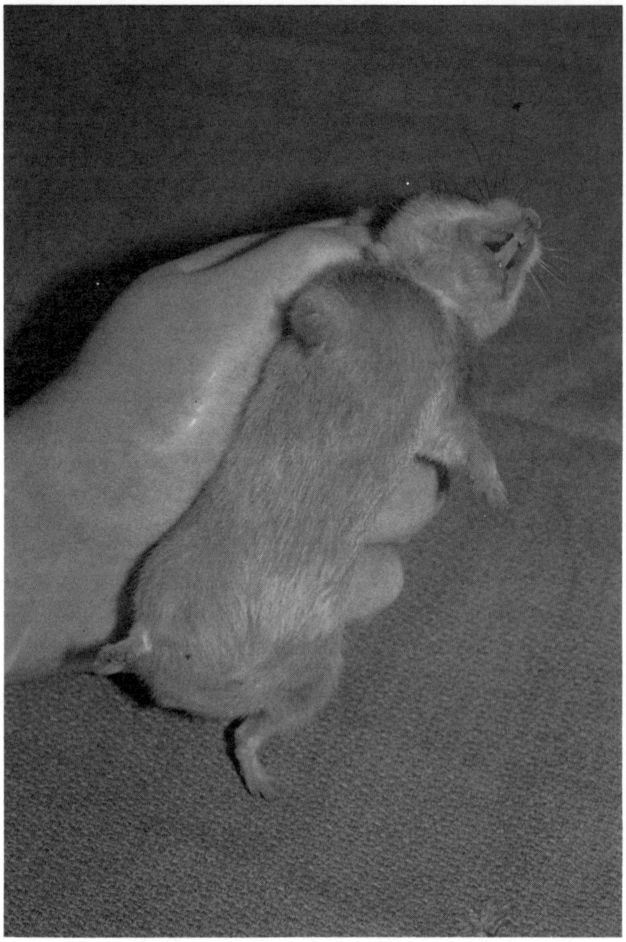

Figure 3—This hamster has been immobilized so that an injection can be given.

Clinical Techniques

A hamster can be handled by cupping the hands gently under it or by picking it up in a small can. It is very important not to surprise a hamster because a startled hamster often bites. After placing the hamster onto a smooth surface, slowly close one hand to allow the loose skin to bunch and then grasp the skin (not the body). The hamster then should be immobilized sufficiently to allow injections to be given (Figure 3).

Several techniques can be used to obtain blood samples. After applying a rubber band tourniquet (Figure 4), the cephalic vein can be used to collect a sample of blood with a 27-gauge needle and a capillary tube (Figure 5). A sample can also be collected with a capillary tube after trimming a toenail. Blood also can be collected through the periorbital sinus by using a microhematocrit tube or directly from the heart by using a 23- to 25-gauge needle on a syringe. Up to 2 ml of blood can be removed safely from a 100-g hamster.[21]

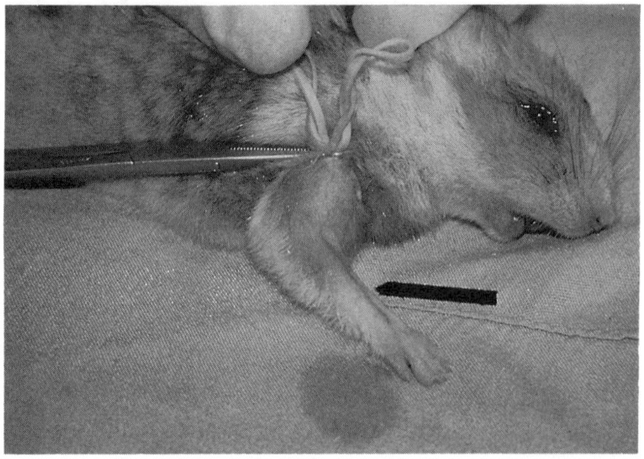

Figure 4—To obtain a blood sample, a tourniquet can be applied to the arm of the hamster. The cephalic vein (arrow) then becomes readily apparent.

Fecal and urinary samples usually can be obtained readily when a hamster is initially handled. Thus, it is wise to have a collection cup, such as a cap from a syringe case, available before handling the hamster.

Medication can be administered orally, intramuscularly, intravenously, or intraperitoneally. The intraperitoneal route is used most often. A 16-gauge, one and one-half to two and one-half-inch, blunt, stainless steel gastric-feeding needle can be used for oral administration. The cephalic or sublingual vein can be used for intravenous injections.[22] Intramuscular injections can be given in the gluteal or lumbar area.

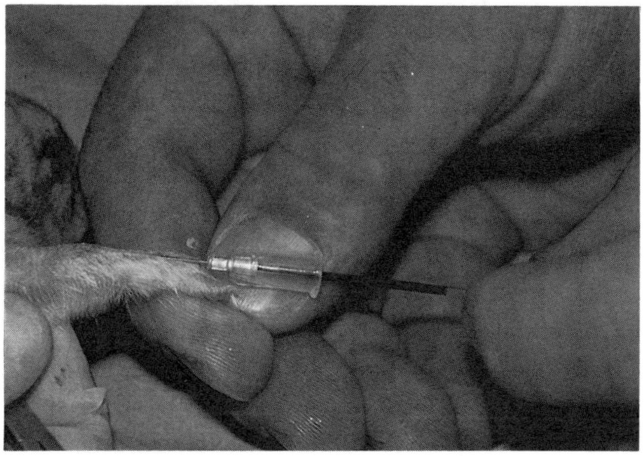

Figure 5—After applying the tourniquet, a 27-gauge needle should be inserted into the cephalic vein and blood collected into a capillary tube.

Pharmaceutic Agents

Antibiotics should be used with caution when treating hamsters because several antibiotics have been associated with induced enterocolitis. Hamsters can develop anorexia, a ruffled haircoat, and diarrhea. There is a reduction of gram-positive flora and a proliferation of gram-negative organisms. *Clostridium difficile* was shown to be a toxin-producing organism that was responsible for lethal enterocolitis.[23]

The use of penicillin, ampicillin, vancomycin hydrochloride, erythromycin, cephalosporin, lincomycin, and oral gentamicin are reported to induce enterocolitis and death in hamsters.[23-25] Other antibiotics also have been reported to induce enterocolitis, but dosage and route may determine whether they are capable of inducing disease. Tetracycline produced no disease when given at an oral dosage of 5 mg every eight hours for five days to hamsters weighing 70 to 90 g. Metronidazole also was reported to produce no disease when it was given at an oral dosage of 7.5 mg every eight hours for five days to hamsters weighing 70 to 90 g.[23] Chloramphenicol palmitate when given at a dose less than or equal to 300 mg/kg did not produce disease.[26]

Chloramphenicol palmitate (50 mg/kg orally) is the antibiotic of choice for treating hamsters. Tetracycline (400 mg/L of water) is also used, but sucrose may need to be added to improve palatability.

The use of ketamine hydrochloride alone has produced variable anesthetic results; however, when combined with xylazine hydrochloride, it has produced satisfactory muscle relaxation and analgesia for abdominal surgical anesthesia. Ketamine (50 to 200 mg/kg) and xylazine (10 mg/kg) produced a longer duration of anesthesia when given intraperitoneally versus intramuscularly. The duration of anesthesia was also dose related. Ketamine (50 mg/kg) and xylazine (10 mg/kg) given intraperitoneally produced anesthesia with a mean duration of 227.3 ± 6.7 minutes. By increasing the dose of ketamine (200 mg/kg), the duration of anesthesia was extended, with a mean of 71.1 ± 4.2 minutes.[27]

Sodium pentobarbital given intraperitoneally at a dose of 50 to 90 mg/kg at a concentration of 10 mg/ml has been suggested for surgical anesthesia lasting 15 to 17 minutes. The minimum lethal dose of pentobarbital is 135 to 150 mg/kg.[28]

Volatile anesthetics, such as methoxyflurane or halothane, when placed on a sponge in a covered container, can anesthetize hamsters for a short period of time. The use of atropine (0.2 to 0.5 mg/kg subcutaneously) is recommended before giving halothane.[28]

Morphine at high doses (150 mg/kg) by intramuscular, subcutaneous, or intraperitoneal injection reportedly results in analgesia without apparent narcosis or respiratory depression. The large volume needed to produce analgesia would limit its clinical usefulness, however. The use of droperidol and fentanyl citrate is not recommended in hamsters because of the effects on the central nervous system.[28]

For short procedures, the use of methoxyflurane has the advantages of safety and speed of recovery. The use of ketamine at a high dose (200 mg/kg) and xylazine for prolonged surgical procedures potentiates the risk of death from anesthesia. Minimal time under anesthesia should be obtained to minimize risk of death.

Infectious Diseases

Proliferative ileitis is the bacterial infection encountered most often in hamsters. It has also been referred to as *wet tail, regional enteritis, terminal ileitis,* and *atypical ileal hyperplasia.* The cause(s) of the disease is not known. *Campylobacter fetus* subspecies *jejuni* has been isolated from hamsters with proliferative ileitis.[29] Pure cultures of *Campylobacter fetus* subspecies *jejuni* did not produce disease when given to healthy hamsters. Ileal extracts from hamsters with proliferative ileitis did produce disease, however, suggesting unknown synergisms or predisposing factors. Stress from a variety of causes may serve as an important factor.[29] Improper diet or change of diet, overcrowding, and familial predisposition are also considered contributory factors. Long-haired and teddy bear hamsters, along with recently weaned hamsters, seem to be highly susceptible.[8]

The infectious agents are spread by a fecal to oral route. Fomites may play a role in transmission. The agent may be passed from weanling to weanling or adult to weanling. The ubiquitous nature of *C. fetus* subspecies *jejuni* has raised the possibility of other animal species being involved as a source of infection. Hamsters have been considered a potential reservoir of human campylobacterosis.[30]

Proliferative ileitis may cause death within one to seven days of onset of clinical signs of watery diarrhea. Signs include matting of fur on the tail or other areas of the body, a hunched stance, irritability, dehydration, and emaciation. If the patient survives the acute attack, ileal obstruction, intussusception, peritonitis, or impaction may occur. Intussusception may be manifested as bloody diarrhea or a prolapsed rectum.

Gross lesions at necropsy include thickening and reddening of the walls of the lower portion of the small intestine. The ileum, jejunum, colon, and rectum contain semifluid yellow material and some gas. In some instances, the bowel mucosa is necrotic and ulcerated. Microscopically there is hyperplasia of crypt epithelium; this results in widening and elongation of the villi. As the disease progresses, abscesses extend through the entire thickness of the gut. Peyer's patches are often obliterated.[29] A silver stain will demonstrate slightly curved bacilli, which are the *Campylobacter* organisms.

Treatment by adding tetracycline to the drinking water at 400 mg/L for 10 days has been used successfully to offset mortality.[31] Prevention is best obtained through selection of hamsters with no familial history of this disease. Avoidance of stress and good husbandry are essential.

Bacterial pneumonia has been reported to be the second most prominent cause of death in hamsters and to be caused by *Pasteurella pneumotropica, Streptococcus pneumoniae,* or other *Streptococcus* spp. Clinical signs are depression, anorexia, and nasal and ocular discharge with respiratory distress. *Mycoplasma pulmonis* has been isolated from the lungs of hamsters, but its role as a pathogen is unknown.[32]

Other bacteria have been reported to produce disease only on rare occasions. Tyzzer's disease caused by *Bacillus piliformis* has been reported; it produced diarrhea and death. Observations at necropsy included white nodules in the heart, dilated cecum and colon containing semiliquid feces, and occasional white spots on the liver.[33] *Escherichia coli* has been reported to produce enteritis without epithelial cell hyperplasia of the villi of the ileum.[34] Bacterial lymphadenitis occurs in the hamster and is similar to that seen in the guinea pig. *Staphylococcus aureus,* β-hemolytic *Streptococcus* Lancefield Group C, and *Streptobacillus moniliformis* have been associated with lymphadenitis. Surgical drainage and antibiotic treatment are indicated. Treatment of well-encapsulated abscesses may be unrewarding.[2,35] Salmonellosis occurs in hamsters but only has been reported rarely. Affected hamsters are depressed and have a rough haircoat. At necropsy, there may be enlargement of the liver, spleen, and lymph nodes as well as patchy hemorrhage of the lungs. Enteritis usually is not present. Prevention is based on good management to minimize introduction of contaminated food or bedding.[36]

Viral infections creating overt clinical signs in hamsters have been reported infrequently. Most viral diseases present as a complicating factor in a production colony or in experimental conditions. Of the viral diseases, lymphocytic choriomeningitis is important because of its zoonotic implications; it is caused by an arenavirus, which is an RNA virus. Clinical signs are rare and depend on the age of the hamster when infected, the strain of the hamster and the virus, the route and dose of infection, and the immunologic competence of the host. If infection occurs congenitally or neonatally, the hamster may show retardation, unthriftiness, weakness, tremors, and prostration. Reproductive impairment has been reported in chronically infected females. Transmission occurs through direct contact, fomites, and aerosols. Findings at necropsy include glomerulonephritis, vasculitis, and lymphocytic infiltration in various organs, including the meninges and brain.[3,37] Prevention and control are based on regular testing of colonies for antibodies.[2]

Sendai virus (parainfluenza I), an RNA virus of the paramyxovirus group, has been reported to result in occasional death of suckling hamsters. Sendai virus is believed to suppress the immunity system.[38] Separate housing from mice, rats, and guinea pigs is suggested for prevention and control.

Parasitic Infections

Protozoa, nematodes, and cestodes are found in the intestinal tract of hamsters. The role of protozoa as a pathogen has not been determined. Protozoa have been found in normal and diseased animals. Both the mouse pinworm, *Syphacia obvelata,* and the rat pinworm, *Syphacia muris,* are capable of infecting hamsters.[39,40] Either can be diagnosed easily by using clear cellophane tape to make an impression smear from the rectum. Both parasites are predominantly located in the cecum. Treatment consists of using piperazine citrate at a dosage of 10 mg/ml of drinking water for seven days, then off for five days, then retreat for an additional seven days.[41]

Hymenolepis nana, a cestode, is an important internal parasite of the hamster because of its zoonotic capabilities.[2] Severe infections may cause intestinal occlusion, impaction, and death. It has a direct or indirect cycle, with flour beetles or fleas as the intermediate host. Diagnosis is made by confirming eggs in the feces or finding them in the adult on postmortem examination. Ground feed containing 0.33% active niclosamide fed ad libitum to hamsters for seven days is safe and effective for eliminating this parasite.[42]

Acariasis is predominantly associated in hamsters with two species of *Demodex* (*D. criceti* and *D. auratus*). Clinically, alopecia of the rump and back with dry scaly skin is present. Pruritus is not usually present.[43] Predisposing factors of malnutrition, concurrent systemic disease, and age are believed necessary for the development of demodectic mange.[44] Mites can be demonstrated by skin scrapings.

Infestation with ear mites (*Notoedres* sp.) also occurs. In females, it usually occurs in the ears only. In males, it occurs on the ears, nose, genitalia, tail, and feet.[8]

Neoplasms

The incidence of spontaneous neoplasms occurring in hamsters is reported to be low (3.7%) compared with the incidence in other rodents. Age, sex, and strain influence the distribution of tumors.[45] The incidence of neoplasms increases in certain strains and in males, which have a longer life span.

Most tumors have been observed after one year of age. Polyps of the intestine, adenomas of the adrenal cortex and thyroid, papillomas of the stomach, and hemangiomas of the spleen are reported to occur. Lymphomas are the most frequently occurring neoplasms in Syrian hamsters and consist predominantly of lymphosarcomas of the lymph gland and small intestine and reticulum cell sarcomas of the lymph nodes.[3] Epizootics of diffuse, poorly differentiated lymphocytic, immunoblastic, or plasmacytoid lymphoma induced by an infectious, horizontally transmitting viroid agent have been reported.[46]

Spontaneous Geriatric Lesions

Compared with other species, Syrian hamsters have a short life span; thus, spontaneous aging diseases are frequently seen. Two of the most common geriatric diseases are amyloidosis and thrombosis. Amyloidosis is frequently associated with thrombosis. Treatment of these geriatric lesions consists of managing clinical signs. A diagnosis of amyloidosis or thrombosis carries a poor prognosis.

Amyloidosis occurs earlier in females and more frequently in certain strains, with an incidence as high as 86%.[47] It occurs in all organs but most often involves the kidneys, spleen, adrenal glands, and liver.[12] Amyloid is produced by reticuloendothelial cells, plasma cells, and histiocytes. The pathogenesis of amyloidosis in hamsters is not understood completely. Amyloid is a protein; three systemic forms presently are recognized. The classification of amyloidosis in hamsters is unclear and needs further study.[48]

A nephrotic syndrome is frequently associated with amyloidosis. Edema, ascites, proteinuria, decreased serum albumin, and increased total globulin are frequently seen in hamsters with amyloidosis.[49,50] Renal failure results from deposits of amyloid. Grossly, the kidneys may appear red-brown, slightly pitted to pale, and misshapened, depending on the degree of involvement.[3]

Microscopically, the renal glomerular capillary tufts may be enlarged and contain amyloid, an amorphous hyaline material (Figure 6). In the liver, amyloid is located adjacent to blood vessels and in portal areas and to a lesser extent around the central veins. Congestion and centrolobular hepatocytic atrophy can occur in a severely affected liver. In the spleen, amyloid replaces the sinusoids, the reticuloendothelial cells, and the macrophages of the red pulp. Replacement of these areas with amyloid causes wide avascular areas. In the adrenal glands, extensive accumulation results in atrophy of cortical cells.[3]

Cardiac thrombosis has been reported to occur as frequently as 73%.[4] The left atrium is the most frequent location, but thrombi may occur in all chambers of the heart (Figure 7). The incidence of thrombosis is equal in both sexes, with females developing lesions earlier in life than males. Consumption coagulopathy and increased fibrinolytic activity have been reported in conjunction with thrombotic disease. Laboratory findings include reduction of activities of factors II, VII, VIII, and X; reduced plasminogen; elevated fibrinogen-fibrin degradation products; and thrombocytopenia.

The process of formation of thrombi in a hamster's

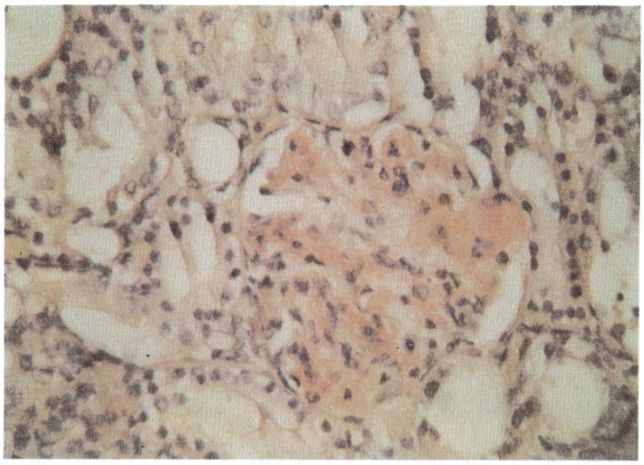

Figure 6—A glomerulus containing amyloid. (Congo red, ×40)

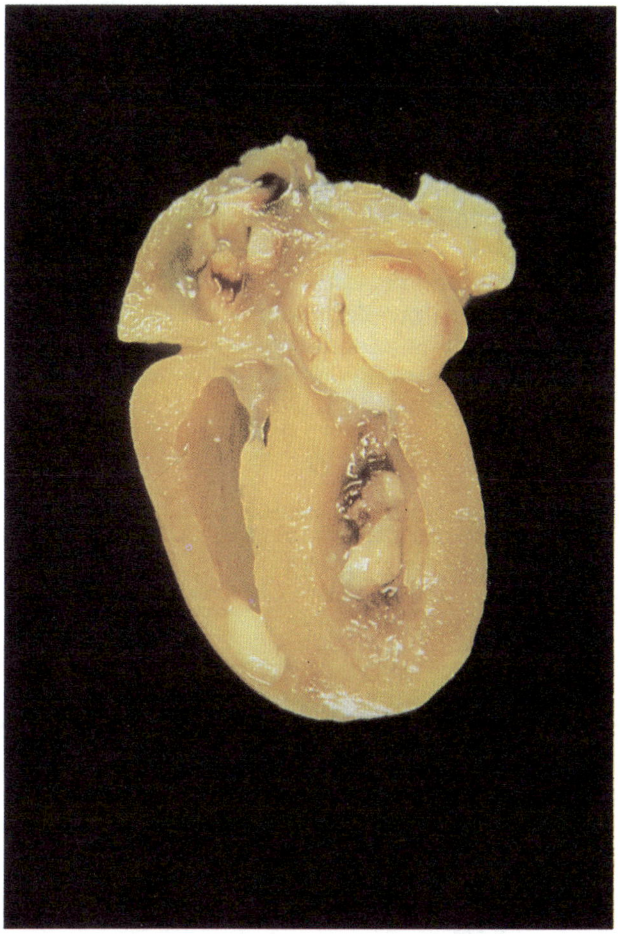

Figure 7—A hamster's heart with thrombi present in all four chambers.

heart is believed to occur not in one stage but with many repetitions of the thrombotic process.[51] Thrombi appear histologically to have varying degrees of organization, suggesting they are formed from more than one episode. The outer fibrotic portion of the older thrombi often contains lymphocyte infiltrates; white, foamy macrophages are found more centrally. Heart failure, vascular injury, septic infections, and amyloidosis have been considered to be inciting factors in the formation of thrombi in hamsters.

Polycystic disease is a developmental or congenital defect seen in hamsters older than one year of age. Cysts are grossly visible and are most often seen in the liver. In the liver, the cysts arise from the biliary duct; histologically the cells resemble biliary epithelium. Grossly, the cysts in the liver can be single or multiple. The wall of the cyst is thin and filled with light-colored fluid. Cystic structures in other organs are histologically similar in that they are dilated and lined with flattened cuboidal epithelium.[52] The condition has not been associated with clinical signs.

Miscellaneous Geriatric Diseases

A calcifying vasculopathy reported to be very common in hamsters is characterized by mild or severe calcification of the vascular walls. The aorta as well as the cardiac, renal, and gastric arteries are affected most often. In advanced cases, the basal laminae of the respiratory epithelium are involved as well as the walls of the alveoli, bronchi, and basal membranes of the renal tubules.[53]

Gastric ulcers occur in older hamsters—more frequently in the glandular stomach than in the forestomach.[54] Liver disease, such as cholangitis, as well as cysts are commonly seen. Cholangitis can be associated with focal or multifocal abscesses.[45] Pyelonephritis and nephrocalcinosis also have been reported in older hamsters.[55] In males, spermatic granuloma, orchitis, prostatitis, prostatic calcification, and seminal vesicular inflammation have been reported in hamsters 62 weeks of age and older. In females, ovarian cysts and endometritis occur. Myocardial fibrosis, myocarditis, pericarditis, and vascular calcinosis have been reported.[56] In the skeletal system, chondrosis (especially of the vertebral joints) is common. The lesions have shown marked extensions toward surrounding soft tissue and resulted in cartilaginous metaplasia of tendons and fascia. These lesions occurred more often in females than in males.[45]

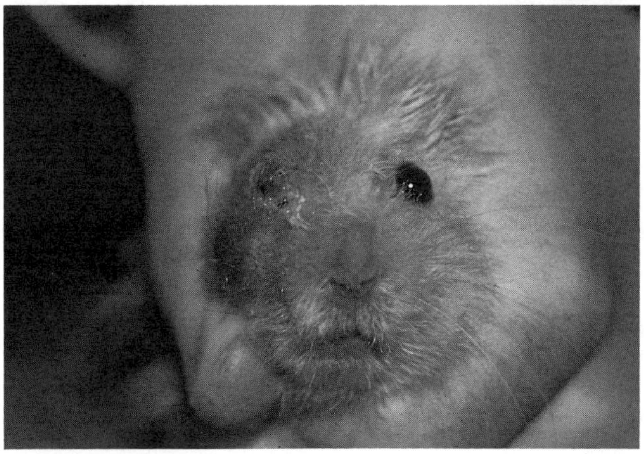

Figure 8—A teddy bear hamster with abscesses of the facial region from periodontitis.

Dental diseases occur more frequently in aged hamsters. In one study, dental caries and periodontitis were the most common nonneoplastic diseases of the digestive system, with an incidence as high as 88%.[45] Periodontitis is associated with abscessation and necrosis extending into the facial region (Figure 8) and involving the harderian glands and brain. The associated vascular thrombosis, especially of the orbital veins, can result in pulmonary emboli.[45] Hamsters have been used experimentally in the study of caries and periodontal disease, both of which can be induced by a finely ground diet or high-carbohydrate concentration. Bacteria play a role in developing plaque that adheres and progressively overgrows the tooth surfaces.[57] The yellowing of the teeth is a normal process of aging and is not related to disease.[7] Malocclusions of the incisors may be a cause of weight loss from inability to eat properly. There is no nerve in the incisor; if overgrowth occurs, the incisors can be trimmed with an instrument (e.g., a canine nail clipper).

Reproductive Problems

Reproductive failures most often are related to errors in management. In one study, starvation for more than one estrous cycle blocked normal follicular development but was reversed by feeding for five days.[58] In another study, exposure to cold temperature (45.5°F [7.5°C]) for two weeks produced anestrus.[59] Male Syrian hamsters, through a pineal-mediated response, developed atrophy of the gonads and accessory sex glands when exposed to a cycle of 22 hours of darkness and 2 hours of light.[60] Sexual receptivity can be blocked when a female hamster is placed in an all-female group.[61] Senescence occurs once the female reaches 15 months of age.[62] Mate incompatibility may also be a cause of mating failures.

Cannibalism resulting from lack of maternal experience and environmental disturbances is a frequent cause of loss of newborn. It is essential that the female not be disturbed 2 days before or 10 days after delivery. If disturbing becomes necessary, feeding the female fresh foods will decrease the probability of cannibalism.[2]

Pregnancy toxemia has been described and was characterized by disseminated thrombi in the kidneys, liver, intestines, and placenta. No pathogenic organisms were found, but stress from shipping was considered a contributing factor. The histologic lesions resembled those seen in guinea pig pregnancy toxemia associated with uteroplacental ischemia.[63]

REFERENCES

1. Hill BF: The Syrian hamster: Its utility in research. *Charles River Digest*: 3(2), 1969.
2. Van Hoosier GL, Ladiges WC: Biology and disease of hamsters, in Fox JG, Cohen BJ, Loew FM (eds): *Laboratory Animal Medicine.* Orlando, FL, Academic Press Inc, 1984, pp 123-147.
3. Schmidt RE, Eason RL, Hubbard GE, et al: *Pathology of Aging Syrian Hamsters.* Boca Raton, FL, CRC Press Inc, 1983.
4. McMartin DM, Dodds WJ: Atrial thrombosis. *Am J Pathol* 107(2):277-279, 1982.
5. Willington M: Observations on the breeding and care of the Chinese hamster. *Lab Anim Care* 15(1):94-101, 1965.
6. Walker EP, Warnick F, Lange KI, et al: *Mammals of the World,* vol 2. Baltimore, The John Hopkins Press, 1964, p 665.
7. Williams CSF: *Practical Guide to Lab Animals.* St. Louis, The CV Mosby Co, 1976, pp 26-34.
8. Harkness JE, Wagner JE: *The Biology and Medicine of Rabbits and Rodents.* Philadelphia, Lea & Febiger, 1983.
9. Warner RG, Ehle FR: Nutritional idiosyncrasies of the golden hamster (*Mesocricetus auratus*). *Lab Anim Sci* 26(4):670-673, 1976.
10. Payne HP: The attractiveness of harderian gland smears to sexually naive and experienced male golden hamsters. *Anim Behav* 27:897-904, 1979.
11. Ohtaki S: Conspicuous sex differences in zona reticularis of the adrenal cortex of Syrian hamsters. *Lab Anim Sci* 29(6):765-789, 1979.
12. McMartin DM: Morphologic lesions in aging Syrian hamsters. *J Gerontol* 34(4):502-511, 1979.
13. Hafez ESE: *Reproduction and Breeding Techniques for Laboratory Animals.* Philadelphia, Lea & Febiger, 1970, p 3.
14. Orsini MW: The external vaginal phenomena characterizing the stages of estrus cycle, pregnancy, pseudopregnancy, lactation, and the anestrus hamster, *Mesocricetus auratus. Proc Anim Care Panel*:193-205, 1961.
15. Musser TK, Silverman J: The hair cycle of the Syrian golden hamster (*Mesocricetus auratus*). *Lab Anim Sci* 30(4):681-683, 1980.
16. Hoffman RA: Hibernation and effects of low temperature, in Hoffman RA, Robinson PF, Magalhaes H (eds): *The Golden Hamster.* Ames, IA, Iowa State University Press, 1968, pp 25-40.
17. Altman PL, Dittmer DS: *Biology Data Book,* vol 3. Bethesda, MD, Federation of the American Association for Experimental Biology, 1974, p 1785.
18. Banta CA, Warner RG, Robertson JB: Protein nutrition of the golden hamster. *J Nutr* 105:38-45, 1975.
19. Harkness JE, Wagner JE, Kusewitt DF, et al: Weight loss and impaired reproduction in the hamster attributable to an unsuitable feeding apparatus. *Lab Anim Sci* 27(1):117-118, 1977.
20. Moreland AF, Barkley WE, Bottigliere NG, et al: *Guide for the Care and Use of Laboratory Animals.* Bethesda, MD, U.S. Department of Health, Education, and Welfare, 1980, p 34.
21. Desai RG: Hematology and microcirculation, in Hoffman RA, Robinson PF, Magalhaes H (eds): *The Golden Hamster.* Ames, IA, Iowa State University Press, 1968, p 185.
22. Ransom JH: Intravenous injection of unanesthetized hamsters. *Lab Anim Sci* 34(2):200, 1984.
23. Bartlett JG, Chang T, Moon N, et al: Antibiotic induced lethal enterocolitis in hamsters: Studies with eleven agents and evidence to support the pathogenic role of toxin. *Am J Vet Res* 39(9):1525-1530, 1978.
24. Ebright IR, Fekety R, Silva J, et al: Evaluation of eight cephalosporins in hamster colitis model. *Antimicrob Agents Chemother* 19(6):980-986, 1981.
25. Small JD: Fatal enterocolitis in hamsters given lincomycin hydrochloride. *Lab Anim Care* 18(4):411-419, 1968.
26. Fekety R, Silva J, Toshniwal R, et al: Antibiotic-associated colitis effects of antibiotics on *Clostridium difficile* and the disease in hamsters. *Rev Infect Dis* 1(2):386, 1979.
27. Curl JL, Peters LL: Ketamine hydrochloride and xylazine hydrochloride anesthesia in the golden hamster (*Mesocricetus auratus*). *Lab Anim Sci* 17:290-293, 1983.
28. Clifford DH: Preanesthesia, anesthesia, analgesia and euthanasia, in Fox JG, Cohen BJ, Loew FM (eds): *Laboratory Animal Medicine.* Orlando, FL, Academic Press Inc, 1984, pp 538-539.
29. Lentsch RH, McLaughlin RM, Wagner JE, Day TJ: *Campylobacter fetus* subspecies *jejuni* isolated from Syrian hamsters with proliferative ileitis. *Lab Anim Sci* 32(5):511-513, 1982.
30. Fox JG, Ackerman JI, Taylor NS: The hamster as a potential reservoir of human campylobacterosis. *J Infect Dis* 147(4):784, 1983.
31. Regina ML, Fales WH, Wagner JE: Effects of antibiotic treatment on the occurrence of experimentally induced proliferative ileitis of hamsters. *Lab Anim Sci* 30(1):38-41, 1980.
32. Renshaw HW, Van Hoosier GL, Amend NK: A survey of naturally occurring diseases of the Syrian hamster. *Lab Anim* 9:179-191, 1975.
33. Zook BC, Huang K, Rhorer RG: *Tyzzer's disease in Syrian hamsters. JAVMA* 171(9):833-836, 1977.
34. Frisk CS, Wagner JE, Owens DR: Hamster (*Mesocricetus auratus*) enteritis caused by epithelial cell-invasive *Escherichia coli. Infect Immun* 31(3):1232-1238, 1981.
35. Ganawy JR: Bacterial, mycoplasma, and rickettsial diseases, in Wagner JE, Manning PJ (eds): *Biology of the Guinea Pig.* New York, Academic Press, 1976, pp 121-135.
36. Innes JRM, Wilson C, Ross MA: Epizootic *Salmonella enteritidis* infection causing septic pulmonary phlebothrombosis in hamsters. *J Infect Dis* 98:133-144, 1956.
37. Parker JC, Igel HJ, Reynolds RK, et al: Lymphocytic choriomeningitis virus infection in fetal, newborn, and young adult Syrian hamsters. *Infect Immun* 13(3):967-981, 1976.
38. Garlinghouse LE, Van Hoosier GL: Studies on adjuvant-induced arthritis, tumor transplantability and serologic response to bovine serum albumin in sendai virus infected rats. *Am J Vet Res* 39(2):297-300, 1978.
39. Taffs LF: Pinworm infections in laboratory rodents: A review. *Lab Anim* 10:1-13, 1976.
40. Ross CR, Wagner JE, Wightman SR, et al: Experimental transmission of *Syphacia muris* among rats, mice, hamsters, and gerbils. *Lab Anim Sci* 30(1):35-37, 1980.
41. Anay ES, Davis BJ: Treatment of *Syphacia obvelata* in the Syrian hamster (*Mesocricetus auratus*) with piperazine citrate. *Am J Vet Res* 41(11):1899-1900, 1980.
42. Ronald NC, Wagner JE: Treatment of *Hymenolepis nana* in hamsters with yomesan (niclosamide). *Lab Anim Sci* 25(2):219-220, 1975.
43. Silveman J, Chavannes J: Balding. *Lab Anim* 12(3):14-15, 1983.
44. Estes PC, Richter CB, Franklin JA: Demodectic mange in the golden hamster. *Lab Anim Sci* 21(6):825-828, 1971.
45. Pour P, Althoff J, Salmasi SZ, Stephan K: Spontaneous tumors and common diseases in three types of hamsters. *J Natl Cancer Inst* 63(3):797-809, 1979.
46. Coggin JH, Bellomy BB, Thomas KO, et al: B-cell and T-cell lymphomas and other associated diseases induced by an infectious DNA viroid-like agent in hamsters (*Mesocricetus auratus*). *Am J Pathol* 110:254-256, 1983.
47. Pour P, Knoch N, Greiser E, et al: Spontaneous tumors and common diseases in two colonies of Syrian hamsters. I. Incidence and sites. *J Natl Cancer Inst* 56(5):931-935, 1976.
48. Mezza LE, Quimby FW, Darham SK, et al: Characterization of spontaneous amyloidosis of Syrian hamsters using the potassium permanganate method. *Lab Anim Sci* 34(4)376-380, 1984.
49. Gleiser CA, Van Hoosier GL, Sheldon WG, et al: Amyloidosis and renal paramyloid in a closed hamster colony. *Lab Anim Sci* 21(3):197-202, 1971.
50. Murphy JC, Fox JG: Nephrotic syndrome in Syrian hamsters. *Abstract of Papers Presented at the Scientific Sessions at the 31st Annual Session of Am Assoc Lab Anim Sci*:80-84, 1980.
51. Dodds JW, Raymond SK, Moynihan AC, et al: Spontaneous atrial thrombosis in ages Syrian hamsters. II. Hemostasis. *Thrombos Haemost* 38:457-465, 1977.
52. Gleiser CA, Van Hoosier GL, Sheldon WG: A polycystic disease of hamsters in a closed colony. *Lab Anim Care* 20(5):923-929, 1970.
53. Pour P, Birt D: Spontaneous diseases of Syrian hamsters—Their implications in toxicological research. Facts, thoughts, and suggestions. *Proj Exp Tumor Res* 24:145-156, 1979.
54. Pour P, Mohr U, Cardesa A, et al: Spontaneous tumors and common diseases in two colonies of Syrian hamsters. II. Respriatory tract and digestive system. *J Natl Cancer Inst* 56:937-949, 1976.
55. Pour P, Mohr U, Cardesa A, et al: Spontaneous tumors and common diseases in two colonies of Syrian hamsters. III. Urogenital system and endocrine glands. *J Natl Cancer Inst* 56:949-961, 1976.

56. Pour P, Mohr U, Cardesa A, et al: Spontaneous tumors and common diseases in two colonies of Syrian hamsters. IV. Vascular and lymphatic systems and lesions of other sites. *J Natl Cancer Inst* 56:963-974, 1976.
57. Keyes PH: Odontopathic infections, in Hoffman RA, Robinson PF, Magalhaes H (eds): *The Golden Hamster*. Ames, IA, Iowa State University Press, 1968, pp 253-282.
58. Printz RH, Greenwald GS: A neural mechanism regulating follicular development in the hamster. *Neuroendocrinology* 7:171-182, 1971.
59. Grineland RE, Folk GE: Effects of cold exposure on the oestrus cycle of the golden hamster (*Mesocricetus auratus*). *J Reprod Fertil* 4:1-6, 1966.
60. Rudeen PK, Rector RJ: Influence of a skeleton photoperiod on the reproductive organ atrophy in the male golden hamster. *J Reprod Fertil* 60:279-283, 1980.
61. Lisk RD, Langenberg KK, Banta JD: Blocked sexual receptivity in grouped female hamsters: Independence from ovarian function and continuous group maintenance. *Biol Reprod* 22:237-242, 1980.
62. Soderwall AL, Britenbaker AL: Reproductive capacities of different age hamsters (*Cricetus auratus*, Waterhouse). *J Gerontol* 10:469-470, 1955.
63. Richter A, Lausen NC, Lage AL: Pregnancy toxemia (eclampsia) in Syrian golden hamsters. *JAVMA* 185(11):1357-1358, 1984.

The Guinea Pig: An Overview Part I

Larry J. Peters, DVM
Post Doctoral Fellow
Division of Laboratory Animal and Wildlife Medicine
College of Veterinary Medicine
University of Florida
Gainesville, Florida

Cavia porcellus, the common guinea pig or cavy, is only rarely seen in private practice, but it is being presented with increasing frequency throughout the United States.

The following article is intended not to convey all details of the guinea pig and its problems, but rather to provide a general overview and a practical aid for the clinician presented with the occasional guinea pig in distress. The subject matter will encompass the most common maladies affecting guinea pigs as family pets, in small backyard breeding enterprises, or in pet shops, and will outline treatment protocols that are practical and economical for both the clinician and client.

The pet cavy differs substantially from its counterpart in the research world, necessitating an equally differing treatment philosophy. Although they are physiologically the same, the emotional value attached to the pet, which exceeds its monetary worth, its atypical environment and diet, and the client's expectations of the doctor all make it more than merely a statistical unit. The emphasis is on treatment of the individual animal rather than population medicine.

History

Today's common pet guinea pig, or *cavy* as it is commonly referred to in show circles, represents the domesticated form of a South American rodent. Grouped taxonomically with chinchillas and porcupines, the creatures exist in nature as vegetarians, living gregariously in burrows. Even now they are raised domestically in rural areas of South America for their tasty flesh. These animals gained recognition first for use in research, and they are still produced primarily for this purpose. They are also quite popular as pets, in which capacity they perform admirably, rarely biting or scratching. Their basic good health and low monetary value have contributed to their infrequent appearance as patients in private practices.

Breeds

The guinea pig exists in three basic varieties, although interbreeding makes possible any combination of characteristics. The three basic varieties, or breeds, are as follows:

1. Shorthair or English—These animals have uniformly short hair with a wide range of color patterns. Inbred strains of this type constitute the typical research animal.
2. Abyssinian—This type is very popular as pets; they have whorls or rosettes in their short rough fur. Many color patterns exist. Criteria for certain show standards are based upon various characteristics of these rosettes.
3. Peruvian—This is the rarest variety, but one of the types most often presented for treatment due to its uniqueness and show value. The hair on these animals often exceeds 6 inches in length.

All three breeds exist in a variety of mono-, bio-, and tri-color patterns.

Anatomy and Physiology

Adult guinea pigs may weigh over 2 lb; obesity is common. Newborns range in weight from 50 to 100 g, depending upon the number in the litter. There have been reported life spans of nine years, but three to six is more realistic as the average in the home environment. Guinea pigs have four toes on each front foot and three on each rear. A diastema is present in the upper lip. All teeth have open roots which grow throughout the life of the animal and must be worn down continually. The ears are moderately large and hairless. The females have only two nipples, one in each inguinal region. The vagina is completely covered by a vaginal membrane except during estrus and parturition. Basic physiological norms are listed in Table I.

TABLE I
PHYSIOLOGICAL NORMS
FOR CAVIAE PORCELLUS

Temperature	38°-39°C
Respiratory rate	70-130/minute
Heart rate	230-300/minute
PCV	40-50%
RBC	$4.5\text{-}7 \times 10^6$
WBC	$5\text{-}15 \times 10^3$ (neutrophils 20-60%) (lymphocytes 35-75%)

Normal urine is thick and white or yellow in color, and it contains many crystals and has an alkaline pH typical of herbivores. The intestinal tract resembles that of the horse, with a large and active cecum.

Neutrophils show red granules with eosin dyes, and mononuclear leukocytes may contain purple or purple-specked vacuoles called *Kurloff's bodies.* These are most noticeable during late pregnancy when estrogen levels are highest.

The cavy, like man, nonhuman primates, the fruit bat, and some other species, requires a dietary source of vitamin C, as it is incapable of endogenous production.

Husbandry

The average guinea pig is a strong, healthy creature capable of tolerating the extremes of weather, housing, and handling to which the normal family subjects it. Even so, it is not invincible, and a great many of the cases presented to the practitioner are the result, directly or indirectly, of improper husbandry or handling.

Handling

Guinea pigs should be grasped firmly and quickly around the thorax from above with one hand. This should be done gently but solidly. The other hand should support the rear limbs and total body weight. Although they seldom bite, guinea pigs will squeal and wiggle until they feel secure. It is difficult, at best, for the small hands of a child to properly restrain a fractious guinea pig. Children can best hold a docile pet supported in their arms next to their bodies.

Guinea pigs are very susceptible to unusually stressful situations. They may go off feed and lose weight when moved from one family to another or even to a new cage. Abortions are not uncommon in late pregnancy following movement or frightening events.

Housing

Housing accommodations provided for pet guinea pigs are limited only by the imagination, ingenuity, and budget of the owners. There is no one specific right way to accommodate the family cavy as long as the family's emotional needs are met without compromising the cavy's physiological needs.

Because of its relatively clean and social nature, the cavy is easily housed. It cannot jump or climb and thus can be kept in an open-topped enclosure at least 10 inches high. Outside hutch-type enclosures are acceptable, but they should provide access to shade and draft-free sleeping and hiding quarters. Temperature ranges of 55 to 90°F are easily tolerated with lower humidities preferred. If the guinea pig is kept outdoors, protection from sudden weather changes is necessary. Young guinea pigs are more susceptible to the cold and do not thrive at temperatures less than 55°F. Adults can tolerate cold better than heat, showing signs of heat stress at higher temperatures and humidity levels, especially if they are deprived of adequate air flow or sufficient shade. Excessive heat has been associated with premature parturition, death of young, and failure to lactate.

Adults do not require a lot of space. Flooring can be solid or wire. Wire flooring provides a cleaner environment and easier maintenance, but the mesh size must be sufficiently large to allow the hocks to be easily retracted should a foot slip through. Foot lesions and fractured hocks are seen more frequently with wire flooring (Figure 1). Solid floors require more effort to keep sanitary, but most people find them, with bedding, more esthetically acceptable. Many types of bedding are acceptable, for example, wood shavings, shredded paper, commercial pellets, and hay. Frequency of bedding changes depends upon the number of animals and type of food fed.

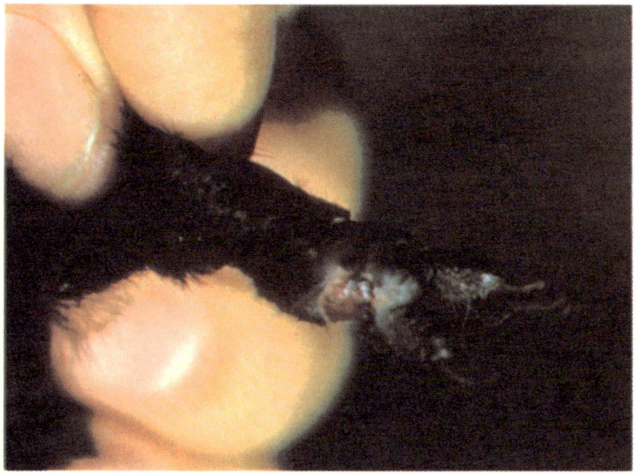

Figure 1—Foot lesion secondary to wire flooring.

Because of their sensitive nature and tendency to panic when frightened, guinea pigs should be housed in a quiet spot away from excitement and noise. Since they are nocturnal, they require periods of light for rest and do poorly if housed for long periods in dark closets or rooms.

More than one animal may be safely housed together and sexes may remain mixed indefinitely. New males may occasionally fight if there is a female nearby. Older, dominant animals may also chew on the ears and hair of subordinate ones.

Feeding and Watering

For a *pig,* the cavy is quite a finicky eater. It may turn up its nose because of changes in the taste or texture of its diet and refuse food or water that has become fouled. A favorite pastime of the cavy is to sit on the edge of its food or water bowl and excrete waste into it. Food should be supplied in hoppers or bins to minimize this occurrence.

The adult guinea pig consumes about 3 oz of water per day. If provided in an open container, the

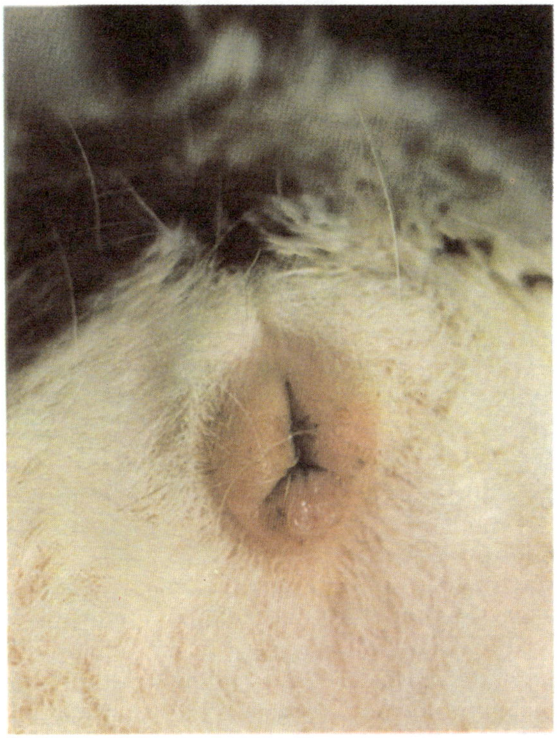

Figure 2—Genitalia of a female guinea pig.

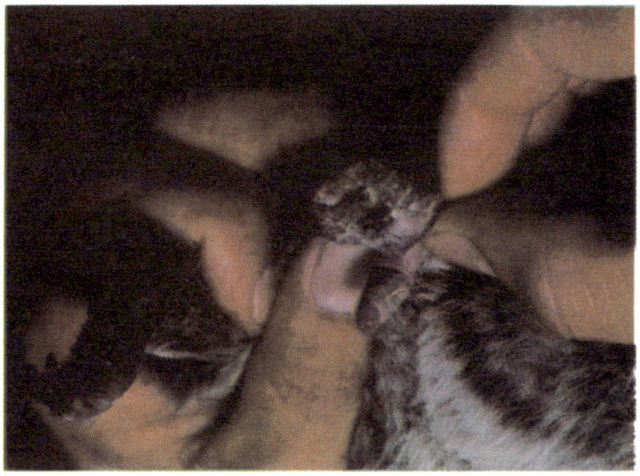

Figure 3—Genitalia of a male guinea pig.

water will be fouled with excreta quickly. Guinea pigs suck from sipper tubes rather than lap like rats; they chew on and blow food back up the tubes, fouling their water within hours. Thus water containers must be cleaned daily.

The most important factor of a guinea pig's diet is the need for vitamin C. This need can be met by feeding commercial guinea pig pellets specially formulated and manufactured to meet the guinea pig's nutritional requirements (with sufficient vitamin C added). However, even under optimum, dry, cool-storage conditions, vitamin C levels remain sufficient for only three months from date of milling. Therefore, unless a pet or feed store sells large volumes of guinea pig food, it may be difficult to obtain fresh, potent pellets, and vitamin C supplementation will still be necessary. The vitamin can be added to the drinking water at 20 mg/day/guinea pig; this solution should be prepared fresh daily, since 50% of the potency is lost within the first 24 hours. Probably the most common means of supplementation is by the addition of fresh greens to the diet. A handful of cabbage or kale or a carrot daily usually suffices. A thorough washing is necessary to insure that no harmful bacteria or pesticide is introduced to the pet. Guinea pigs will graze on lawns and grass clippings; large amounts of luscious greens may cause loose stools. Rabbit chow is often fed successfully instead of guinea pig pellets. Its physical appearance is similar and it is accepted by the cavy, but it is lower in protein and inadequate in vitamin C. The medicated type should never be used, as fatal disruption of the guinea pig's intestinal flora can result.

Roughage is not necessary if the guinea pig is on a good diet, but the animals enjoy burrowing into it, and a good-quality grass hay to nibble on appears to decrease barbering and hair pulling. It has also been reported to decrease hair thinning often associated with late pregnancy.[1]

Breeding

Only the basic essentials of guinea pig reproduction will be covered here since the majority of the clinical situations presented involve complications of pregnancy rather than lack of sufficient productivity.

The breeding age of males (boars) is four to six months and of females (sows) is three to five months, although puberty can occur as early as three to four weeks. Females have an estrous cycle of 14 to 19 days; estrus lasts for about 50 hours, during which time the vaginal membrane is open. The male is only accepted for about 15 hours during this time. A postpartum heat occurs about three to five hours following birth, and conception rates at this ovulation exceed 70%.

Although efficient, males are not particularly aggressive breeders. Copulation time is short and ejaculation is immediate. One to two days following copulation, a light-colored tubular mass of coagulated semen about an inch long called a *vaginal plug* falls from the vagina. This verifies that copulation, but not necessarily conception, has occurred.

Females should be bred, if pregnancy is desired, before nine months of age. In older virgin females the pubic symphysis becomes fused and fat has accumulated in the pelvic area, increasing chances of dystocia.

Guinea pigs may be bred in harems, as permanent pairs, or a male may be temporarily placed with the female during her estrus. Harems usually consist of one male and 10 to 12 females, with the animals left together continually. Problems are unusual, and young will often nurse from other than their own dams. Care should be taken not to excite the group or the young may be trampled by the frightened herd as it stampedes in circular fashion around its pen. Rectangular rather than square enclosures help to lessen this tendency.

Sexing

The female displays a Y-shaped vaginal opening between the urethral orifice and the anus (Figure 2). This opening is closed by the vaginal membrane except during estrus and parturition. The urethral orifice in the female is external and ventral to the vaginal opening.

The male has no opening between the orifice at the tip of the penis and the anus (Figure 3). A slitlike structure, which is often mistaken for a vaginal opening, is evident in this area. It is merely the fold between the two halves of the scrotum following retraction of the testicles. The penis can be palpated just ventral to this *slit* and can be everted by gentle pressure. The anourethral distance is the same in both sexes. Internally the male possesses very large Y-shaped seminal vesicles. These structures, which resemble bicornuate uteri, lie anterior to the prostate and are very noticeable at necropsy.

Pregnancy

Gestation in the guinea pig is relatively long. Depending upon the litter size, it ranges from 60-70 days, being longer with small litters and shorter with larger ones. Average litter size is about three young, but up to eight have been reported. Litters greater than five are often born dead. Commercial breeders are usually satisfied with 10 to 12 young reared annually per female, but some sows will produce 18 if the postpartum heat is utilized.

Embryos can be palpated easily by four to five weeks or as early as two to three weeks with practice. Because of the sensitive nature of the pregnant sow, the wisdom of transporting her to the clinic for palpation is debatable.

The pubic symphysis will begin to open 10 days prior to delivery and will be ¾ inch wide at parturition. This can be easily palpated from beneath with the forefinger and is indicative of impending birth.

Babies weigh 50 to 100 g at birth; those less than 50 g usually do not survive. A 10% stillbirth and weaning mortality rate is not uncommon under even the best of conditions. The sow is not very motherly; she makes no nest and even remains in the sitting position while nursing. The young are born precocious, i.e., fully haired, with teeth, and with their eyes open. They are thus able to survive without nursing, although they are usually not weaned until they are three weeks old or 150 g. Cannibalism is rare, but fatal trampling is not uncommon in large groups. The mother and young can be removed from the group for awhile if necessary.

Clinical Techniques

Blood Sampling

Routine blood sampling presents a problem in that there are no readily accessible, large, superficial veins. Small amounts of blood for capillary tubes can be obtained from the dorsolateral penile or the saphenous veins with light syringe pressure and a small-gauge needle. Direct capillary tube filling can be done by incising the saphenous vein of a leg previously smeared with petroleum jelly or by incising a toenail, or it can be obtained from the orbital sinus under anesthesia.

Larger volumes of blood can be obtained from the femoral triangle or by direct cardiac puncture while under light anesthesia. The latter procedures for diagnostic purposes may appear radical, but individuals have been so bled repeatedly at weekly intervals without adverse incidence.

Drug Administration

Intramuscular injections may be given into the posterior lateral thigh 0.5 to 1 cm above the stifle or into the lumbar musculature. Subcutaneous injections are easily made into any dorsolateral location from the flank to the nape of the neck. Small amounts of drug can sometimes be injected into the dorsolateral penile veins or the larger ear veins, or one can do a cutdown on the saphenous vein above the hock as it turns inward and upward. Intraperitoneal injections are made slightly to the right of midline about 1 inch anterior to the pubic bone while elevating the rear of the animal. Beware of this procedure in heavily pregnant sows.

The oral route is by far the simplest. Medication can be mixed in food or water, passed through a stomach tube, or dropped into the mouth. A makeshift speculum is helpful when attempting to pass a stomach tube.

REFERENCE

1. Williams CSF: *Practical Guide to Lab Animals.* St. Louis, CV Mosby Co, 1976.

The Guinea Pig: An Overview Part II

Larry J. Peters, DVM
Post Doctoral Fellow
Division of Laboratory Animal and Wildlife Medicine
College of Veterinary Medicine
University of Florida
Gainesville, Florida

The guinea pig is susceptible to a vast array of diverse organisms, the majority of which are not encountered in the typical pet. The literature on the iatrogenic diseases and research-related problems is voluminous; they will not be discussed here. This article will be limited to those problems that are most likely to be encountered in a pet in a household environment. Even though the guinea pig is physiologically a hardy animal, it is very sensitive to stress associated with temperature, feeding, handling, etc., and many of its health problems are related to primary problems in these areas.

The Anamnesis

A complete history can be the best diagnostic tool available. The anamnesis should cover the following items: source of the pig; clinical signs; onset of signs; previous illnesses; type, source, and age of diet; type of feed and water containers used; bedding type; humidity, temperature, airflow, and light cycle of pet's environment; method and frequency of cage cleaning; new animals introduced to the household; and other pets or local wildlife.

Common Diseases and Health Problems

Cutaneous

Differential diagnoses of some of the more commonly seen cutaneous or externally evident problems in the guinea pig are listed in Table I.

Suppurative cervical lymphadenitis, or *lumps,* is an infection and abscessation usually of the cervical lymph nodes, but involvement of any node is possible. This condition is caused by a Lancefield group C, gram-positive, beta-hemolytic streptococcus normally contracted through mucous membrane abrasions.[1-3] The involved nodes form abscesses containing a thick, yellowish white suppurative exudate. Cellulitis and arthritis may be present, but animals often display no apparent discomfort. Small abscesses are sometimes noted in the visceral organs, and uterine infections have caused abortions. Treatment varies from surgical excision or drainage with lavage in severe cases to conservative therapy utilizing an appropriate antibiotic in less involved situations.

TABLE I

CUTANEOUS OR EXTERNALLY EVIDENT PROBLEMS

Clinical Sign	*Differential Diagnosis*
Open lesions	Bite wounds Trauma from sharp objects Draining abscesses Thermal or caustic burns Self-trauma
Cutaneous or subcutaneous swelling	Abscesses Aberrant parasite larvae Mastitis Arthritis (Vitamin C deficiency)
Dermatitis	Fungal infection (*Trichophyton* spp.) Bacterial infection Parasites: Mites, *Trixacarus caviae*; lice, *Chirodiscoides caviae, Gliricola porcelli*
Alopecia	Nutritional Mites Barbering (nibbling hair from each other) Mechanical (rubbing on feeders or cage parts) Fungal Unknown (diffuse loss over flanks and backs is common during pregnancy)

Another form of *chronic abscessation* of the cervical lymph nodes has been attributed to a gram-negative organism, *Streptobacillus moniliformis.* This condition is usually not lethal, but it causes encapsulated, often unilateral swellings similar to those of suppurative cervical lymphadenitis. It can be acquired through breaks in the oral mucous membrane and is found as a normal respiratory inhabitant in the rat.[2] Treatment of these abscesses is the same as that for suppurative cervical lymphadenitis.

Superficial fungal infections on the guinea pig are frequently encountered. The most common causative agent is *Trichophyton mentagrophytes.* With this condition, scaley, scabby lesions usually begin around the face, and they may later spread to other parts of the body. Diagnosis should be by fungal culture, because this organism does not fluoresce under UV light.[2] Treatment consisting of 25 to 100 mg/kg griseofulvin PO for four weeks has been successful.

Septicemia

A fulminating septicemia with or without pneumonia has been associated with a Lancefield group C streptococcus. Hematuria, hemoglobinuria, depression, fever, and death (acutely or within three to four days) often occur with the condition.[2,4,5]

Naturally occurring *pseudotuberculosis* caused by *Yersinia pseudotuberculosis* is not uncommon in the pet cavy. This gram-negative coccoid- to bacillary-shaped organism survives and multiplies in feces, necessitating good sanitation. This condition is generally chronic, manifesting itself as emaciation, diarrhea, nodules in the lymph nodes and viscera, and death in three to four weeks. A more acute death can occur from miliary lesions in the lungs and liver. The primary lesions in chronic cases often begin in the mesenteric nodes, which become palpably enlarged. Necrotic white or yellow nodules containing thick, smooth, caseated pus can also occur in the gastrointestinal tract and mammary tissues. Nonfatal cases exhibiting only enlarged nodes have been reported. Spread is through oral ingestion; it is believed that the organism might be acquired from greens contaminated by the feces of wild birds and rodents.[6] Treatment of this condition is difficult and, except in very early cases, the prognosis is poor. Thorough washing of greens before feeding is important in prevention.

Salmonellosis (paratyphoid) is one of the most lethal infections that can be contracted. It is caused by the bacilli *Salmonella typhimurium* and *Salmonella enteritidis,* and it can remain latent until exacerbated by stress. Salmonellosis often occurs acutely, causing sudden death, but it can also be chronic, with emaciation and diarrhea. Conjunctivitis is common. The more chronic cases show granulomatous lesions in the spleen, liver, and lymph nodes. Acute cases show liquid gut contents composed of purulent exudate in the lumen of the intestines. Lymph nodes will be grossly increased in size within 48 hours postinfection. The route of infection is oral or conjunctival. Salmonellosis closely resembles syndromes caused by *Yersinia pseudotuberculosis* and *Corynebacterium pyogenes.* It can be latent or it can be acquired from feedstuffs and bedding contaminated with rodent excreta.[6] Treatment is usually unsuccessful unless it is begun very early in the case.

Respiratory System

Differential diagnoses of the more commonly seen respiratory syndromes are listed in Table II.

Guinea pigs are susceptible to *pneumonia* caused by a variety of pathogens. The pigs are usually predisposed by stressful situations, i.e., weather change and exposure, shipping, or following purchase from a group colony. Subclinical vitamin C deficiency can also be a predisposing factor.

Streptococcal pneumonia is a devastating disease in the guinea pig that can reach epizootic proportions.[2,4,5] It can be manifested clinically as an acute or chronic condition. The acutely affected animal may be found dead. Any of the following signs may be noted in longer-term illnesses: pleuritis, peritonitis, pericarditis, arthritis, localized abscesses, emaciation, respiratory distress, rise in temperature, coughing, sneezing, blood-stained crusts around the nose, purulent conjunctivitis, hemoglobinuria, and hematuria. Since all

TABLE II

RESPIRATORY SYNDROMES

Clinical Sign	*Differential Diagnosis*
Conjunctivitis	Bacterial infection Chlamydial neonatal conjunctivitis Foreign body Trauma
Nasal discharge/ dyspnea	Pregnancy toxemia Heat stress Allergy Dry hay as bedding Bacterial rhinitis Bacteria pneumonia Foreign body

of these signs except hematuria are manifested in acute salmonellosis, detection of hematuria is valuable in making a differential diagnosis.[4,5] Streptococcal pneumonia is often noted in sows shortly following parturition. Streptococcus is a common surface organism of humans and animals and is contracted via the respiratory system.[2]

Bordetella bronchiseptica, a small, gram-negative bacillus or coccobacillus, often seen in pairs, has been isolated from the respiratory tract of clinically normal animals and is a normal inhabitant of the respiratory tract of rabbits.[2] Disease caused by this organism often occurs secondary to stress, resulting in sudden death or typical bronchopneumonic signs including dyspnea, congestion, consolidation, and purulent bronchial exudate. The source of infection is often other guinea pigs or rabbits, and it is contracted by contact or airborne routes.[4]

A *gram-positive diplococcus* has been implicated in some cases of severe pneumonia, causing hemorrhagic lungs, pulmonary abscesses, purulent otitis, pleuritis, and pericarditis.[2]

There is a *naturally occurring pneumonia* caused by a filterable virus which results in an acute illness approximately one week following inhalation.[2] Congestion and consolidation of the lungs are the primary signs. Treatment entails early diagnosis, use of an appropriate antibiotic, and intense supportive measures.

Reproduction

Differential diagnoses of the common reproductive syndromes are listed in Table III.

TABLE III

REPRODUCTIVE SYNDROMES

Clinical Sign	*Differential Diagnosis*
Infertility	Nutritional deficiency Environmental stress Genital infections Immature or old age Feed toxins or hormone contaminations Seasonal phenomena
Perinatal mortality	Nutritional deficiency Bacterial diseases Pregnancy toxemia Environmental stress Aflatoxin in feed
Dystocias	Large fetuses Uterine torsion Sick, malnourished, or weakened sow Fused pubic symphysis Obese female
Litter desertion or cannibalism	Maternal inexperience Environmental disturbances Mastitis

Vaginitis of diverse etiologies can occur in guinea pigs. Various bacteria, often secondary to bedding or other foreign bodies, have been isolated from such infections.[2] Treatment of vaginitis consists of thorough examination of the vagina for foreign matter and therapy with appropriate antibiotics. Vaginoscopy is more easily accomplished during estrus, when the vaginal membrane is relaxed.

Mature boars may accumulate a mass of sebaceous material in the folds of skin between the two halves of the scrotum; this is called a *scrotal plug.* It can be up to 1 inch in diameter and is often confused with an external rectal impaction at first glance.[5] Treatment consists of thorough cleaning with soap and water.

Obstetrical problems such as stillbirths and abortions are not uncommon in guinea pigs, and often no cause can be incriminated. Stress of pregnancy can be great upon the sow. Often the total fetal mass may weigh more than the mother, prohibiting her from walking the last few days prior to delivery.[5] If this occurs, food and water should be made easily accessible.

Fusion of the pubic symphysis, excess fat in the pelvic cavity, too large a fetus, and uterine inertia can all contribute to *dystocia.* The only solution for the first three problems is a cesarean section. To overcome uterine inertia, one unit of oxytocin can be injected IM.[4,5] Surgery is indicated if no positive results are achieved within 15 minutes.

Situations such as dual presentation of fetuses, uterine torsion, and dystocia in immature, old, and weak sows can be occasionally corrected via external manipulation.

The pressure of the gravid uterus upon the liver can cause bile blockage and hepatic dysfunction, resulting in a vitamin-K-deficient *hemorrhagic syndrome.* This can cause complications during cesarean sections and even following vaginal deliveries.

Pregnancy toxemia is fairly common in the guinea pig. It is typically seen in stressed, heavily pregnant sows that are 56 or more days into gestation and carrying three or more fetuses. Acute deaths can occur within 24 hours with no history of clinical illness. Treatment is usually too late and ineffective; however, 1 to 2 ml 50% dextrose in 3 to 5 ml saline IV or IP can be tried.[5] The condition can also be chronic, beginning with a ruffled hair coat, lethargy, and anorexia three to five days prior to death and progressing to a reluctance to move, prostration, and coma. The eyes are dull, yellow crusts form along the eyelids, and abortion may occur. A similar syndrome can occur 7 to 11 days postpartum. It is nearly 100% fatal despite treatment. Hyperlipemia and ketone-positive urine with high protein and a pH of 5 or less are consistent findings. The etiology of pregnancy toxemia is unknown, but obesity is an important factor. Stress should be kept to a minimum and the animal should not be transported or fasted during the latter periods of gestation. A genetic predilection may exist.

TABLE IV

CNS and Musculoskeletal Disorders

Clinical Sign	*Differential Diagnosis*
Incoordination/convulsions	Guinea pig paralysis Trauma Pregnancy toxemia Toxicity Toxoplasmosis
Paralysis or reluctance to move	Guinea pig paralysis Fractures Luxations Vitamin C deficiency Arthritis Vitamin E deficiency Urinary calculi Prostatitis Late, heavy pregnancy Toxoplasmosis Imbalance of Ca:P
Torticollis	Otitis interna Encephalitis Trauma

CNS and Musculoskeletal Systems

Table IV is a listing of differential diagnoses of some CNS and musculoskeletal disorders found in the guinea pig.

A syndrome called *guinea pig paralysis* is noted occasionally. A filterable agent has been incriminated. Urinary incontinence is the first sign, with gradually increasing hindlimb hypotonia and weakness progressing to complete posterior paralysis. A mild fever and weight loss also occur during the course of the disease. There is no known treatment, and it does not appear to be readily, if at all, transmissible between animals.

Parasites

Endoparasites are not common in the guinea pig. Cysts of the ciliate *Balantidium coli* or *Balantidium caviae* may be noted in direct smears.[2,5] There are usually no clinical signs, and the endoparasites are usually considered nonpathogenic.

The coccidian *Eimeria caviae* is sometimes found in the guinea pig; it also is usually not pathogenic. Extremely heavy infestations, though, can result in colitis, mucoid diarrhea without blood, loss of appetite, emaciation, and occasionally, death from complications. The sporulation time of this coccidium is 6 to 12 days. Good sanitation will break the cycle of reinfestation—reinfestation is via ingestion. The greatest losses occur in the four- to eight-week-old age groups following stress. Regular cleaning and keeping no open water or feed containers are the best preventive measures. Treatment has been undertaken with sulfamethazine, sulfaquinoxaline, and sulfathiazole added to the drinking water to make a 0.05% solution or with succinyl sulfathiazole in a 0.1% solution for at least two weeks.[5]

Eggs of the *cecal pinworm Paraspidodera uncinata*, an ascarid of the cecum and colon, are occasionally noted on fecal exam. This parasite is normally nonpathogenic and nonzoonotic, but it can cause diarrhea and unthriftiness in heavy infestations. It has a direct life cycle, with eggs infective within one week after passing and mature worms present two weeks postingestion. Treatment with piperazine and proper cleaning of the premises usually alleviate the problem.[2,5]

External parasitic infestations are normally of minor significance in guinea pigs. *Chirodiscoides caviae*, the guinea pig fur mite, generally causes no clinical manifestations. Repeated infestations have been reported to cause skin lesions. The fur mite can usually be treated effectively with any flea powder suitable for use on cats. The cages should be cleaned thoroughly twice weekly for at least three weeks.

Trixacarus caviocoptes caviae, a sarcopticlike mite causing typical mange-type lesions, has only recently been recognized in this country.[8] It can cause alopecia, epidermal scaling, pruritus with self-trauma, and, in extreme cases, anorexia, emaciation, and death (Figures 2 and 3). Details concerning its life cycle are not known. It appears that the mite is capable of existing subclini-

TABLE V

Gastrointestinal Problems

Clinical Sign	*Differential Diagnosis*
Diarrhea	Nonspecific Acute cecitis Antibiotic toxicity Salmonellosis Coccidiosis Parasitism Toxicosis
Hypersalivation	Dental malocclusion[7] Vitamin C deficiency Adrenocortical insufficiency Oral foreign body Rectal impaction (Figure 1)
Constipation/vomiting	Calcification of stomach or colon Tumor Impacted cecum Torsion Intussusception

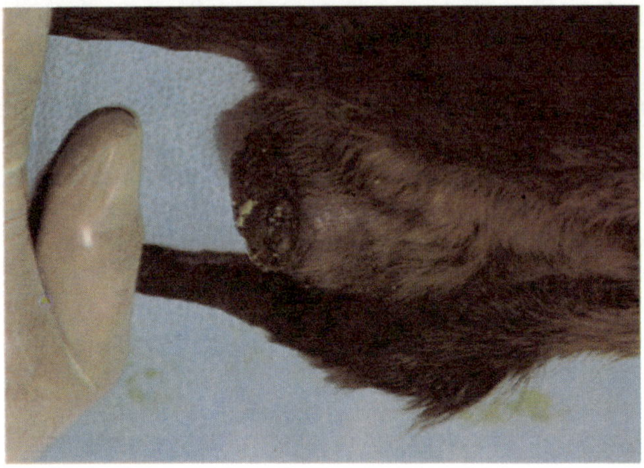

Figure 1—One gastrointestinal problem in the guinea pig is rectal impaction.

cally, becoming active with stresses such as shipping or pregnancy. Young guinea pigs may acquire the mite from the sow before weaning but show no signs until maturity. The mite is sometimes extremely difficult to demonstrate by scrapings. A negative scraping does not rule out the possibility of the condition if clinical signs are consistent with the diagnosis. Treatment with lime sulfur or benzene hexachloride has been reported to be effective if repeated two to three times at three-week intervals.[8,9] No species cross-infestation has been demonstrated.

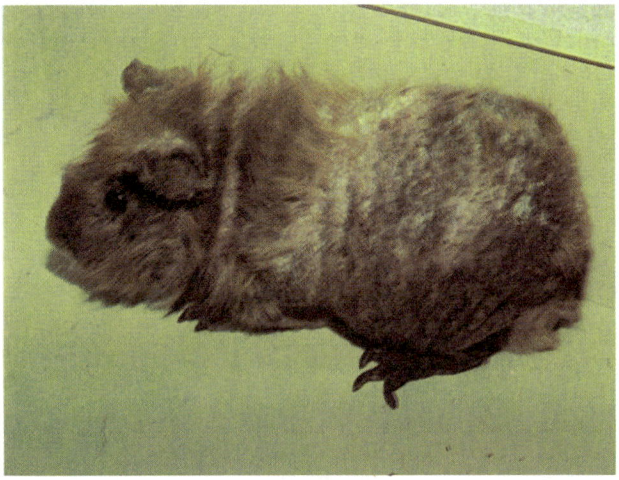

Figure 2—*Trixacarus caviocoptes caviae* mange is commonly seen in the guinea pig.

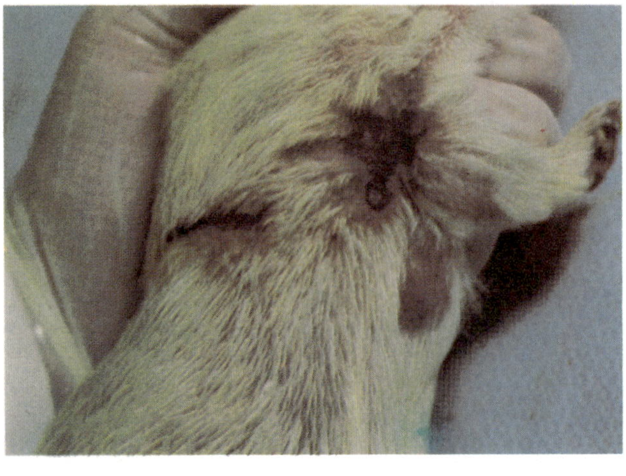

Figure 3—Self-trauma secondary to *Trixacarus caviocoptes caviae* mange.

The guinea pig lice *Gyropus ovalis* and *Gliricola porcelli* are common. There are usually no clinical signs associated with their presence, but the owner may become alarmed by the visible mites on the animal. Treatment with a feline flea powder is usually successful.

Miscellaneous Conditions

Miscellaneous guinea pig problems and their differential diagnoses are listed in Table VI.

Pododermatitis is manifested as a chronic, fibrous granuloma on the ventral surface of the foot (Figure 4). Staphylococci are often isolated from the lesions. The lesions occur more commonly in animals kept on wire flooring. Treatment consists of moving the animal to dry, soft bedding and administering antibiotics if necessary. The feet seldom return to normal following disfigurement.

Overgrowth of nails is another frequent condition in animals kept on wire or smooth flooring (Figure 5). Routine clipping is necessary.

A mild to severe exudative *conjunctivitis* has been attributed to an unnamed viral agent. It appears to be self-limiting, and treatment is symptomatic.[2]

TABLE VI

MISCELLANEOUS GUINEA PIG PROBLEMS

Clinical Sign	*Differential Diagnosis*
Weight loss	Nutritional deficiencies Anorexia Metastatic calcification Chronic disease Malocclusion Ectoparasitism Endoparasitism Tumors Inability to reach food Aflatoxicosis
Sudden death	Acute enteritis Pregnancy toxemia Hemorrhagic syndrome Starvation/dehydration Lymphosarcoma Trauma Antibiotic toxicity Dystocia Urinary calculi Septicemia Toxemia Chilling/overheating Aflatoxicosis Toxoplasmosis

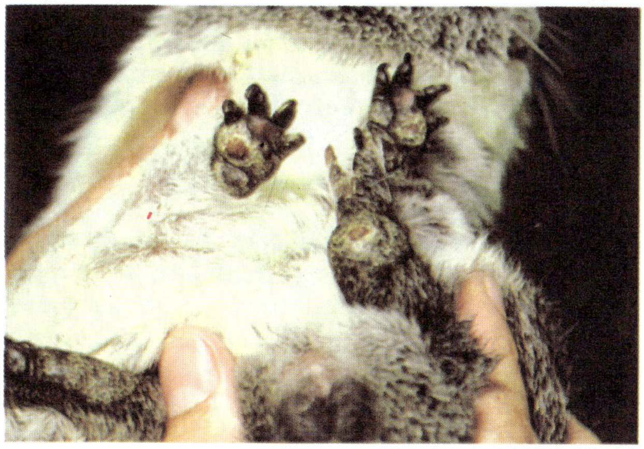

Figure 4—Pododermatitis is one of the miscellaneous conditions seen in the guinea pig.

Vitamin C deficiency is not a common problem in well-cared-for pets, because they normally receive plenty of greens in their diets. It becomes a problem if rabbit food alone or outdated guinea pig chow is fed as the sole diet. An anorexic animal should always receive forced supplementation of some form. A normal animal needs 10 to 20 mg/kg/day. Two weeks on a deficient ration can cause lameness. The first clinical signs of a vitamin C deficiency are a depressed, anorexic animal with ruffled fur. Hemorrhage into joints and muscles subsequently occurs causing lameness and a stiff posture. If treatment at 50 mg/day PO or parenterally is initiated at this stage, the animal can usually be saved. Fast-growing young and pregnant sows die first. Subclinical or marginal deficiencies often predispose animals to many other diverse problems.

Slobbers is really a clinical sign of a condition of unknown etiology. The fur under the jaws and down the neck remains wet from the constant drooling of saliva. The saliva is sometimes green or yellow colored. Overgrowth of teeth due to a selenium excess has been incriminated, but often the teeth are normal. Treatment is symptomatic at best. Teeth should be trimmed if overgrown and a well-balanced ration should be provided.

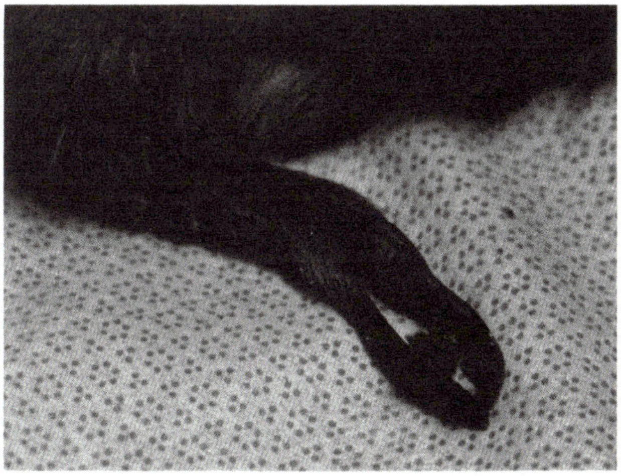

Figure 5—Overgrown toenails in the guinea pig should be clipped.

Animals in the 12- to 18-month age range have been noted to develop *calcification of* various *soft tissues,* especially of the stomach and colon. This can lead to steady emaciation and death if severe enough; it is usually a postmortem finding.

The guinea pig appears to be particularly susceptible to *anaphylaxis.* This condition is often marked by severe respiratory distress because of a well-developed smooth muscle coat around the bronchial tree and pulmonary vessels.[2] Sensitivity testing is generally impractical, so clients should be made aware of the potential of reactions prior to any injection.

Antibiotics do not usually adversely affect guinea pigs immediately via anaphylaxis, as is often thought. Rather, the animals develop problems later subsequent to the antimicrobial effects of the drugs. The gastrointestinal tract of the guinea pig is populated predominately by gram-positive organisms. Antibiotics that attack principally gram-positive organisms, allowing a secondary increase in gram-negative organisms, may cause diarrhea, enterotoxemia, coliform bacteremia, and, possibly, death in three to five days. Thus, antibiotics specifically affecting gram-positive bacteria are contraindicated. Broad-spectrum antibiotics that affect both gram-positive and gram-negative organisms lessen this risk of harmful bacterial overgrowth.

Neoplasms are rare in guinea pigs less than three years of age. In older animals, neoplasms occur most often in the pulmonary system.

Treatment

Most conditions diagnosed in the pet cavy can be handled similarly to the way the equivalent entity is handled in the more common pet species. Sound medical common sense is used while making special considerations of specific anesthetic, antibiotic, and handling needs. The treatment of any condition should always include alleviating the cause as well as the presenting signs.

Antibiotic Therapy

Antibiotics in the guinea pig, as in many species should be chosen with consideration given to the bacterial sensitivity of the organism, ease of administration, cost, toxicity, and public health implications of the disease. Antibiotics of choice should be broad spectrum. Table VII lists some antibiotics and their doses that have been used effectively in guinea pigs.[4]

Anesthesia

Anesthesia in the guinea pig has long presented a major problem in proper care and treatment. The animal's small size, high metabolic rate, sensitivities, lack of superficial veins, inaccessible glottis, and respiratory system that is very sensitive to anesthetic-induced suppression all combine to complicate anesthesia.

TABLE VII

ANTIBIOTICS COMMONLY USED IN THE GUINEA PIG

Antibiotic	*Dose*	*Route of Administration*	*Period of Administration*
Chloramphenicol palmitate[4,5]	50 mg/kg	PO	Daily for 5 to 7 days
Chloramphenicol sodium succinate[4,5]	30 mg/kg	IM	Daily for 5 to 7 days
Cephaloridine[3,4]	10-30 mg/kg	IM	Daily for 10 days to 2 weeks
Sulfamethazine[4,5]	4 ml of 12.5% stock solution in 500 ml drinking water	PO	1 to 2 weeks
Carbenicillin[12]	200 mg/kg	PO	Divided doses daily for 1 to 2 weeks

Some of the more commonly utilized anesthetic regimes are described below.

Ether has classically been used as an inhalant by dropping the animal into ether vapor in a closed container. Ether gives good analgesia and muscle relaxation, but it is sporadically unsafe. The animals tend to salivate profusely, so they should be given atropine. Also, they hold their breath at first exposure and often succumb thereafter with one fatal gasp.[4]

Halothane has proved to be a satisfactory drug for induction and maintenance of anesthesia when used at 1% concentration. A 35 to 40% decrease in blood pressure has been reported with its use. Chamber induction with face-mask maintenance is a common technique with halothane anesthesia.

Methoxyflurane, at a concentration of 3% for induction and 1% for maintenance, has proved to be an excellent anesthetic. Induction is slow—up to 15 minutes—but relaxation is good and recovery is within 10 minutes. Atropine should be given prior to induction. Methoxyflurane should be administered the same as halothane.[2,4,5]

Sodium pentobarbital is administered at 30 to 40 mg/kg IP. Its effects last 30 minutes but are unpredictable.[5]

Sodium thiopental has been used with success at 55 mg/kg IP.

Innovar-Vet™[a] is administered at 0.22 to 0.88 ml/kg IM. Its effects range from tranquilization to surgical anesthesia.[10] Anesthesia is very good, but IM injection causes a severe inflammatory reaction in the surrounding tissues, causing nerve, vessel, and muscle necrosis and, sometimes, sloughing of extremities. Self-mutilation of the affected area has been noted.[2,4]

Ketamine hydrochloride is administered at 44 to 100 mg/kg. It produces good sedation but only poor to good anesthesia even at higher dosages.[4] Excellent results have been obtained by using ketamine for induction and methoxyflurane for maintenance.

A combination of 20 mg *acepromazine added to* 100 mg *ketamine* given at 0.2 to 0.4 ml/kg has produced good results.[11] Xylazine 14 mg plus 100 mg ketamine given at 0.4 ml/kg has also been used successfully.[4]

With any anesthesia, the guinea pig should be fasted for 12 hours prior if possible to prevent vomiting and/or dose miscalculations. The heart beat, respiration, muscle relaxation, mucous membrane color, and reflexes should be monitored to determine depth of anesthesia. The pedal reflex is not a reliable indicator in this species.

In case of respiratory arrest, ventilation is sometimes possible by blowing into a plastic syringe cover or cupped hand held over the nose.[4] Tracheal intubation is difficult to accomplish.

Signs of anesthetic overdose include dilatation of pupils, protrusion of eyeballs, and cyanosis.

Surgery

Surgery in the guinea pig is not unlike that in the more common pet species after adequate anesthesia has been achieved. Aseptic technique should be strictly adhered to because of the stress-sensitive nature of the animal and the desirability of minimal antibiotic usage.

Commonly encountered surgical cases include traumatic lacerations and bite wounds, cesarean sections, fractures, cystotomies, tumor and abscess removals, ovariohysterectomies, and castrations.

Radiology

Radiology is a useful tool in the diagnosis of guinea pig maladies, and there are no normal contraindications for its use. It has been used as an aid in diagnosing such diverse conditions as arthritis, malocclusions, fractures, luxations, otitis media, pyometra, neoplasms, and abscesses.

[a]Pitman-Moore, Inc., Washington Crossing, NJ 08560.

Vaccinations

There are no vaccinations indicated for the pet guinea pig.

Public Health

Some problems of potential importance to humans can exist in guinea pigs. Guinea pigs have long been incriminated as offenders in human allergies. They are very susceptible to both the human and bovine type of tuberculosis and can transmit the disease to humans as well. Owners should thus be directed to consult their physicians should one of these conditions be confirmed in their pets. Other human pathogens rarely harbored by guinea pigs include bordetella, salmonella, pasteurella, streptococcus, and diplococcus. Rabies virtually never occurs in pet rodents in the United States.

Euthanasia

Placing the guinea pig in a closed container with a supersaturated atmosphere of ether, chloroform, or halothane is an acceptable method for euthanasia. An overdose of pentobarbital, 80 mg/kg, given IP is, however, probably the most acceptable and convenient method.

REFERENCES

1. Henderson JD: Cervical lymphadenitis in the guinea pig. *VM SAC* 71:462-463, 1976.
2. Wagoner JE, Manning PJ: *The Biology of the Guinea Pig*. New York, Academic Press, 1976.
3. Diaz, J, Soave DA: Cephaloridine treatment of cervical lymphadenitis in guinea pigs. *Lab Anim Dig* 8:60, 1973.
4. Wagoner JE, Harkness JE: *The Biology and Medicine of Rabbits and Rodents*. Philadelphia, Lea & Febiger, 1977.
5. Williams CSF: *Practical Guide to Lab Animals*. St. Louis, CV Mosby Co, 1976.
6. Townsend J: The guinea pig: General husbandry and nutrition. *Vet Rec* 96:451-454, 1975.
7. Olson GA: Malocclusion of the cheek teeth of a guinea pig. *Lab Anim Dig* 7:12-14, 1971.
8. McDonald SE, Lavvipierre MJ: *Trixacarus caviae* infestation in two guinea pigs. *Lab Anim Sci* 30(1):67-70, 1980.
9. Henderson JD: Treatment of cutaneous acariasis in the guinea pig. *JAVMA* 163:591-592, 1973.
10. Rubright WC, Thayer CB: Innovar-Vet, a surgical anesthetic for the guinea pig. *Pract Vet* 43(3):15-25, 1971.
11. Mulder JB, Johnson HB: Anesthesia with ketaset plus in guinea pigs and hamsters. *VM SAC* 74:1807-1808, 1979.
12. Jacobson E: Personal communication, University of Florida, 1980.

A Clinical Guide to the Pet Ferret

Lennox M. Ryland, DVM
Halecrest Veterinary Hospital
Seattle, Washington

Susan L. Bernard, MS
John R. Gorham, DVM, PhD

Animal Disease Research Unit
Agricultural Research Service, USDA
Washington State University
Pullman, Washington

Man's association with ferrets can be traced back as far as the fourth century BC, when the long-bodied, supple descendants of the European polecat were first domesticated and used for exterminating snakes and rodents, and later, for hunting rabbits. The domestic ferret (*Mustela putorius furo*) should not be confused with the native North American black-footed ferret (*Mustela nigripes*), now nearly extinct.[1] Unlike its fellow Mustelidae (e.g., skunks, otters, mink, weasels, badgers), the domestic ferret is not a wild animal, and it has survived for generations only in captivity. Long raised as a laboratory animal for studies in reproductive physiology, pharmacology, and virology, the ferret is becoming increasingly popular today as a household pet. For the veterinary practitioner unfamiliar with the care and management of a pet ferret, the following is intended to be a guide to routine prophylactic, diagnostic, and therapeutic procedures.

Species Characteristics

There are two varieties of ferrets, based on coloration: fitch ferrets are buff with black masks, feet, and tails (Figure 1); albino ferrets are white with pink eyes. The albino phenotype and color mutants (e.g., Siamese, silver, and silver mitt) are recessive to the fitch. Female ferrets are called *jills* and males, *hobs*. Baby ferrets are *kits*.[2]

Kits are born deaf and blind after 42 days gestation. The average litter size is 8 (range, 2 to 17). Their eyes and ears open at 21 to 37 days of age, and their deciduous teeth begin to erupt at 14 days, at which time kits begin to eat solid food. Their permanent canines erupt at 47 to 52 days of age, and kits are weaned by the time they are 8 weeks old. They reach their adult weight at 4 months of age.[3] Males are typically twice as large as females (range, 600 to 2000 g), but both sexes undergo photoperiodic weight fluctuations of 30 to 40% of their body weight, adding subcutaneous fat in the fall and losing this fat in the spring.[4]

Ferrets reach sexual maturity in the spring following their birth (or at 9 to 12 months of age).[3] The female is seasonally polyestrous, with a normal breeding season from March to August, though females may remain in heat for up to 6 months if copulation does not occur. Onset of estrus can be recognized by enlargement of the vulva (Figure 2), which

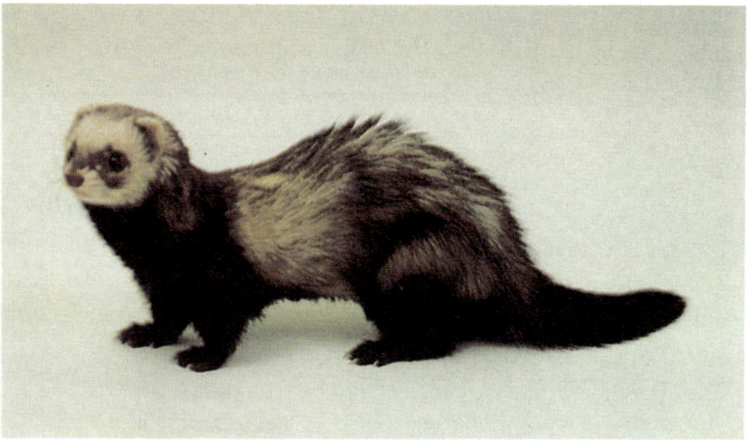

Figure 1—Typical fitch ferret.

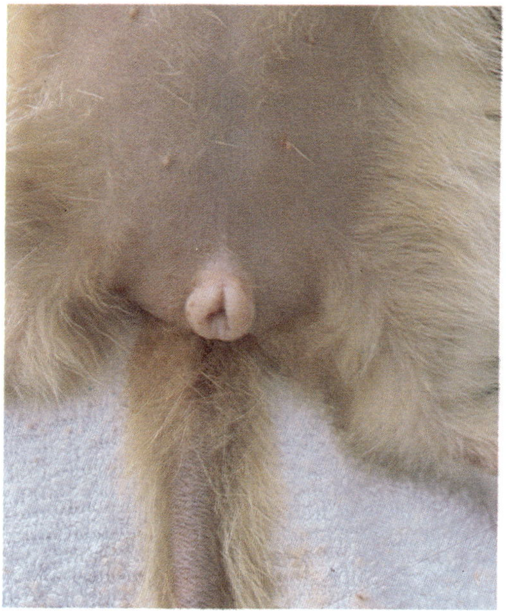

Figure 2—*(Right)* Swollen vulva indicative of estrus. Note alopecia of ventral abdomen and tail.

regresses to normal size within 2 to 3 weeks after coitus. Ovulation is induced by copulation, and if fertilization fails to occur, a pseudopregnancy of 42 days will ensue. Male ferrets' breeding readiness is signaled by descent of the testes into the scrotum. Two litters per year can be obtained if the females are bred early in the breeding season.

Gross anatomic features of the ferret include the absence of a cecum, appendix, and prostate gland (male).[5] Ferrets have a vertebral formula of $C_7T_{14}L_6S_3Cd_{14-18}$ with 14 pairs of ribs.[6] The ferret's permanent dental formula is $2(I^3/_3\ C^1/_1\ P^4/_3\ M^1/_2)$.[7] Supernumerary incisors are common in adults.[8] Ferrets do not have well-developed sweat glands and are prone to heat prostration at a temperature approaching 32°C (90°F). The average life span in laboratory colonies is 5 to 6 years, but pet ferrets commonly live 9 or 10 years.

Ferrets typically have genial personalities and adapt well to human companionship, particularly if they are raised from infancy in close human contact. They are inquisitive and playful animals by nature, and when given supervised freedom in which to satisfy their innate curiosity and inclination to burrow, they need no special exercise equipment. Because they tend to urinate and defecate in habitual places, they can be easily trained to use a litter box. Some pet ferrets have even been trained to walk on a leash and harness. There is no natural animosity between ferrets and cats or dogs.

Diet

The nutritional requirements of ferrets have not been determined. For more than 25 years at Washington State University (WSU), ferrets have been maintained adequately on a standard wet feed mink diet (30% fat, 35% protein, 5 to 6% ash). Pet ferrets are maintained with commercial cat food supplemented with table scraps. At WSU, because nutritional deficiencies have never been recognized in the colony and because there are few reports in the literature, the nutritional requirements of ferrets are assumed to be similar to those of cats and mink. The National Research Council requirements for mink and cats are listed in Table I.[9,10] Since ferrets will eat to their caloric requirement, they can eventually get into a situation of low protein intake on cat food. This can result in poor reproductive performance.[38] Milk is a good source of supplemental calcium, but may cause loose feces. The ferret has little, if any, capacity to digest fiber. Small bones should be withheld from the diet to prevent their becoming lodged in the mouth or gastrointestinal tract. Ferrets do not need to eat mice or other rodents. Fresh water, in either a cup or drinking bottle, should be available at all times.

Restraint

The ferret is best restrained when grasped above the shoulders, with one hand gently squeezing the forelimbs together, the thumb under the animal's chin. A handler may choose to wear a leather glove, as even the best trained ferret becomes apprehensive in strange surroundings.

The drugs and dosages commonly used to provide chemical restraint and sedation in ferrets are summarized in Table II. At WSU, a simultaneous intramuscular injection of xylazine HCl (1 to 4 mg/kg) and ketamine HCl (20 to 30 mg/kg) is used routinely for short periods of chemical restraint (10 to 20 minutes). If longer periods of anesthesia are needed, gas anesthesia (methoxyflurane or halothane) delivered by mask works well. The use of barbiturates is limited due to the relative inaccessibility of peripheral veins. Intramuscular and subcutaneous injections are given as with the cat or dog, with due regard to the increased fat layer present in autumn or winter.

Vaccinations

Ferrets must be protected against canine distemper by

TABLE I

RECOMMENDED NUTRIENT ALLOWANCES FOR CATS AND MINK[9,10] (PERCENTAGE OR AMOUNT/KG DIET, DRY BASIS[a])

Nutrient	Unit	Amount: Mink	Amount: Cat
Protein	%	25–32	28
Fat	%	6–20	9
Linoleic acid	%	ND[b]	1
Minerals			
Calcium	%	0.3	1.0
Phosphorus	%	0.3	0.8
Potassium	%	ND	0.3
Sodium chloride	%	0.5	0.5
Magnesium	%	ND	0.05
Iron	mg	114	100
Copper	mg	ND	5
Manganese	mg	ND	10
Zinc	mg	ND	30
Iodine	mg	ND	1
Selenium	mg	ND	0.1
Vitamins			
Vitamin A	IU	10,000	10,000
Vitamin D	IU	ND	1,000
Vitamin E	IU	25	80
Thiamine	mg	1.2	5
Riboflavin	mg	1.5	5
Pantothenic acid	mg	4–8	10
Niacin	mg	20	45
Pyridoxine	mg	1.1	4
Folic acid	mg	0.5	1.0
Biotin	mg	ND	0.05
Vitamin B_{12}	mg	30	0.02
Choline	mg	1,000	2,000

[a]Based on a diet with metabolizable energy concentration of 4 kcal/g of dry matter (cat) and 4.25 kcal/g of dry matter (mink).
[b]Not determined.

vaccination with modified live virus of chick embryo tissue culture origin. The first dose of vaccine should be administered at six to eight weeks of age (four to six weeks if kits are from unvaccinated dams) and a booster given two weeks later; thereafter, boosters should be given every three years. Killed vaccine provides only short-term immunity that is slow to develop and that is not effective in all ferrets.[11] Distemper vaccine prepared from ferret cell culture should not be used, because attenuated virus may possibly retain its virulence for its natural host.

Rabies vaccine, killed only, should be administered annually, beginning at three months of age. The ferret is assumed to be highly susceptible to rabies and capable of transmitting the virus. Two cases of ferret rabies have been reported in the United States since 1954, and in one of those, the possibility exists that clinical disease followed vaccination with modified live rabies virus.[12]

Ferrets are not susceptible to disease produced by feline panleukopenia, mink virus enteritis, canine hepatitis, feline rhinotracheitis, or feline calicivirus, and do not require vaccination against these diseases. There is no definitive evidence that ferrets are susceptible to disease produced by canine parvovirus; therefore, vaccination is probably not warranted. Because clinical trials have never been conducted on the safety or efficacy of the commonly used four- and five-way canine vaccines, the authors are hesitant to recommend them for use in ferrets. A schedule of vaccinations and prophylactic procedures is outlined in Table III.

TABLE II

DRUGS USED FOR CHEMICAL RESTRAINT AND SEDATION IN FERRETS

Drug	Dosage	Route
Sedatives		
Acepromazine	0.2–0.5 mg/kg	IM, SQ
Xylazine	1.0 mg/kg	IM, SQ
Preanesthetics		
Atropine	0.05 mg/kg	IM, SQ
Acepromazine	0.1–0.25 mg/kg	IM, SQ
Anesthetics		
Ketamine (9 parts:1 part acepromazine)	20–35 mg/kg (ketamine) 0.2–0.35 mg/kg (acepromazine)	IM, SQ
Xylazine (followed by ketamine)	1–4 mg/kg (xylazine) 20–30 mg/kg (ketamine)	SQ
Halothane		Mask
Methoxyflurane		Mask
Pentobarbital	30 mg/kg	IP

Routine Surgical Procedures

Female ferrets not intended for breeding purposes should be spayed at six to eight months of age. Estrous

TABLE III

SCHEDULE OF VACCINATIONS AND ROUTINE PROPHYLACTIC CARE

Age	Plan
6–8 weeks (4–6 weeks if dam unvaccinated)	First CDV;[a] fecal
9–12 weeks	Second CDV; fecal
12 weeks	Rabies[b] vaccination
6–8 months	Spay/castrate; fecal Remove musk glands (optional)
1 year	Rabies booster (annual)
3 years	CDV booster (triennial)

[a]CDV = canine distemper vaccine (nonferret origin).
[b]Killed.

females have high endogenous estrogen levels which cause a greater than 50% prevalence of fatal bone marrow depression (see *metabolic diseases*).[13] The use of one intramuscular injection of 100 IU of human chorionic gonadotropin (HCG) 10 or more days after onset of estrus will cause ovulation. Females will cycle out of heat in 20 to 25 days and remain in anestrus for 40 to 50 days.[13] The use of megestrol acetate to delay or prevent estrus in ferrets greatly increases the risk of subsequent pyometra and should be avoided.

Male ferrets not intended for breeding should be castrated at six to eight months of age to reduce their aggressiveness and desire to roam and to remove some of the musky odor resulting from sebaceous secretions. The testes are present in the scrotum only during the breeding season; from July to December, they are located in the subcutis of the caudoventral abdomen.

Ferrets have paired musk-producing glands lateral to the anus which secrete when the animal is angry, excited, or in estrus. These may be removed at the time of neutering or spaying. Standard procedures for canine anal sac excision may be followed. A modified protocol designed specifically for ferret musk gland resection has been published.[14] Excision of these paired glands will reduce, but cannot eliminate, the ferret's musky odor.

Physiologic and Laboratory Data

Blood samples for clinical laboratory procedures may be obtained by toenail clipping (≤0.5 ml), caudal tail venipuncture, or by jugular venipuncture. Cardiac puncture is possible by both transthoracic and transdiaphragmatic approaches but represents additional risk.

Hematological values for ferrets are presented in Table IV[5] and are generally similar to those of the cat. Notable exceptions include the ferret's higher hematocrit (mean, 52.3%), more numerous erythrocytes (mean, $9.17 \times 10^6/mm^3$), and higher percentage of reticulocytes (mean, 4.6%). Estrous females will tend to have lower platelet and leukocyte counts.

Normal serum chemistry values for ferrets are given in Table V. No major differences between these values and those of the cat or dog are apparent. Mild to moderate proteinuria is a consistent finding in normal ferrets and is postulated to result from the ferret's relatively high systolic blood pressure.[5] The naturally dark urine of the male may give false positive values for ketonuria when colorimetric determinations are used.

The ferret's normal heart rate approximates 250 beats/minute.[5] Electrocardiographic (ECG) measurements of wave amplitude are similar to those of the normal feline ECG, although the height of the ferret's R wave may approach but should not exceed 2.0 mV. Radiographically, the cardiac silhouette may be interpreted incorrectly as having dilatation of the left ventricle.

The ferret's normal respiratory rate is 33 to 36 breaths/minute and its body temperature varies between 38 and 40°C (100.8 to 104°F).

Common Parasites and Fungi

Ferrets are subject to most of the external parasites of domestic dogs and cats. Infestation with *Sarcoptes scabiei* may take two forms. In cases in which skin lesions predominate, focal to generalized alopecia and intense

TABLE IV

HEMATOLOGIC VALUES OF NORMAL FERRETS OF BOTH SEXES[a]

Hematology	*Mean*	*Range*
Hematocrit (%)	52.3	42–61
Hemoglobin (g/dl)	17.0	15–18
Erythrocytes ($10^6/mm^3$)	9.17	6.8–12.2
Leukocytes ($10^3/mm^3$)	10.1	4.0–19
Leukocytes		
Lymphocytes (%)	34.5	12–54
Neutrophils (%)	58.3	11–84
Monocytes (%)	4.4	0–9.0
Eosinophils (%)	2.5	0–7.0
Basophils (%)	0.1	0–2.0
Reticulocytes (%)	4.6	1–14
Platelets ($10^3/mm^3$)	499	297–910
Total protein (g/dl)	6.0	5.1–7.4

[a]From Thornton PC, Wright PA, et al: The ferret, *Mustela putorius furo*, as a new species in toxicology. *Lab Anim* 13:119-124, 1979. Adapted with permission.

TABLE V

SERUM CHEMISTRY VALUES OF NORMAL FERRETS OF BOTH SEXES[a]

Parameter	*Unit*	*Mean*	*Range*
Glucose	mg/dl	136	94–207
BUN	mg/dl	22	10–45
Albumin	mg/dl	3.2	2.3–3.8
Alkaline phosphatase	IU/L	23	9–84
Aspartate aminotransferase (SAST; SGOT)	IU/L	65	28–120
Total bilirubin	mg/dl	<1.0	
Cholesterol	mg/dl	165	64–296
Creatinine	mg/dl	0.6	0.4–0.9
Sodium	mmol/L	148	137–162
Potassium	mmol/L	5.9	4.5–7.7
Chloride	mmol/L	116	106–125
Calcium	mg/dl	9.2	8.0–11.8
Phosphorus	mg/dl	5.9	4.0–9.1

[a]From Thornton PC, Wright PA, et al: The ferret, *Mustela putorius furo*, as a new species in toxicology. *Lab Anim* 13:119-124, 1979. Adapted with permission.

pruritus are associated with the mite, which can be found in a skin scraping. In cases in which sarcoptic lesions are confined to the toes and feet, the feet are swollen, scabby, and if untreated, clawless. Treatment consists of cutting back the claws and removing the scabs after softening them in warm water. The mites may be eliminated by application of sulfur ointment or lime and sulfur dips and washes. Organophosphates and carbamates should be used with caution, as safe levels for ferrets have not been established. However, at WSU, sarcoptic mange has been treated successfully with carbaryl (0.5%) shampoos applied weekly for three weeks. Pruritus may be reduced by concomitant administration of corticosteroids (2 mg/kg prednisone). Ferrets may also be infested with fleas (*Ctenocephalides* spp.) and ear mites (*Otodectes cyanotis*) which may be treated with rotenone or pyrethrin products.[15]

Less is known about the susceptibility of the ferret to the common internal parasites of the dog and cat, although coccidiosis and toxoplasmosis have been reported. The ferret is undoubtedly also susceptible to a variety of gastrointestinal helminths (including *Toxascaris leonina*) and protozoa (including *Giardia* spp.[39]). Guidelines for cats should be followed whenever treatment is initiated. Natural infections with *Dirofilaria immitis* have been reported in ferrets.[16] Because of the small size of its heart, 6 to 10 adult worms are sufficient to produce severe respiratory distress, ascites, and death. Avermectins are very effective against *Dirofilaria* in ferrets.[17]

Ringworm (*Microsporum canis*) has been reported in young ferrets and may be transmitted by cats. Lesions are similar to those in other species (Figure 3). Affected ferrets may be treated orally with griseofulvin (25 mg/kg), although clinical signs often regress without treatment.

Bacterial Diseases

Ferrets are moderately susceptible to botulism (*Clostridium botulinum*) types A and B, and they are highly susceptible to botulism type C. Signs of dysphagia, ataxia, and paresis appear 12 to 96 hours after eating contaminated foods. Death follows with paralysis of respiratory muscles. There is no successful treatment, although the disease can be prevented by excluding from the diet ingredients of questionable origin or freshness, or by prophylactic annual use of type C toxoid.

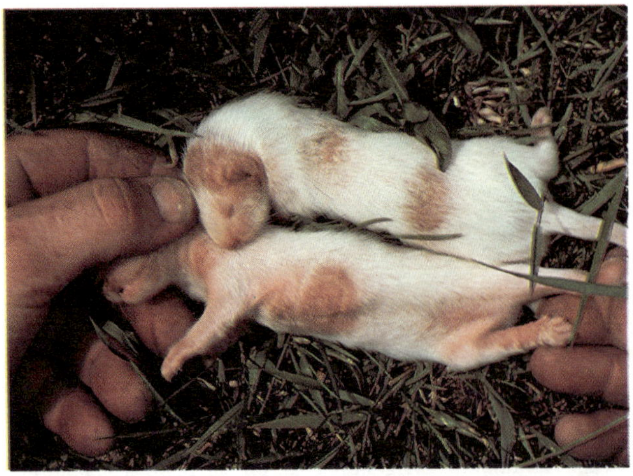

Figure 3—Lesions caused by *Microsporum canis* in a young kit. These lesions regressed without treatment.

Avian, bovine, and human strains of mycobacteria cause tuberculosis in ferrets. Lesions are seen primarily in the alimentary tract and abdominal lymph nodes. Signs may not appear until the late stages of active infection, when the animal becomes emaciated and may exhibit paralysis of the pelvic adductor muscles. Paralysis later affects all four limbs.[18] Massive accumulations of histiocytes in abdominal organs and intracellular acid-fast bacilli are diagnostic. Tuberculosis may be suspected if the animal gives a thermal response to the subcutaneous tuberculin test or if it has palpably enlarged mesenteric lymph nodes.

Staphylococcal, streptococcal, and corynebacterial abscesses and localized infections of the mammary glands (in nursing jills), uterus, vulva, infected bite wounds incurred during mating, and oral injuries caused by ingested bones are common. Group C streptococcal pneumonia and septicemia may lead to valvular endocarditis. Treatment should be similar to that used in cats, based on results of culture and antibiotic susceptibility testing. However, ferrets should be given no more than 50 mg of streptomycin at 12-hour intervals, because it is toxic in higher doses.[15]

Campylobacter fetus subsp. *jejuni* has been isolated from six of nine ferrets with proliferative colitis. Clinical signs of proliferative colitis included green mucohemorrhagic feces, rectal prolapse, anorexia, and dehydration.[19] Supportive fluid therapy combined with broad-spectrum antibiotics (chloramphenicol or gentamicin) did not alleviate the condition. All affected ferrets died or were euthanatized when moribund.[19]

Viral Diseases

Ferrets are highly susceptible to canine distemper. Moreover, because the case fatality rate approaches 100%, ferrets are used as test animals for the detection of the virus. The initial signs of disease appear 7 to 10 days after exposure and include anorexia and mucopurulent ocular and nasal discharges (Figure 4). A rash appears commonly under the chin and in the inguinal area 10 to 12 days following exposure (Figure 5). The foot pads may swell and become hyperkeratotic. The animal continues to deteriorate until death, 12 to 16 days after exposure with ferret-adapted strains (21 to 25 days with canine strains). Ferrets that survive the catarrhal phase may die during a central nervous system phase of distemper, signs of which include hyperexcitability, excess salivation, muscular tremor, convulsions, and coma. Because the signs of distemper are so typical, the disease is rarely confused with other conditions. Clinical diagnosis can be confirmed with fluorescent antibody techniques or histopathology. In the authors' experience with over 1000 cases of distemper, not a single ferret has survived, suggesting that euthanasia is a practical alternative to symptomatic, supportive treatment.

Ferrets are susceptible to infection with several strains of human influenza virus, which may cause initial signs similar to those of distemper. Within 48 hours of exposure, the affected ferret becomes listless, febrile, and anorectic, and its nose becomes moist. Sneezing attacks may develop, accompanied by a purulent nasal discharge. Congestion may be relieved by antihistamines suitable for use in other small animals. Recovery usually occurs within five days of onset of signs and the ferret is immune for at least five weeks against the homologous influenza strain. Vaccination with attenuated live virus affords protection of a similar duration, but it is not recommended routinely.[20]

Aleutian disease is usually subclinical in ferrets, but affected animals may become hypergammaglobulinemic and cachectic, with black, tarry feces. They may eventually succumb as long as 200 days after infection. Stressed animals may die unexpectedly even though in good flesh.[21] The disease may be differentiated from acute episodes of nonspecific enteritis and should be suspected if the ferret's gamma globulin fraction exceeds 20% of total serum protein. The diagnosis can be confirmed by counter immunoelectrophoresis. Lesions include lymphocytic and plasmacytic infiltration of liver, spleen, lungs, and kidneys, and follicular hyperplasia of lymph nodes. There appears to be a biological difference between Aleutian disease virus of mink or ferret origin.[22]

Feline leukemia virus (FeLV) does not appear to produce clinical disease in ferrets. The authors have recognized FeLV-positive, clinically healthy, ferrets.[40] It is possible that ferrets have their own retrovirus which cross reacts with the FeLV assay.[a]

Ferrets are susceptible to pseudorabies and infectious bovine rhinotracheitis. However, natural outbreaks of these diseases have not been reported.

Metabolic Diseases

One of the most common clinical problems seen in pet ferrets is bone marrow depression associated with prolonged estrus.[13,23] There is a greater than 50% prevalence of this disorder during the months of April through July in intact nonbred females. Bone marrow depression is due to high endogenous estrogen levels during estrus, producing pancytopenia. Clinical signs include pale mucous membranes, bilaterally symmetrical alopecia, melena, petechial hemorrhages, anorexia, and depression (Figure 6). Pale (fatty) bone marrow which floats in formalin is the most consistent finding. Pancytopenia predisposes animals to secondary bacterial infections and bleeding disorders. Treatment of bone marrow depression is difficult, as most animals have a packed-cell volume (PCV) of less than 10% and a platelet count under 20,000/mm². Two animals are known to have survived this condition using two different treatment regimens. One female was ovariohysterectomized despite a PCV of 6%.[41] The other ferret was treated successfully with ovariohysterectomy and 15 intravenous blood transfusions (10 ml each) over a five-month period, coupled with anabolic steroids, corticosteroids, force feeding, and oral vitamin supplementation.[24] A bone marrow transplant was also done but is of questionable value. The use of whole blood transfusions (if available) and surgery may be the most logical treatment. If surgery is not elected, the animal can be cycled out of heat with HCG, as described previously. During this period, anabolic steroids, vitamins, and transfusions are recommended.

Posterior paralysis accompanied by incontinence may appear in an otherwise healthy animal. This paralysis may be due to hemivertebrae, vertebral fractures, intervertebral disk disease, hematomyelia, or myelitis.[13,25,26] Ferrets with no radiographic lesions and ferrets with intervertebral disk problems have responded favorably to steroid therapy. This condition can recur.

Urolithiasis is fairly common in ferrets. It is manifested by urinary incontinence and malaise and can be fatal.[27] Males and females are affected equally. Renal and cystic calculi composed of magnesium ammonium phosphate (struvite) have been reported. Therapy is similar to that for feline urolithiasis and cystitis. Limiting dietary ash and providing adequate water may aid in decreasing the recurrence of uroliths.

Pregnant and postparturient females are predisposed to several nutrition-dependent diseases, such as eclamptogenic toxemia and *nursing sickness*. Vitamin and mineral supplementation suitable for use in cats should be instituted during pregnancy and lactation. Insuring that the dam's dietary needs are met during these critical times will help reduce preweaning deaths among kits due to lactational failure or cannibalism. Cannibalism is more pronounced in certain families and may be an undesirable genetic trait, though normally most dams or kits will consume a dead neonate.

Ferrets are subject to a variety of spontaneous and congenital malformations that may be hereditary. These include anencephaly, neuroschisis, gastroschisis, cryptorchidism, amelia, corneal dermoids, and cataracts.[28,29]

Endocrine imbalances similar to those of dogs and cats have been reported in ferrets. At least one ferret has been treated satisfactorily for diabetes mellitus with insulin[b] (1 to 2 units/kg).[30]

A bilaterally symmetrical alopecia of the tail and/or ventral abdomen is common in estrous females and has been observed in males during the normal breeding season (Figure 2). The cause of the alopecia is unknown but a hormonal basis is suspected. Hair returns to normal once the breeding season ends or if the female goes out of heat (either by breeding or HCG injection). Avidin

[a]Leukassay F®, Pitman-Moore, Inc., Washington Crossing, NJ 08560.

[b]NPH Iletin®, Eli Lilly and Co., Indianapolis, IN 46285.

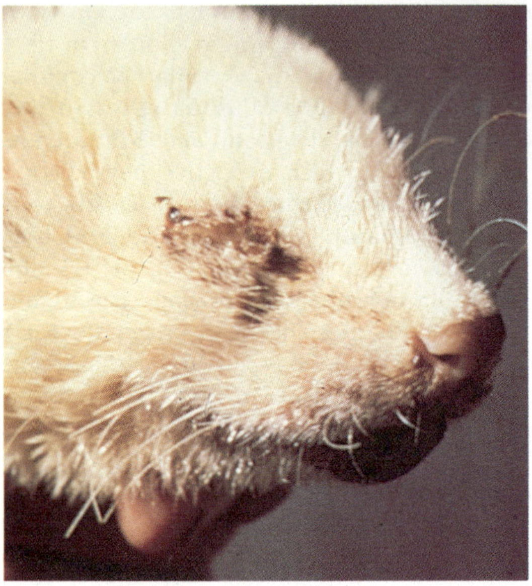

Figure 4—Nasal and ocular discharge associated with canine distemper in ferrets.

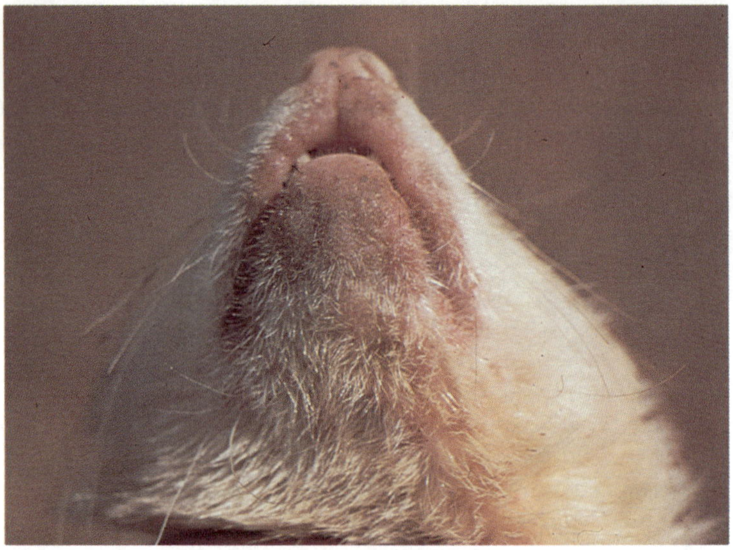

Figure 5—Chin rash in a ferret with canine distemper.

(present in raw eggs) binds up biotin and can cause alopecia.[15] Biotin deficiency can be avoided by decreasing the number of raw eggs in the diet, by boiling the eggs for 15 minutes, or by supplementing the feed with additional biotin.

Zinc toxicity in ferrets causes a diffuse nephrosis manifested by cachexia and macrocytic, hypochromic anemia.[31] Diets contaminated with high levels of zinc are associated with these toxic signs.[32] Treatment includes removal of the cause and supportive therapy.

Neoplastic Diseases

A variety of spontaneous epithelial and mesenchymal neoplasms have been reported in ferrets. Two cases of lymphosarcoma have been reported.[8,33] Affected animals were not tested for FeLV; therefore, the relationship between FeLV and ferret lymphosarcoma is not known.

Ovarian leiomyomas are common in ferrets. These neoplasms do not appear to interfere with ovulation and pregnancy and are incidental findings at necropsy.[34] Bilateral ovarian thecomas with endometrial hyperplasia have been reported in one ferret as an incidental finding.[33] An estrogen-secreting adrenal adenoma reportedly caused an ovariectomized female to exhibit signs of estrus.[33] No other apparent hormonal imbalance was recognized in this female.

Cutaneous squamous cell carcinomas have been reported in ferrets. One tumor was removed successfully, with no evidence of metastasis four months later.[33,35] Cutaneous collections of mast cells have been reported. These mast cell tumors are not considered aggressive.[36]

Adenocarcinoma in two ferrets has been described. One was pancreatic and was considered an incidental postmortem finding.[33] The second was hepatocellular and was from a cachectic ferret with a chronic draining abdominal fistula.[8]

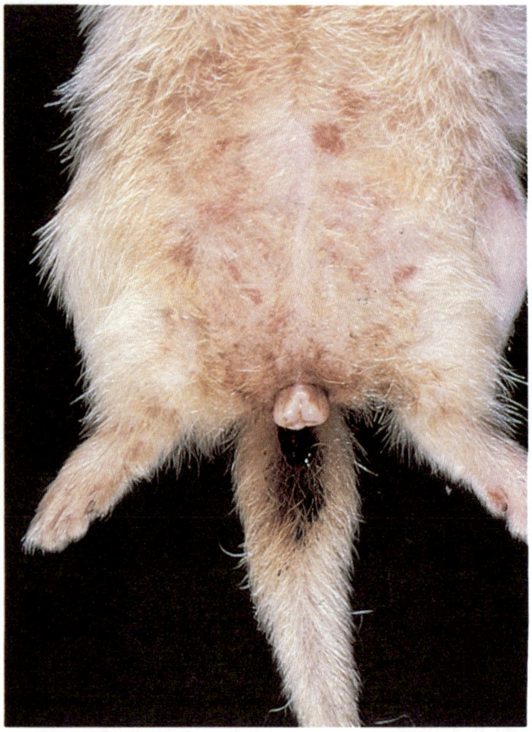

Figure 6—Estrous female that succumbed to bone marrow depression. Cutaneous petechiae, melena (staining tail), and alopecia are common.

Malignant megakaryocytic myelosis was reported in a lethargic, anorectic four-year-old female ferret.[37] Systemic metastases were reported.

These examples of confirmed diagnoses are given to underscore the similarities between ferrets and more familiar companion animal species. Judicious use of diagnostic tools (history, physical examination, clinical pathology, radiology) is as relevant to ferrets as to the dog or cat. Once a diagnosis has been reached, medical therapy, where appropriate, should follow guidelines established for cats unless experience dictates otherwise.

Acknowledgment

The authors wish to thank Dr. C. W. Leathers for his critical review of this article.

REFERENCES

1. *Threatened Wildlife of the United States*, Publication 114, US Government Printing Office, Washington, DC, US Dept. of the Interior, Bureau of Sport Fisheries and Wildlife, 1973, p 289.
2. Roberts MF: *All about Ferrets*. Neptune City, NJ, TFH Public Inc, Ltd, 1977.
3. Shump AV, Shump KA: Growth and development of the European fitch (*Mustela putorius*). *Lab Anim Sci* 28:89-91, 1978.
4. Hammond J. *The Ferret: Some Observations on Photoperiod and Gonadal Activity, and Their Role in Seasonal Pelt and Bodyweight Changes*. Cambridge, Heffer & Sons Ltd, 1974, pp 3-11.
5. Thornton PC, Wright PA, et al: The ferret, *Mustela putorius furo*, as a new species in toxicology. *Lab Anim* 13:119-124, 1979.
6. Owen R: *On the Anatomy of Vertebrates*, vol 2. New York, AMS Press, 1973.
7. Owen R: *On the Anatomy of Vertebrates*, vol 3. New York, AMS Press, 1973.
8. Andrews PL, Illman O, et al: Some observations of anatomical abnormalities and disease states in a population of 350 ferrets (*Mustela furo L.*) *Z Versuchstierkd* 21:346-353, 1979.
9. *Nutrient Requirements of Cats*, vol 13. Washington, DC, National Academy of Sciences, 1978.
10. *Nutrient Requirements of Mink and Foxes*, vol 7. Washington, DC, National Academy of Sciences, 1968.
11. Ott RL, Svehag SE, et al: Resistance to experimental distemper in ferrets following the use of killed tissue vaccine. *West Vet* 6:107-111, 1959.
12. *Veterinary Public Health Notes*, US Dept. of Health and Human Services. Public Health Service, Centers for Disease Control, Atlanta, GA, 30333. Oct. 1980.
13. Bernard SL, Leathers CW, et al: Estrogen induced bone marrow depression in ferrets. *Am J Vet Res*, in press.
14. Creed JE, Kainer RA: Surgical extirpation and related anatomy of anal sacs of the ferret. *JAVMA* 179:575-577, 1981.
15. Ryland LM, Gorham JR: The ferret and its diseases. *JAVMA* 173:1154-1158, 1978.
16. Miller WR, Merton DA: Dirofilariasis in a ferret. *JAVMA* 180:1103-1104, 1982.
17. Blair LS, Campbell WC: Trial of Avermectin B_1a, mebendazole and Melarsoprol against pre-cardiac *Dirofilaria immitis* in the ferret (*Mustela putorius furo*). *J Parasitol* 64:1032-1034, 1978.
18. Symmers WS, Symmers C, et al: Observations on tuberculosis in ferrets (*Mustela furo L.*). *J Comp Pathol* 63:20-30, 1953.
19. Fox JG, Murphy JC, et al: Proliferative colitis in ferrets. *Am J Vet Res* 43:858-864, 1982.
20. Potter CW, Oxford JS, et al: Immunity to influenza in ferrets. I. Responses to live and killed virus. *Br J Exp Pathol* 53:153-167, 1972.
21. Ohshima K, Shen DT, et al: Comparison of the lesions of Aleutian disease of mink and hypergammaglobulinemia in ferrets. *Am J Vet Res* 39:653-657, 1978.
22. Porter HG, Porter DD, et al: Aleutian disease in ferrets. *Infect Immun* 36:379-386, 1982.
23. Kociba GJ, Caputo CA: Aplastic anemia associated with estrus in pet ferrets. *JAVMA* 178:1293-1294, 1981.
24. Ryland LM: Remission of estrus-associated anemia following ovariohysterectomy and multiple blood transfusion in a ferret. *JAVMA* 181:820-822, 1982.
25. Fredrick MA: Intervertebral disc syndrome in a domestic ferret. *VM SAC* 76:835, 1981.
26. Padgett GA, Alexander JE: Posterior paralysis in mink. *North-eastern Mink Farms* 110:20-21, 1966.
27. Nguyen HT, Moreland AF, et al: Urolithiasis in ferrets (*Mustela putorius*). *Lab Anim Sci* 29:342-345, 1979.
28. Willis LS, Barrow MV: The ferret (*Mustela putorius furo L.*) as a laboratory animal. *Lab Anim Sci* 21:712-716, 1971.
29. Utroska B, Austin AL: Bilateral cataracts in a ferret. *VM SAC* 74:1176, 1979.
30. Carpenter JW, Novilla MN: Diabetes mellitus in a black footed ferret. *JAVMA* 171:890-893, 1977.
31. Straube EF, Schuster NH, et al: Zinc toxicity in the ferret. *J Comp Pathol* 90:355-361, 1980.
32. Straube EF, Walden NB: Zinc poisoning in ferrets (*Mustela Putorius furo*). *Lab Anim* 15:45-47, 1981.
33. Chesterman FC, Pomerance A: Spontaneous neoplasms in ferrets and polecats. *J Pathol Bacteriol* 89:529-533, 1965.
34. Cotchin E: Smooth-muscle hyperplasia and neoplasia in the ovaries of domestic ferrets (*Mustela putorius furo*). *J Pathol* 130:169-179, 1980.
35. Zwicker GM, Carlton WW: Spontaneous squamous cell carcinoma in a ferret. *J Wildl Dis* 10:213-216, 1974.
36. Symmers SC, Thomson APD: Multiple carcinomata and focal mast cell accumulations in the skin of a ferret (*Mustela furo L.*) with a note on other tumors in ferrets. *J Pathol Bacteriol* 65:481-492, 1953.
37. Chaudhung KA, Shilinger RB: Spontaneous megakaryocytic myelosis in a four-year-old domestic ferret (*Mustela furo*). *Vet Pathol* 19:561-564, 1982.
38. Evans RH: Personal communication, Ralston Purina Co, St. Louis, MO.
39. Kaufman J: Personal communication, Fort Collins, CO.
40. Strother M: Personal communication, Washington State Univ.
41. Ranta L: Personal communication, Desert Veterinary Clinic, Richland, WA.

UPDATE

Since the original publication of this article in 1983, numerous reports describing various clinical disease syndromes have appeared in the literature. The reader is referred to *Biology and Diseases of the Ferret*, by James G. Fox (Lea & Febiger, 1988) for a comprehensive list of published articles to 1988. Of particular interest are the increasingly common reports of pancreatic islet cell tumors (insulinomas), FeLV-unassociated lymphosarcomas, and cardiomyopathies. The signs, diagnosis, and treatment of these conditions are similar to those in other affected species. While the incidence of estrogen-induced bone marrow suppression has declined with increased public awareness, the aforementioned use of HCG is unreliable for inducing ovulation in estral females. Owners should be encouraged to spay jills; but, where feasible, sterile matings with vasectomized hobs will terminate estrus effectively without pregnancy.

Vaccination recommendations remain unchanged, but practitioners should note that, as of this writing, Imrab (Pitman-Moore, Inc.) is the only rabies vaccine approved for use in ferrets. While controlled studies have never been conducted, it is this author's opinion (LMR) that multivalent canine vaccines with modified life distemper virus of nonferret origin are both safe and effective.

Canine Distemper Virus (CDV) Vaccination

First injection, 8 to 10 weeks of age; second injection, 10 to 12 weeks of age; booster injections, every 3 years.

Although ferrets are not susceptible to disease caused by canine parvovirus type 2 (CPV-2), canine parainfluenza virus (CPI), or the other diseases mentioned in the article, vaccination with four- or five-way canine vaccines is not harmful. Ferrets in our colony that were vaccinated with these products resisted disease when challenged with virulent CDV.

Prolonged Estrus

Jills in prolonged estrus may be cycled out of estrus and into pseudopregnancy by 20 μg gonadotropin-releasing hormone (GnRH).

Deep Mycoses

Cryptococcus neoformans,[1] *Blastomyces dermatitidis*,[2] and *Actinomyces*[3] spp. have been reported in ferrets.

Bacterial Diseases

Escherichia coli may cause gangrenous mastitis in nursing jills. Gentamicin given intramuscularly at 1 mg/kg daily for one week (or gentamicin injected directly into the affected gland) plus procaine penicillin G given intramuscularly daily for one week may be efficacious in controlling the disease if it is diagnosed early.

Viral Diseases

Many ferrets of various ages reported by clinicians to have enlarged spleens (or idiopathic hypersplenism, reported initially by Ferguson[4]) are FeLV-positive. It is possible that there is a ferret-host retrovirus, as in some cases the histopathologic diagnosis was splenic lymphosarcoma. Removal of the affected spleen may be curative.

1. Greenlee PG, Stephens E: Meningeal cryptococcosis and congestive cardiomyopathy in a ferret. *JAVMA* 184:840–841, 1984.
2. Lenhard A: Blastomycosis in a ferret. *JAVMA* 186:70–72, 1985.
3. Skulski G, Symmers WStC: Actinomycosis and torulosis in a ferret. *J Comp Pathol* 64:306–311, 1954.
4. Ferguson DC: Idiopathic hypersplenism in a ferret. *JAVMA* 186:693–695, 1985.

Lennox M. Ryland
Renee C. Pearson
John R. Gorham

Canine Distemper Virus Infection in the Domestic Ferret

Michael Davidson, DVM
Department of Companion Animal and Special Species Medicine
School of Veterinary Medicine
North Carolina State University
Raleigh, North Carolina

The domestic ferret (*Mustela putorius furo*) is used extensively in biologic research and, in recent years, has become increasingly popular as a pet. Excellent general reviews of the routine care and management of the ferret appear in the recent veterinary literature; the reader is referred to these for a detailed discussion of this animal and its diseases.[1-3]

One of the most common and devastating infectious diseases affecting the domestic ferret is canine distemper virus (CDV). Infection from this virus is, by far, the single most important disease threat to ferret research colonies. This threat is no less substantial to pet ferrets, especially those allowed contact with dogs.

Distemper was first described in the ferret by Dunkin and Laidlaw in 1926 during their initial investigations of distemper virus in dogs.[4,5] Because of its extreme susceptibility to the disease, the ferret has since been used widely to characterize the disease in the dog and was instrumental in the development of effective vaccines for use in dogs. Canine distemper virus vaccine was originally formulated by serial passages of the virus in susceptible ferrets. This so-called *Green's distemperoid strain* lost most of its pathogenicity for the dog and was used as an effective vaccine in the species in the 1930s and 1940s.[6,7] Since that time, distemper virus has been adapted to chick embryo and canine cell lines in vitro; and ferret-adapted strains of the virus are now used only rarely. The ferret, however, remains a popular means to study distemper infection experimentally.

Causative Agent and Host Range

Canine distemper virus is a member of Paramyxoviridae and is closely related to the rinderpest and measles viruses. The virus is susceptible to ultraviolet light, heat, and drying conditions and survives outside the host for only short periods. Commonly used disinfectants are effective in destroying the virus.[8,9] The natural host range of canine distemper virus includes many species of terrestrial carnivores, including Ailuridae (lesser panda), Canidae (dog, dingo, fox, coyote, jackal, wolf), Hyaenidae (hyena), Procyonidae (raccoon, kinkajou, coati, bassariscus), Viverridae (binturong), Mustelidae (weasel, ferret, mink, skunk, badger, otter, stoat, marten), and possibly some members of Felidae.[8,10,11] The species within Mustelidae, including the domestic ferret and mink, are considered to be among the most susceptible to infection by and the effects of canine distemper virus.

Epizootiology

Transmission of canine distemper virus to ferrets occurs by contact with infected dogs, ferrets, or (theoretically) wild carnivores. The virus is shed in the nasal exudate and saliva of infected animals and readily spread by aerosolization of the viral particles.[12-14] Excretion of virus by ferrets begins on the fifth day after inoculation, and viral shedding continues until the death of the animal.[14,15] Once the infection has been established in a susceptible colony, it is probable that the entire stock will be affected.[4,13] Immunity to infection is of long duration, probably lifelong. Because recovery from natural infection is exceedingly unusual, however, immune animals are rarely encountered. For the same reason, recovered carrier animals are not a significant source of infection for other ferrets.[4,5,16]

Pathogenesis

Naturally acquired infection in ferrets follows an initial course similar to that occurring in dogs. Two days after aerosol exposure via the upper respiratory tract, viral replication initially occurs in the regional lymph nodes of the respiratory tract. The virus quickly spreads to the mediastinal and mesenteric lymph nodes, spleen, Kupffer's cells of the liver, and leukocytes of the peripheral blood. Viremia occurs on the fourth or fifth day after exposure, as evidenced by the presence of viral antigen in mononuclear cells. After approximately one week, further hematogenous spread of the virus occurs, affecting the epithelium of the respiratory tract, gastrointestinal tract, cutaneous tissues, urinary tract, and superficial ocular tissues.[17-19]

The respiratory tract, along with lymphoid tissue, is a major site for viral replication, with antigen concentration reaching a maximum on Day 12 after inoculation.[14,20] At this time, cellular destruction of lymphoid tissue (lymph nodes and lymphatic nodules of the spleen) is apparent.[20] Viral antigen persists in the infected tissues until the death of the animal.[17] Central nervous system invasion and replication can also occur.[4,20,21] In the ferret (as in the dog), certain strains of the virus are neurotrophic and central nervous system infection is more commonly seen.[21,22] Secondary bacterial infection of the respiratory, gastrointestinal, cutaneous, or superficial ocular tissues may complicate the disease process.

Clinical Findings

Clinical signs of distemper in the ferret reflect the fact that the virus is pantrophic (capable of replicating in a wide variety of cells). Unlike in the dog, however, the course of the disease is fairly constant, with a predictable progression of findings. The incubation period usually ranges from 4 to 10 days, with the onset of clinical signs typically occurring 7 to 9 days after exposure. Consistent findings during this period include anorexia, fever (body temperature of up to 105 °F [40.5 °C]), and a mucopurulent conjunctivitis (Figure 1). The ocular discharge is often the first sign noted; and the eyelids may stick together with dry, purulent crusts. Additional ocular findings can include severe blepharitis, keratoconjunctivitis sicca, and corneal ulceration. Several days after the ocular signs are evident, erythematous cutaneous rashes develop in the inguinal area (Figure 2), beneath the chin (Figure 3), and on the foot pads. Small vesicles may form in these areas, with a secondary pyoderma commonly occurring. Pruritus often accompanies the epidermal infection and may be the presenting sign. Hyperkeratosis of the foot pads is highly suggestive of distemper (Figure 4). Clinical findings related to the respiratory tract vary from catarrhal rhinitis to severe, fulminating pneumonia, often complicated by secondary bacterial pathogens. Gastrointestinal infection is evidenced by loose stools or diarrhea, which may be dark and tarry. Anorexia and fever persist throughout the course. Animals surviving the acute catarrhal phase may develop central nervous system infection with associated myoclonus, paresis, muscular tremors, hyperexcitability, convulsions, or coma.[1,2,4,14,17,20-23]

Ferrets usually succumb to the effects of the disease within one week from onset of clinical signs; however, this time interval varies with the virus strain. Death has been reported as soon as 2 days[22] and as late as 35 days[1,2,23] after inoculation. Exposure to massive doses of the virus results in a shorter course. The mortality associated with distemper is believed to be related to several factors, most notably widespread replication and necrosis in lymphoid tissue and circulating lymphocytes, with associated immunosuppression.[18,20,24]

Initial investigators of distemper in ferrets reported a mortality of approximately 90%.[4] Other researchers reported the mortality varied with the virus strain; and, with some strains, the death rate was only 50%.[21] These infections were laboratory induced, however, and may have been influenced by experimental techniques or design. Most reports consider natural infection with distemper to be a highly fatal disease, with mortality approaching 100%.[1,2,8,11,19,23]

Diagnosis

Clinical signs of distemper are highly suggestive of the disease; however, other viral infections of the ferret, most notably human influenza virus infection, produce a nasal and ocular discharge that might be confused with distemper. For this reason and because canine distemper virus has such significant implications for pet owners or research colonies, prompt diagnosis is required.

Rapid antemortem diagnosis is usually possible through the use of fluorescent antibody techniques on blood smears or conjunctival scrapings. Despite the fact that less than 1% of the circulating leukocytes contains viral antigen, mononuclear cell fluorescence is found two to three days after experimental inoculation and is invariably positive by the sixth day. Conjunctival epithelial fluorescence occurs slightly later, usually becoming positive by the ninth day of infection. Conjunctival epithelium and leukocytes are reported to continue to exhibit a positive fluorescence throughout the course of the disease.[17,25] False-negative results may be encountered if leukopenia is present. Serum antibody levels to canine distemper virus can aid in diagno-

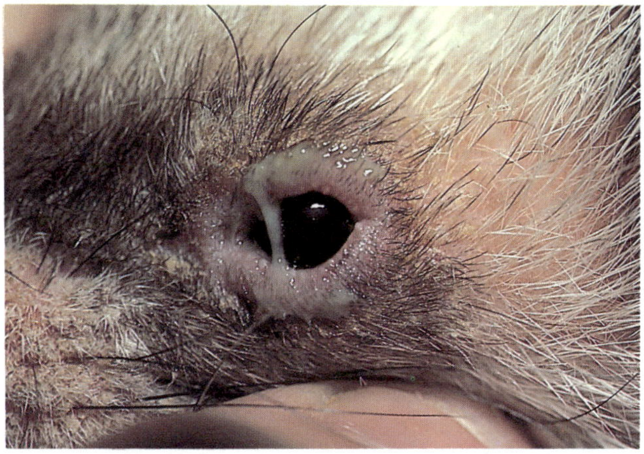

Figure 1—Blepharitis and conjunctivitis with mucopurulent ocular discharge in a one-year-old ferret with distemper.

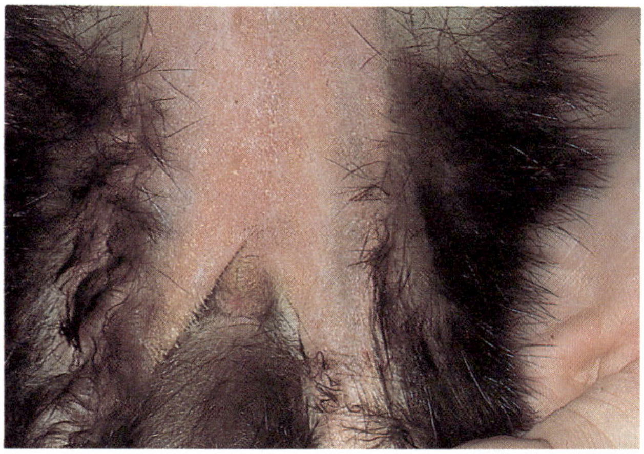

Figure 2—Erythematous, seborrheic dermatitis in the inguinal region (area has been clipped).

sis. Because naturally immune ferrets are rarely encountered, the presence of serum antibody to canine distemper virus in an unvaccinated animal suggests infection is likely. Lymphopenia may be found[24] but is nonspecific for canine distemper virus.

Postmortem diagnosis is usually no challenge, as widespread distemper inclusions are present (see Pathologic Findings). Viral isolation, although time-consuming, is an additional means of confirming infection. The ferret is the traditional test animal for viral inoculation when isolating canine distemper virus from any species. Intraperitoneal administration of suspensions of spleen, liver, or lung of infected ferrets to test ferrets results in typical signs and course of the disease. The virus can also be isolated in vitro on canine lung macrophages or ferret kidney cells, both of which exhibit characteristic cytopathic effects when infected.[8,9,19]

Pathologic Findings

Gross pathologic findings are often limited to the cutaneous and ocular abnormalities noted on physical examination. A catarrhal and/or hemorrhagic tracheitis or bronchitis may be present. Secondary bacterial pneumonia is

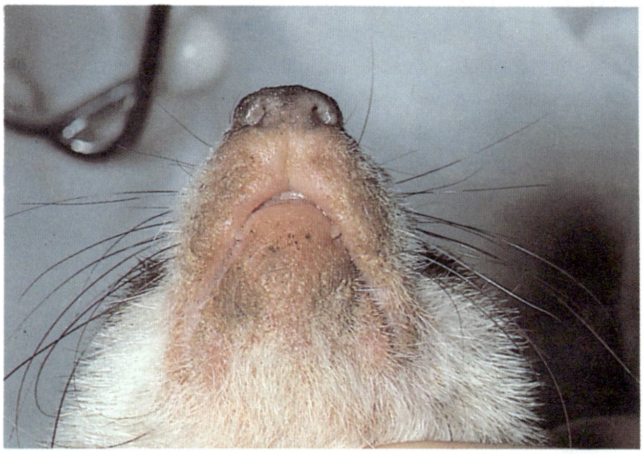

Figure 3—Characteristic chin rash often seen in ferrets with distemper.

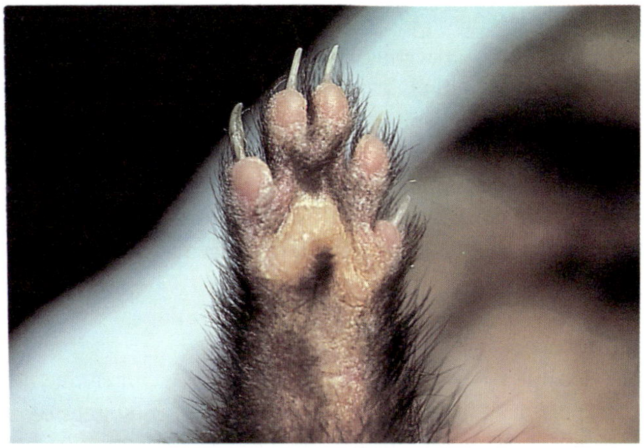

Figure 4—Hyperkeratosis and swelling of the foot pads in a ferret. This finding is extremely suggestive of canine distemper virus infection.

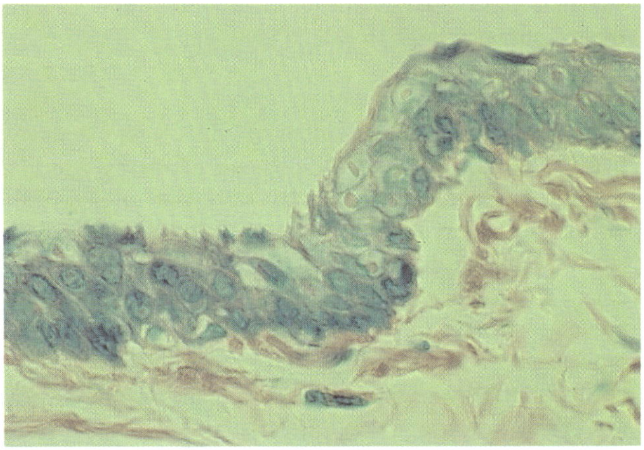

Figure 5—Conjunctiva in a ferret with canine distemper virus infection. Numerous acidophilic, cytoplasmic, viral inclusions are present in the conjunctival epithelium. (Courtesy of Dr. Robert Peiffer, University of North Carolina)

present in a minority of cases. Splenomegaly is common. When the central nervous system is infected, the meninges may appear inflamed and congested.

Inclusion bodies are the most remarkable diagnostic feature on histopathologic examination. Distemper inclusions are eosinophilic or acidophilic rounded structures more commonly found in the cytoplasm but also present in nuclei. They represent viral particles and cellular components associated with the virus. The more widespread nature of inclusion formation in the ferret compared with that of the dog correlates with the extreme virulence of canine distemper virus in ferrets. Inclusions are easily identified in the epithelium of the bronchi, renal pelvis, urinary bladder, stomach, biliary ducts, and conjunctiva (Figure 5). Inclusions are present but less numerous in the skin epithelium, hair follicles, reticulum cells of the spleen, small intestinal epithelium, corneal epithelium, and glia and neurons of the central nervous system.

Widespread necrosis of the lymph nodes and lymphatic nodules of the spleen is apparent. Hyperkeratosis and parakeratosis of the epidermis (including the foot pads), hair follicles, and sebaceous glands are often identified. Other microscopic findings can be related to secondary bacterial infection of the respiratory, cutaneous, and superficial ocular tissues. Reports of pathologic findings in the central nervous system are limited because of the acute fulminating nature of the disease. Scattered neuronal degeneration has been described with central nervous system infection.[4,8,17,19-22]

Therapy

Because of the high mortality associated with canine distemper virus in ferrets, euthanasia has been suggested as an acceptable alternative to symptomatic care.[1,2,23] This is certainly recommended in the colony setting, where further exposure to susceptible ferrets is catastrophic. Should therapy be attempted for pet ferrets, it should be entirely supportive and should include maintenance of hydration with subcutaneous fluids, parenteral bactericidal antibiotics, and topical antibacterial ophthalmic ointments.

Prevention

Vaccination to canine distemper virus with attenuated live virus strains is the only effective means by which to prevent the disease in susceptible ferrets or to control the disease during an outbreak. While the ferret was used extensively in the development of an effective vaccine for dogs, no product has been specifically designed and approved for use in ferrets. Canine distemper virus vaccines propagated on chick embryo tissues were investigated extensively in ferrets in the 1950s during the development of that product for use in dogs. These studies indicate that use of the vaccine in ferrets is safe and is capable of eliciting an effective immune response.[16,26-33] Similar studies on vaccines of canine cell origin are limited; however, they suggest less effectiveness in inducing the production of protective antibody than chick embryo products do.[34] In addition, canine cell products may be associated with a higher incidence of vaccine-induced disease.[24] No studies, to the author's knowledge, have been conducted on the safety and efficacy of the multivalent vaccines commonly used in dogs. For this reason, use of these vaccines in ferrets cannot be recommended. Killed vaccine elicits only short-term immunity and is not effective in producing a response in some ferrets.[4,35] Canine distemper virus vaccines propagated on ferret cell lines should be avoided because they may retain their pathogenicity for this species.[1,2,6,7,15]

Maternal antibody is passively transferred from vaccinated dams to their offspring, and an effective immune response cannot occur until the antibody concentration decreases below a certain level. The majority of kits from immune dams are capable of responding to a vaccine by 7 weeks of age, and all evidently are responsive by 10 weeks of age.[28,36] A schedule that includes vaccination at 7 and 10 weeks is therefore recommended for young ferrets. Kits from unvaccinated dams should receive their first vaccine at 4 to 6 weeks of age and again in 3 weeks.[1,2] The duration of immunity to chick embryo vaccines in ferrets is reported to be as long as 5½ years.[16] Therefore, booster vaccines are recommended at one year and every three years thereafter. Pregnant ferrets can be vaccinated without endangering the embryo.[37] Although the dose of egg-adapted distemper virus required to immunize ferrets is reported to be only 1/50 of that required for dogs,[34,38] the standard canine dose apparently has no detrimental effects and is therefore commonly used.[26,27,29,38]

Several routes of vaccine administration are possible in ferrets. Subcutaneous or intramuscular injections are equally effective.[38] Large numbers of animals, as in a colony setting, are routinely immunized by aerosolization of the vaccine.[29,36] Jet injection using air propulsion to deliver the vaccine subcutaneously is another means of administration.[39]

In the event of an outbreak of distemper in a colony, immediate steps must be taken to prevent spread of the disease. Ferrets exhibiting clinical signs of distemper should be isolated or destroyed. Remaining animals should be immediately vaccinated. A single administration of chick embryo vaccine solidly protects ferrets against the disease within 24 to 72 hours. The protection in this case may result from interference with the replication or establishment of infection rather than a true immune response.[27]

In settings where vaccination of ferrets is not possible because of experimental concerns, strict measures should be taken to ensure that the animals are not exposed to the virus. Prevention of contact with dogs or possible fomites of the virus is essential.

The use of canine distemper virus vaccines in exotic animals for which they were not designed is not without risk. Distemper infection has been reported to have been induced by modified live chick embryo vaccines in several species of carnivores, including the black-footed ferret (the North American wild counterpart of the domestic ferret)[40] and the mink.[41] Canine cell products have been documented as the cause of disease in a lesser panda,[11] gray foxes,[42] and domestic ferrets.[24] The severity of these infections varied from mild distemperlike signs to fatal disease indistinguishable from the natural infection. The author has observed ferrets exhibiting typical signs of distemper with a nonfatal course after administration of vaccines of canine cell origin.

Difficulty arises in differentiating natural infection from vaccine-induced disease. Distinguishing the two has significant implications, as the latter is associated less often with a fatal outcome. Vaccination followed by signs of distemper is suggestive of vaccine-induced disease; however, experimentally, attenuated virus vaccines will not protect against virulent distemper virus when the two are injected simultaneously.[27] This finding would imply that ferrets exhibiting clinical signs of distemper after vaccination in a veterinary clinic may be suffering from a vaccine break or may have been exposed at the time of vaccination.

Specific studies have not been conducted to determine whether a positive fluorescent antibody test is found after vaccination of ferrets with modified live virus. Because viral antigen of attenuated virus replicates in tissues following vaccine administration,[32] however, a positive test (although weaker than that seen with natural infection) might be expected. Replication of the virus is certainly expected in cases in which attenuated virus has retained its pathogenicity for the recipient, as occurs in vaccine-induced disease. The use of in vitro isolation techniques by tissue-suspension inoculation of susceptible ferrets is necessary for confirming possible vaccine breaks.[11,42] These, unfortunately, are postmortem techniques and may be subject to some interpretation.[43] Survival from a course of distemper might suggest vaccine-induced disease, as this is fatal less often than natural infection. Treatment of these cases would be similar to that for natural infection and includes supportive care and prophylactic antibiotics.

While vaccine-induced disease may occur, its frequency is no doubt rare; and excellent studies on the safety and efficacy of chick embryo vaccines in ferrets have been conducted. The benefits derived from their use therefore greatly outweigh any associated risks.

Summary

The host range of canine distemper virus spans many species of carnivores, including the domestic ferret. Infection usually occurs through contact with infected ferrets or dogs and is characterized by specific cutaneous, ocular, and respiratory signs. Antemortem diagnosis of infection is based on clinical signs, fluorescent antibody studies on blood smears or conjunctival scrapings, and serum antibody levels. Widespread viral inclusions are noted on histopathologic examination. The use of chick embryo vaccines at 7 and 10 weeks of age, at 1 year, and every 3 years thereafter is effective in prevention of the disease and is recommended despite reports of vaccine-induced disease in some wild carnivores.

REFERENCES

1. Ryland LM, Gorham JR: The ferret and its diseases. *JAVMA* 173(9):1154-1158, 1978.
2. Ryland LM, Bernard SL, Gorham JR: A clinical guide to the pet ferret. *Compend Contin Educ Pract Vet* 5(1):25-32, 1983.
3. Moody KD, Bowman TA, Lang CM: Laboratory management of the ferret for biomedical research. *Lab Anim Sci* 35(3):272-279, 1985.
4. Dunkin GW, Laidlaw PP: Studies in dog distemper: I. Dog-distemper in the ferret. *J Comp Pathol Ther* 39:201-212, 1926.
5. Laidlaw PP, Dunkin GW: Studies in dog distemper: IV. The immunization of ferrets against dog distemper. *J Comp Pathol Ther* 41:1-7, 1927.
6. Green RG, Swale FS: Vaccination of dogs with modified distemper virus. *JAVMA* 95(750):469-470, 1939.
7. Green RG: Modification of distemper virus. *JAVMA* 95(750):465-466, 1939.
8. Appel M, Gillespie JH: Canine distemper virus, in Gard S, Hallauer C, Meyer KF (eds): *Virology Monographs*, no. 11. Vienna, Austria, Springer-Verlag, 1972, pp 1-93.
9. Greene CE: Canine distemper, in Greene CE (ed): *Clinical Microbiology and Infectious Diseases of the Dog and Cat.* Philadelphia, WB Saunders Co, 1984, pp 386-406.
10. Keymer IF, Epps HBG: Canine distemper in the family Mustelidae. *Vet Rec* 85(7):204-205, 1969.
11. Bush M, Montali RJ, Brownstein D, et al: Vaccine-induced canine distemper in a lesser panda. *JAVMA* 169(9):959-960, 1976.
12. Gorham JR, Brandly CA: The transmission of distemper among ferrets and mink. *Proc 90th Annu Meet AVMA*:129-141, 1953.
13. Shen DT, Gorham JR: Contact transmission of distemper virus in ferrets. *Res Vet Sci* 24(11):118-119, 1978.
14. Crook E, Gorham JR, McNutt SH: Experimental distemper in mink and ferrets. I. Pathogenesis. *Am J Vet Res* 19(73):955-957, 1958.
15. Gorham JR: The epizootiology of distemper. *JAVMA* 149(5):610-618, 1966.
16. Gorham JR: Egg-propagated distemper virus. *Vet Med* 52(7):339-346, 1957.
17. Lui C, Coffin DL: Studies on canine distemper infection by means of fluorescein-labeled antibody. I. The pathogenesis, pathology, and diagnosis of the disease in experimentally infected ferrets. *Virology* 3:115-131, 1957.
18. Appel MJG: Pathogenesis of canine distemper. *Am J Vet Res* 30(7):1167-1182, 1969.
19. Gorham JR: Canine distemper, in Brandly CA, Jungherr EL (eds): *Advances in Veterinary Science*. New York, Academic Press, 1960, pp 287-351.
20. Crook E, McNutt SH: Experimental distemper in mink and ferrets. II. Appearance and significance of histopathological changes. *Am J Vet Res* 20(75):378-383, 1959.
21. Larin NM: Canine distemper virus in the ferret. *J Comp Pathol Ther* 65:325-333, 1955.
22. Kilham L, Habermann RT, Herman CM: Jaundice and bilirubinemia as manifestations of canine distemper in raccoons and ferrets. *Am J Vet Res* 17(62):144-148, 1956.
23. Bernard SL, Gorham JR, Ryland LM: Biology and diseases of ferrets, in Fox JG, Cohen BJ, Loew FM (eds): *Laboratory Animal Medicine*. Orlando, FL, Academic Press, 1984, pp 386-397.
24. Kauffman CA, Bergman AG, O'Connor RP: Distemper virus infection in ferrets: An animal model of measles-induced immunosuppression. *Clin Exp Immunol* 47:617-625, 1982.
25. Samol S, Gorski J: Detection of distemper virus infection in ferrets by the fluorescent antibody technique. *Medycyna Weterynaryjna* 34(2):98-101, 1978.
26. Baker GA, Leader RW, Gorham JR: Immune responses of ferrets to vaccination with egg-adapted distemper virus. I. Time of development of resistance to virulent distemper virus. *Vet Med* 47(11):463-466, 1952.
27. Cabasso VJ, Stebbins MR, Cox HR: Onset of resistance and duration of immunity to distemper in ferrets following a single injection of avianized distemper vaccine. *Vet Med* 48(4):147-150, 1953.
28. Ott RL, Gorham JR: The response of newborn and young ferrets to intranasal administration with egg adapted distemper virus. *Am J Vet Res* 16(61):571-572, 1955.
29. Morris JA, Coborn DR, O'Connor JR: Rapid protection of ferrets

against fully virulent distemper virus with nebulized attenuated distemper virus. *Cornell Vet* 44(2):198-207, 1954.
30. Bosgra O, Hoogendoorn H: Vaccination and immunity to distemper and "hard pad" disease in ferrets. *Tijdschr Diergeneesk* 81:649-658, 1956.
31. Gorham JR, Ott RL: Transplacental and neonatal attempts to immunize ferrets against distemper. *Vet Res* 76(16):434-435, 1964.
32. Gorham JR, Farrell RK, Ott RL, Parisot T: Multiplication of attenuated egg-adapted distemper virus in the vaccinated host. *Vet Med* 52(6):289-292, 1957.
33. Cabasso VJ, Cox HR: A distemper-like strain of virus derived from a case of canine encephalitis: Its adaptation to the chick embryo and subsequent modification. *Cornell Vet* 42(1):96-107, 1952.
34. Rockborn G, Norby E, Lannek N: Comparison between the immunizing effect in dogs and ferrets of living distemper vaccines, attenuated in dog tissue culture and embryonated eggs. *Res Vet Sci* 6(4):423-427, 1965.
35. Ott RL, Svehag SE, Burger D: Resistance to experimental distemper in ferrets following the use of killed tissue vaccine. *West Vet* 6:107-111, 1959.
36. Farrell RK, Skinner SF, Gorham JR, Lauerman LH: The aerosol and subcutaneous administration of attenuated egg adapted distemper vaccine to ferret kits from distemper immune females. *Res Vet Sci* 12(5):392-393, 1971.
37. Hagen KW, Goto H, Gorham JR: Distemper vaccine in pregnant ferrets and mink. *Res Vet Sci* 11(5):458-460, 1970.
38. Shen DT, Gorham JR, Evermann JF, McKeirnan AJ: Comparison of subcutaneous and intramuscular administration of a live attenuated distemper virus vaccine in ferrets. *Vet Rec* 114(2):42-43, 1984.
39. Shen DT, Gorham JR, Ryland RM, Strating A: Using jet injection to vaccinate mink and ferrets against canine distemper, mink enteritis, and botulism type C. *VM SAC* 76(5):856-859, 1981.
40. Carpenter JW, Appel MJG, Erickson RC, et al: Fatal vaccine-induced canine distemper virus infection in black-footed ferrets. *JAVMA* 169(9):961-964, 1976.
41. Menchaca ES, Martin AM, Moras EV: Distemper in mink caused by vaccine virus. *Revista de Medicina Veterinaria, Argentina* 55(3):241-249, 1974.
42. Hallbrooks RD, Swango LJ, Schnurrenberger PR, et al: Response of gray foxes to modified live-virus canine distemper vaccines. *JAVMA* 179(11):1170-1174, 1981.
43. Pearson GL: Letter to the editor. *JAVMA* 170(2):103-109, 1976.

An Introduction to Diseases of Nonhuman Primates

Theresa Y. Parrott, DVM
Pembroke Park Animal Clinic
Pembroke, Florida

During the past 12 years, laws restricting the importation of nonhuman primates into the United States have drastically reduced the numbers of primates appearing in the pet trade. Import bans have forced many private and public institutions to increase captive breeding efforts. An awareness of nutritional and medical problems in primate species can increase reproductive potentials and life expectancy.

Types of Nonhuman Primates Commonly Encountered

New World nonhuman primates are maintained in zoos and research facilities commonly. These animals also are the most frequent pet monkeys encountered in private veterinary practice. Distinguishing characteristics of New World primates include the presence of a prehensile tail and imperfectly opposable thumbs.[1,2] Sizes range from 150-g marmosets (*Callithrix*) (Figure 1) to 12-kg Woolly monkeys (*Lagothrix*). Other New World primates include the squirrel (*Saimiri*), spider (*Ateles*), and capuchin (*Cebus*) (Figure 2) monkeys.

Old World primates common in research and in private facilities include rhesus (Figure 3), pig tail, crab eating, and Japanese monkeys (*Macaca* spp.) as well as green monkeys (*Cercopithecus* spp.) and Patas monkeys (*Erythrocebus* spp.). These monkeys have ischial callosities and cheek pouches. On rare occasions, chimpanzees (*Pan*), baboons (*Papio*) and orangutans (*Pongo*) are seen outside zoologic institutions.

Examination Techniques

Examination procedures on smaller simian species can be conducted with minimal restraint. A pair of leather welder's gloves is excellent for marmosets and squirrel monkeys. The larger species can be handled with a pair of primate gloves.[a] Tranquilization will be necessary if the patient cannot be handled safely (i.e., if it exceeds 5 kg in weight) or if an adequate examination cannot be performed (Table I).

Respiratory rates and heart rates will be increased when the patient is restrained. If blood sampling is required, the femoral vein is easily accessible in an awake animal. Directing the needle slightly downward in the femoral triangle, the clinician can obtain enough blood to run a complete blood count and panel. Clipping the patient's nails to obtain blood smears is painful and

[a]Primate Imports Inc., PO Box 416, Port Washington, NY 11050.

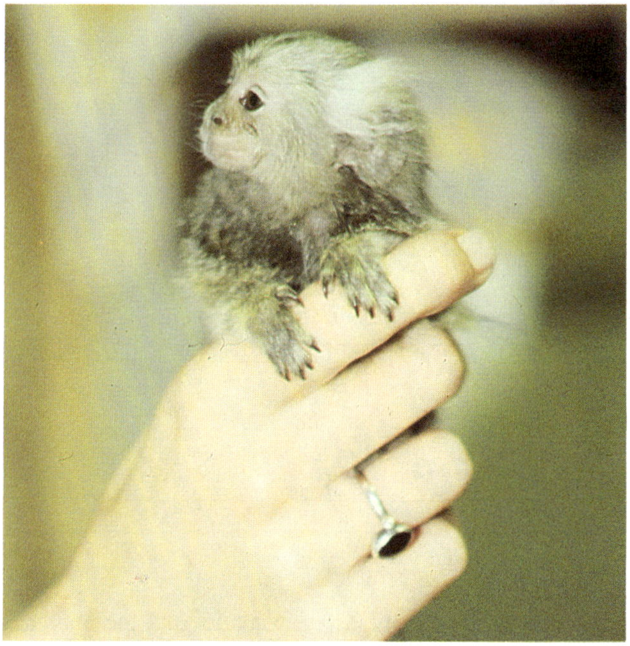

Figure 1—A marmoset (*Callithrix*).

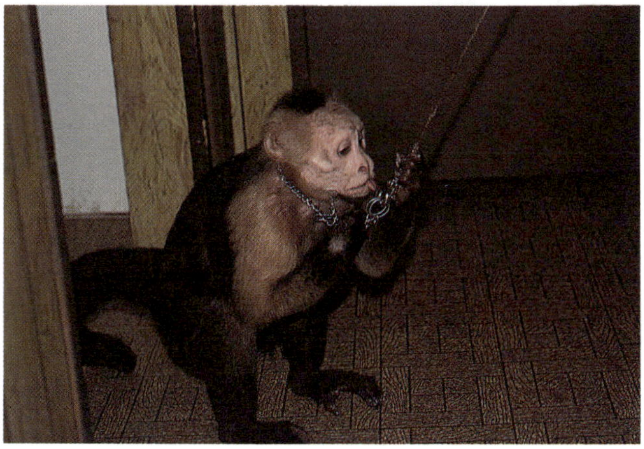

Figure 2—A capuchin (*Cebus*).

should be avoided. The cephalic veins might be difficult to expose for venipuncture because of the heavy forearm musculature and the relatively small vessels in nonhuman primates. In certain instances, lateral cephalic and saphenous veins are used to take small to moderate amounts of blood from tranquilized patients, especially in smaller primates. Normal physical and hematologic values are listed in Table II.

Common Ailments

Vitamin C Deficiency

Patients with vitamin C deficiency present with poor haircoats, bleeding mucous membranes, and general debilitation. A history of a diet lacking in vitamin C is common. Oral vitamin C given at 15 to 25 mg/kg of body weight daily will correct the deficient state. Ascorbic acid can be given by injection at an initial rate of 7 to 10 mg/kg.[3,4]

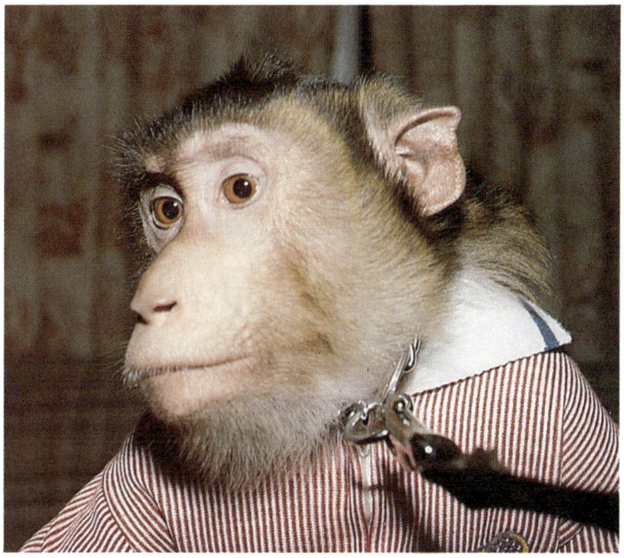

Figure 3—A rhesus monkey (*Macaca*).

Calcium/Vitamin D_3 Deficiency

Deficiency of calcium and/or vitamin D_3 will cause rickets and osteomalacia in young nonhuman primates.[4,5] Acute lameness is the most common complaint made by owners. Radiographs show skeletal demineralization, and scoliosis/kyphosis often is evident. Folding fractures also are common. A chronically deficient state will induce fibrous osteodystrophy of the mandible, with loss of dentition. Correction of the diet and oral calcium and vitamin D_3 are indicated. Because New World monkeys do not synthesize vitamin D_3, it must be given daily as a dietary additive.[3,4] Calcium carbonate is preferable to bone meal because of the unwanted phosphorus in the latter.

Inadequate Caloric Intake

Inadequate caloric intake can cause chronic catabolism and hypoglycemia.[5] When a depressed or comatose primate is presented, this should be one of the primary working diagnoses. An intravenous catheter should be inserted; the author prefers sites in the following order: lateral saphenous, metatarsal/metacarpal, and cephalic veins. The size of the smaller primates can restrict the clinician's access to the larger vessels. Intravenous dextrose should be given in addition to lactated Ringer's solution for treatment of shock. Intravenous prednisolone should be given at a dose of 3 to 5 mg/kg. Blood should be drawn, and the blood glucose level should be determined (normal is 60 to 110 mg/dl).[5] Rectal temperature should be taken; if it is below normal, treatment for hypothermia is initiated. If the intravenous set must be maintained for more than a few hours, the patient's hands should be wrapped and a restraining collar applied around its neck. This will prevent removal of the set by the patient.

Gastrointestinal Disorders

Internal Parasites

Among the most common internal parasites encountered

TABLE I
Common Immobilizing Agents for Primates[a]

Agent	*Route*	*Dose*	*Induction and Duration*
Ketamine hydrochloride	Intramuscular	10–30 mg/kg	3–10 min induction, 30–50 min duration
Diazepam	Intramuscular	1–3.5 mg/kg	15–30 min induction, 60–90 min duration
Promazine hydrochloride	Intramuscular	5 mg/kg	3–8 min induction, 40–80 min duration
Meperidine hydrochloride	Intramuscular	12 mg/3.5–10 kg	3–10 min induction, 30–90 min duration
Fentanyl citrate and droperidol (Innovar)	Intramuscular	1 ml/18 kg	3–15 min induction, 30–60 min duration

[a]Other agents are available, but most require intravenous use. Halothane and methoxyflurane are inhalation agents.

in captive nonhuman primates are *Strongyloides* spp.[4,6,7] An animal with chronic diarrhea, dull haircoat, and weight loss should be suspected of being parasitized with this genus. Other parasites encountered include ascarids, acanthocephalans, and *Dipetalonema* spp.[4,6,7] Table III lists worming agents and dosages.

Dietary Indiscretion

The usual clinical presentation of dietary indiscretion is acute onset of diarrhea with a history of recent ingestion of substances normally not included in the patient's diet. Foods incriminated most commonly include cooked or processed meats, milk, and abundant greens. Treatment should include fluid replacement therapy in dehydrated patients, parenteral antibiotics, and withholding of food for a period of 24 hours.

Bloat

Ingesting moderate to large amounts of fluids after eating monkey biscuits or other water absorbent substances can lead to gastric dilatation. The patient will present depressed or comatose, with shallow, rapid respirations. The mucous membranes might be cyanotic, and the abdomen usually is distended. (Woolly monkeys commonly have a potbellied appearance; care should be taken not to confuse this with gastric dilatation.) Treatment consists of passage of a gastric tube to relieve vascular and respiratory compromise. Gastric lavage using warmed lactated Ringer's solution often is rewarding. Treatment for shock should include intravenous prednisolone, replacement fluids, and dextrose. Solid food should not be offered for at least 48 hours. Fruit juices and oral electrolyte mixtures can be given.

Infectious Diseases

Influenza

Signs of influenza in primates include depression, emesis, diarrhea, and fever.[4,5,7] A careful history might show that the handler or the owner also has been ill recently. Treatment should be symptomatic, and care should be taken to maintain the patient's hydration.

Herpes Simplex

Herpes simplex usually is transmitted from the handler

TABLE II
Physical and Hematologic Values of Primates[4,5,6]

	Weight	*Rectal Temperature (°C)*	*Respiratory Rate (breaths/min)*	*Heart Rate (beats/min)*	*Packed Cell Volume (%)*	*White Blood Cell Count (10 × 3/mm³)*	*Red Blood Cell Count (10 × 6/mm³)*
Marmoset	235–250 g	35.4–39.7	20–50	240–350	36.1–60.7	7.1–14.7	4.04–7.70
Squirrel monkey	750–1000 g	33.5–38.8	20–50	225–350	42.0–57.0	5.0–16.0	7.4–11.3
Capuchin	1.7–4.0 kg	37.0–38.5	30–50	165–225	40.0–63.0	6.3–34.3	4.15–6.68
Woolly monkey	6–8 kg	36.0–39.0	15–30	80–180	35.0–40.0	11.0–14.0	—
Spider monkey	6–8 kg	36.0–39.0	18–35	210	34.0–47.0	8.9–31.2	3.50–4.92
Rhesus monkey	10–25 kg	36.0–40.0	10–25	150–333	37.0–42.0	8.64–15.50	5.0–6.0

TABLE III
Worming Agents Used in Primates in Clinical Practice[4,5,6]

Agent	*Spectrum*	*Dosage*
Thiabendazole (Mintezol®—Merck Sharp & Dohme)	Intestinal nematodes	50–100 mg/kg
Mebendazole	Intestinal nematodes	3 mg/kg for 10 days or 15 mg/kg for 2 days
DDVP (Task®—Solvay Veterinary)	Intestinal nematodes and *Trichuris* spp.	16–20 mg (active ingredient)/kg—two doses 24 hours apart
Diethylcarbamazine citrate	Filarids (*Dipetalonema* spp.)	6–20 mg/kg for 6–15 days

to the nonhuman primate. Acute depression and death are the usual clinical signs.[5,7] Treatment is symptomatic. Strict hygiene methods are essential.

Measles and Pox

Natural outbreaks of measles and pox have been reported in primates.[4-6] The clinical signs and course resemble that of humans. A vaccine for measles is available (Attenuated live measles—Merck Sharp & Dohme). Measles virus is important because it has an immunosuppressive effect and can cause a false-negative tuberculin reaction. Pox virus can be transmitted to the handler.

Infectious Hepatitis

Infectious hepatitis has been reported in chimpanzees and can be transmitted to man.[4,5] Gloves always should be worn by people working with soiled materials from these animals. Precautions also should be taken with sharp objects (e.g., needles and scalpel blades) contaminated with blood or other body fluids.

Tuberculosis

All newly acquired primates should be tested with 0.1 ml of Old Tuberculin (the Tine test®—American Cyanamid, or the Mantoux test®—Coopers Animal Health); human purified protein derivatives can show only an obscure reaction compared with mammalian tuberculin. Intradermal test sites include the ventral forearm, the chest, and the eyelid. The test should be read at 48 and 72 hours[5,6]; reactions should be investigated. Clinical signs include chronic debilitation and cough. Old World primates are more susceptible to tuberculosis than New World primates are.

Salmonella

Various *Salmonella* spp. cause violent diarrhea and vomiting, with leukocytosis usually present. The feces should be cultured; the patient can be started on antibiotics (sulfonamides or cephalosporins) while the culture is pending. With diarrhea caused by *Salmonella*, as well as other infectious diarrheas, fluid therapy is as important as antibiotic therapy.

Surgery

Lacerations

Nonhuman primates housed in groups commonly fight among themselves. Most of the superficial wounds will heal by second intention without complications. Deep cuts or punctures need to be thoroughly cleaned and debrided. As with other animals, closure of the wound should follow normal tissue tension planes. Buried sutures are managed more easily in primate patients. The hardest part of wound management is patient cooperation. To ensure wound healing, the primate probably will need to be kept away from the surgical site for at least three to five days after closure. Collars, bandages, and tranquilization have been used successfully.

Dental Procedures

Removing or blunting the canine teeth in nonhuman primates often is requested for safety. In blunting, the canines are cut off to be even with the incisors. The pulp is removed, and the pulp cavity is filled with amalgam. Maintenance can be a problem with this procedure. The filling often will fall out, and the patient will need to be tranquilized again for repair work. This can be a major problem in large colonies of captive primates. Tooth extraction is permanent. The teeth must be elevated adequately before removal is attempted. Care must be taken when extracting canine teeth. Dental flap techniques are recommended and resemble those used in dogs. The roots on the canine teeth of primates are long, and fracture of the tooth or the alveolar bone is common if elevation and removal is not done carefully. Removing canine teeth from the great apes can be difficult and disfiguring. When properly performed, canine cutting followed by partial pulpectomy gives good results.

Rectal Prolapse

Primates with acute diarrhea, colitis, and obstipation commonly prolapse their rectums. Reduction of the prolapsed portion can be accomplished with corn starch, sugar, or sulfa-urea granules. After replacement, a purse-string suture using a nonabsorbable suture material is placed in the mucocutaneous junction. The suture ends should not protrude because of the risk of picking by the patient. The purse-string suture should be slack enough to allow feces to pass. It should be removed after 7 to 14 days.

Sterilization

Sterilization is not performed routinely in nonhuman primates. Neoplasia, metritis, or intractable hormone problems usually are the reasons for castration or ovariohysterectomy. The anatomy of the female nonhuman primate is similar to that of a woman; surgery should not be attempted without first studying the specific anatomy of the primate. Castration of the male can be performed as it is in canids. Care must be taken to inhibit self-mutilation after surgery.

UPDATE

Wormers: ivermectin for intestinal nematodes at a dose of 200 μg/kg

Immobilizing Agents: Telazol® (A. H. Robins) 100 mg/ml at 0.1 ml per 10 lb

Tuberculosis: The Tine test® (American Cyanamid) is not accurate.

Nutrition: vitamin D_3 is vital as a supplement in marmosets, especially when kept indoors. In addition to that supplied in a commercial diet, vitamin D_3 can be provided at 10,000 IU/6 oz water or 10,000 IU per 1000 g food.

REFERENCES

1. Chiarelli AB: *Taxonomic Atlas of Living Primates*. New York, Academic Press, 1972, pp 10–30.
2. Napier JR, Napier PH: *Handbook of Living Primates*. New York, Academic Press, 1967, pp 3–7.
3. *Nutrient Requirements of Nonhuman Primates*, ed 14. Washington, DC, National Research Council, National Academy of Sciences, 1978.
4. Johnson D, Russell RJ, Stunkard JA: *A Guide to Diagnosis, Treatment and Husbandry of Nonhuman Primates*. Edwardsville, KS, Veterinary Medicine Publishing Co, 1981, pp 6–20.
5. Wallach JD, Boever WJ: *Diseases of Exotic Animals*. Philadelphia, WB Saunders Co, 1983, pp 3–123.
6. *UFAW Handbook on the Care and Management of Laboratory Animals*, ed 4. Baltimore, The Williams & Wilkins Co, 1972, pp 374–423.
7. Griner LA: *Pathology of Zoo Animals*. San Diego, Zoological Society of San Diego, 1983, pp 332–337.

General Principles of Fracture Repair in Raptors

Stephen J. Withrow, DVM
Diplomate, ACVS
Associate Professor
Colorado State University
Fort Collins, Colorado

Fracture repair in raptors is both challenging and frustrating in many cases. This is due to inherent problems with these birds as well as poorly documented experimental and clinical experiences from which the surgeon may formulate the best therapy. Although some variations exist, the general principles of orthopedics apply to birds: (1) rigid fixation; (2) anatomic alignment; and (3) early return to function.

The common problems encountered in raptors with fractures include the following.

1. *Restraint.* Simply trying to catch and examine the bird can lead to systemic stress and strain as well as local increase in forces at the fracture site. The falconry technique of hooding the bird may lessen stress.
2. *Anesthesia.* Safe and effective inhalation anesthesia is available but requires practice for proficiency.[1] Short procedures may be accomplished with ketamine[a] and/or xylazine.[b]
3. *Conditioning.* Many birds are debilitated upon presentation. All raptors should be considered dehydrated and in a negative nitrogen balance. Immediate correction of these deficits is vital to safe anesthesia, fracture healing, and long-term convalescence. Definitive fracture repair should often be delayed several days until the bird is eating or, if necessary, until after force-feedings. Weight gain is usually indicative of adequate nutrition.
4. *Housing.* Small, dark, and warm cages should be available for the initial rehabilitation and healing time.[2]
5. *Infection.* Many fractures are open and infected on presentation. Good general wound cleansing and debridement is important. Infected fractures are at greater risk for osteomyelitis even though the fracture may heal if stability and preservation of blood supply can be achieved. Gentamicin (8 mg/kg BID) has been suggested for open fractures.[3]
6. *Equipment constraints.* Much of the well-established orthopedic

---

[a]Vetalar®, Parke, Davis & Co., Morris Plains, NJ 07950.
[b]Rompun®, Haver-Lockhart, Shawnee, KS 66201.

instrumentation was developed for larger mammals and does not have sufficient variability to treat all species of raptors.

7. *Bone strength.* Because the bones of raptors are designed for light-weight strength, the cortices are often too thin and brittle (especially of the humerus) to accept and hold implants (especially the Kirschner-Ehmer [KE] apparatus and plates).[4,5]
8. *Location of fracture.* Many fractures occur near or through a joint. If return to normal function is the goal, arthrodesis or ankylosis of the joint, which is often acceptable in mammals, will not do. Rotational deformities of humeral fractures result in magnification of the deformity at the wing tip. Generally, the closer the fracture is to the wing tip, the better the prognosis.
9. *Experience of the surgeon.* Few surgeons have the time, dedication, expertise, or case load to become proficient in raptor orthopedics. This leads to little uniformity in case management and poor follow-up.
10. *Aftercare.* The postoperative rehabilitation is vital to total case care. Reliable information is scanty on this aspect of raptor care even though it will often ultimately be the deciding factor between success and failure.[6] Gradual increases in range of motion and exercise must be encouraged if return to the wild is anticipated. The assistance of an experienced falconer may be indispensable in rehabilitation.
11. *Adhesions.* Even though the fracture may heal clinically and radiographically, adhesions of ligaments and tendons may totally limit flight and/or function. This is especially true when joints are immobilized for prolonged periods as with casts, splints, or tape.
12. *Nature of fractures.* Many fractures are highly comminuted, making reduction and stabilization more difficult. Although healing may take place, the prolonged hospitalization requires extensive rehabilitation.
13. *Multiplicity of injuries.* Many wild birds suffer severe trauma (e.g., those hit by a car or gunshot) that may result in several fractures. It is often wise to take whole-body radiographs with the possibility of multiple injuries in mind.

Normal Bone Healing in Birds

Good experimental work has been published on healing of fractures in pigeons.[7] Bird bones heal in a fashion similar to that of mammalian bones. The endosteal callus contributes slightly more to healing than does the periosteal callus, but both are involved in the process.

Avian fractures heal at a similar rate to that of mammalian fractures, with a range of three to eight weeks being commonly quoted.[3,8,9] This rate varies with stability, blood supply, and infection.

The radiographic changes seen during healing closely parallel those expected for mammals. Callus is usually visible on radiographs in two to three weeks. Xeroradiography has been suggested as a more precise method of assessing healing.[5,8]

Pneumatic bones (especially the humerus) heal slightly slower than medullary bones (radius and ulna) but will heal.[5,9] The old wive's tale of fractured pneumatic bones releasing contaminated air into the tissues and causing osteomyelitis is unfounded. Humeral fractures do result in subcutaneous emphysema, but this resolves in 24 hours and healing commences normally. Closed fractures appear to be at low risk for infection.[9]

Healing in Infected Bone

Even when the bone is infected, there can be recovery. Many infected fractures will heal, although often with a central medullary sequestrum. This sequestrum can be removed later, and then final healing will commence.[7] Birds often show little or no systemic signs of infection with osteomyelitis. Exudate in avian species tends to be yellow white and caseous. It should be removed prior to definitive repair or at final debridement.

Preparation of the Surgery Site

Aseptic technique should be attempted. Antibiotics, circulating at the time of surgery, are probably helpful. Feathers immediately adjacent to the proposed incision should be gently plucked and not cut off. Large primary feathers should be preserved if possible. A water-soluble jelly on surrounding feathers may keep them from blowing into the incision. Skin preparation is done in a standard fashion with caution against overzealous scrubbing of friable skin. Transparent adhesive plastic drapes allow better visualization than standard drapes and are lighter.

Approaches to the Bones

The approaches to avian bones have been well described in the literature.[10] Whatever approach is used, it must be atraumatic. Excessive manipulation of soft and bony tissues leads to increased infection rates, more adhesions, and avascular nonunions.

Closure should be with small-sized absorbable suture (3-0, 4-0). Excessive tension should be avoided because of the tendency for the skin to tear.

Means of Repair

All the general principles of orthopedics apply to raptor fracture repair. Ingenuity and adaptation of existing techniques is often needed, however.

Fractures to Treat Closed

Almost all fractures of the pectoral girdle (scapula, clavicle, coronoid) and pelvis should be left alone without support. Greenstick or minimally displaced

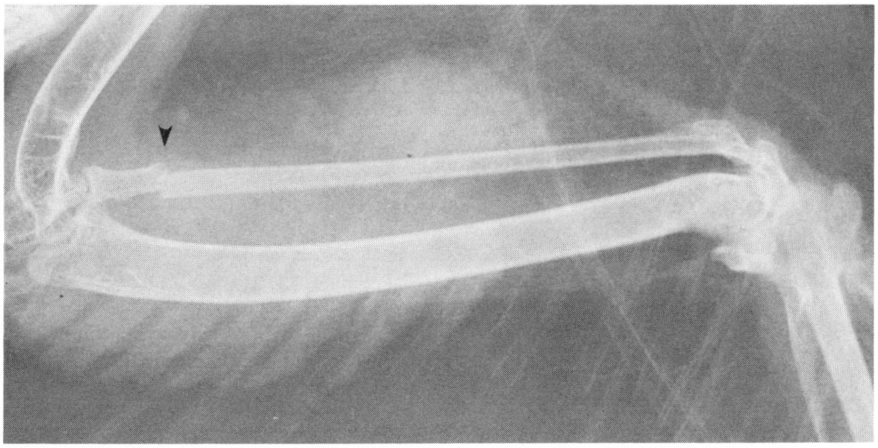

Figure 1A

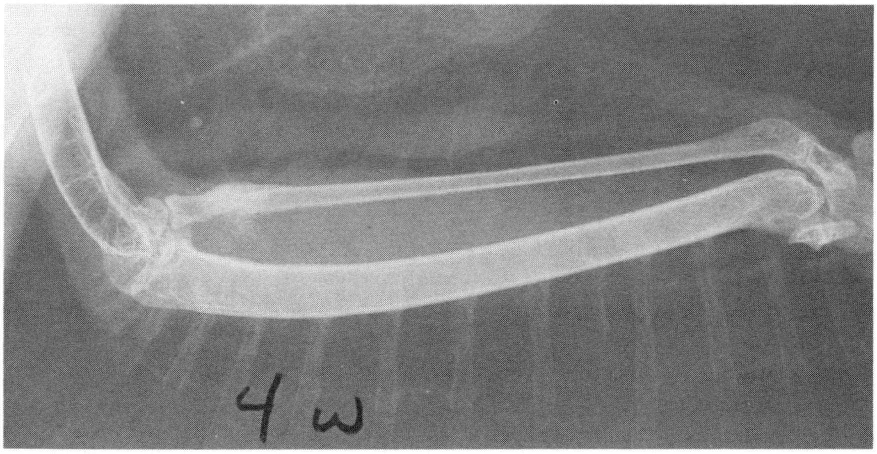

Figure 1B

Figure 1—(**A**) Fracture of the proximal radius (*arrow*) in a prairie falcon. Fracture was managed with cage rest alone. (**B**) Well-healed fracture at three weeks. Rehabilitation began at two weeks and the bird was released at four weeks.

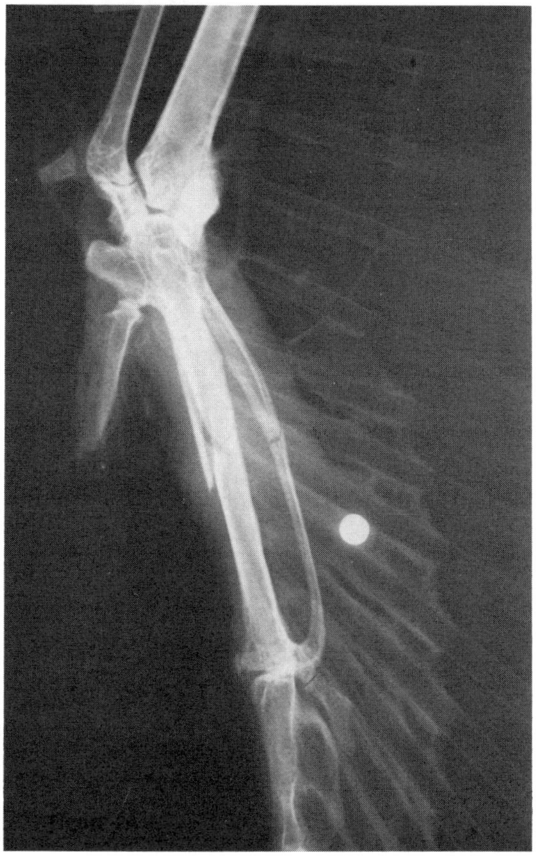

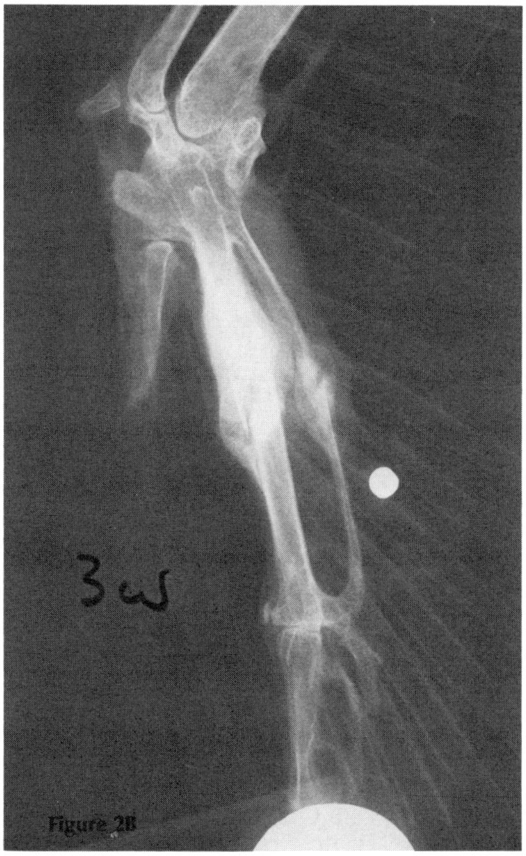

Figure 2—(**A**) Well-aligned fracture of metacarpals 3 and 4 in a rough-legged hawk. Fracture was managed by taping the wing to the body for nine days. (**B**) Fractures have completely united at three weeks with a periosteal callus although final remodeling will require more time. Early rehabilitation can start at this time.

fractures (especially in a two-bone system) can also be left alone (Figure 1). Selected coronoid fractures with severe displacement may be pinned.

Closed Reduction and Support

Partially healed or reasonably stable fractures can often be splinted or taped to the body for two weeks or less (Figure 2). The disadvantages of splinting are that balance is disrupted and some birds thrash and fight it. More importantly, joint motion is stopped which can result in ankylosis.

Fractures of the tibia can be cast with plaster or fiberglass.[11] Only the tibia is immobilized, leaving the proximal and distal joints to move. Many variations of this technique have been tried including the use of syringe cases (Figure 3), through-and-through pins imbedded in plaster, or aluminum casts.[3,12]

Slightly more callus forms with external than with internal coaptation, because of increased motion. This does not outweigh its benefits (e.g., fast, easy, cheap, safe, less infection, short anesthesia) when indicated, however.

Intramedullary Pins

One of the more popular methods of repair is intramedullary pinning. The major problem encountered with this method is in the humerus, where the bone has a large medullary cavity with thin cortices. Because a pin does not counteract rotation, rotation must be stopped by means of hemicerclage, full cerclage, external support, or external pin splints (e.g., KE apparatus) (Figure 4).

The anatomy of each bone must be carefully studied to ensure that pin placement does not interfere with joint motion. Pins can be inserted in a retrograde or normograde manner as long as the joint is missed. All implants in wings (except wire) should be removed before aerodynamically sound flight can be expected.

Guidelines for Pin Placement[13]

The guidelines for pin placement are given in Table I. Pins must be cut short enough to not damage soft tissue but long enough so that they can be removed. Shuttle pins should not be placed since they cannot be removed.

External Pin Splints (Figure 5)

External pin splints can be used in larger birds. The advantages are (1) the implant is not in the fracture site; (2) the ease of application and removal; and (3) they have no effect on range of motion in joints. A good description of splinting techniques has been published.[3] Because of the brittle nature of avian bone external pin splints may create further fractures and therefore must be used cautiously. Small Kirschner wires may be utilized when held together with methylmethacrylate or dental acrylic.

TABLE I

GUIDELINES FOR PIN PLACEMENT

Bone	*Method of Pin Placement*
Femur	Normograde from medial and/or lateral epicondyle
Tibia	Normograde from the craniomedial tibial plateau or normograde from the medial and/or lateral malleoli
Metatarsal	Very hard to pin
Humerus	Retrograde or normograde from the lateral or medial epicondyle; retrograde out cranial proximal humerus
Ulna	Retrograde or normograde at the elbow
Radius	Very hard to pin because of its small size and proximity to joints

Plates

Little good information is available on plates. The screw-holding power of avian bone makes plating difficult, and plates are rarely used except in some leg fractures. Lighter plastic plates, however, warrant further evaluation.

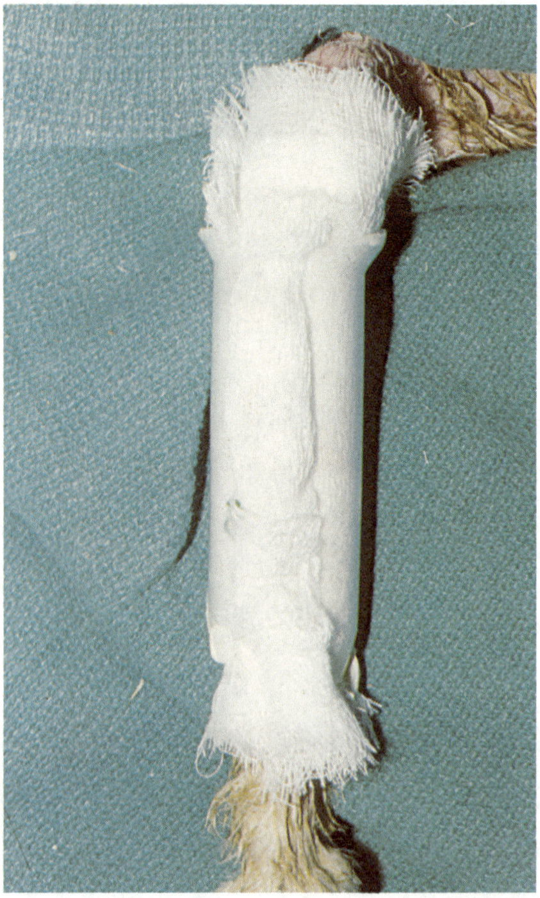

Figure 3—Bird with fractured tibia (tibiotarsus). After padding with gauze, an appropriate-sized plastic syringe case is slit longitudinally and placed over the bone. This is an easy, inexpensive, well-tolerated, and readily removable form of external fixation.

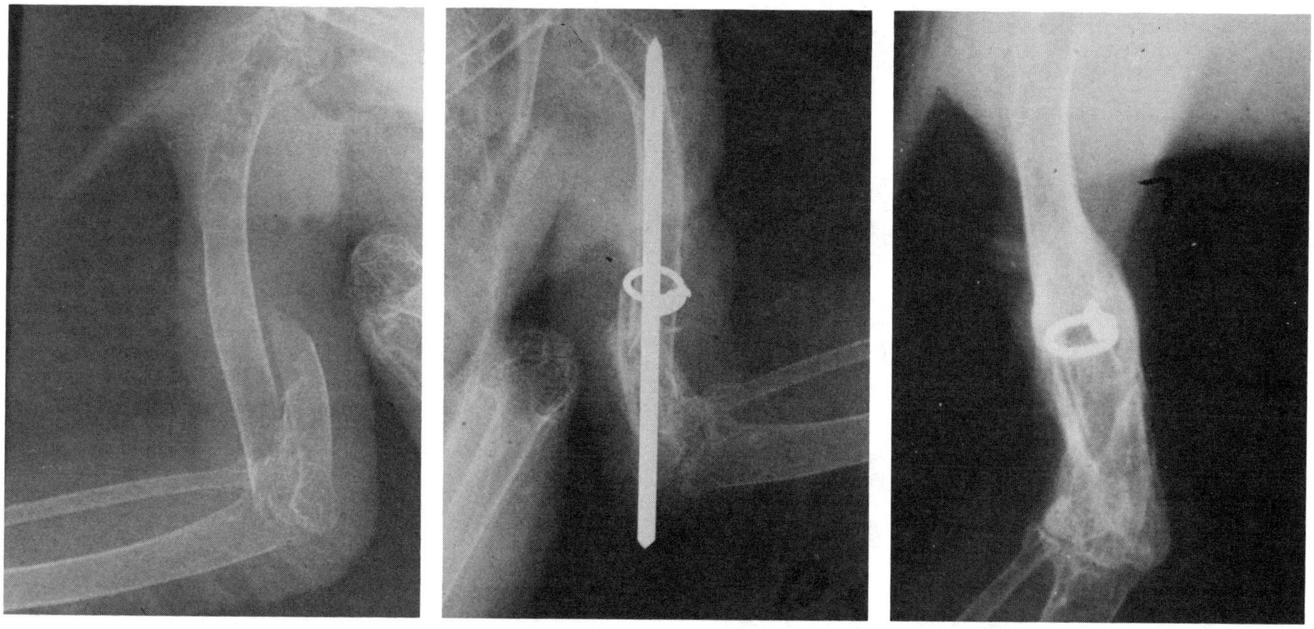

Figure 4A **Figure 4B** **Figure 4C**

Figure 4—**(A)** Spiral oblique fracture of distal humerus in a sparrow hawk. **(B)** Postoperative reduction of fracture with a small intramedullary pin (Kirschner wire) and single full-cerclage wire. Fracture is slightly impacted. **(C)** Seven-week postoperative radiograph of well-healed fracture. Intramedullary pin was removed at four weeks. Dense central cortex should remodel with time. No clinical signs of infection existed and the bird was rehabilitated and released.

Luxations

Most luxations are serious injuries, and return to useful function is unlikely, especially if more than two days elapse between the injury and attempt at treatment.[13]

Amputation

Amputation of a badly injured wing or leg can be done if there is a place for the bird in a zoo or suitable sanctuary. The result of a wing amputation is usually cosmetic and the birds do well. Leg amputation, however, can lead to foot problems on the remaining leg.

Prognosis

Many of the comments above apply to more or less perfect reduction and ultimate return to nature. If other suitable functions for the bird are available, many fractures will heal well enough for the bird to survive. At Colorado State University less than 20% of the birds with operated wing fractures fly again, although many of the leg fractures, even though not perfect, are functional. Greater success with closed reductions is common because the easier fractures are usually treated this way. Rehabilitation is critical and is undertaken by experienced falconers.[14]

The greatest problem for the avian orthopedist is the severe lack of information on the ultimate outcome of surgery and return to the wild. Only two documented cases were found where banding and follow-up revealed successful return to the wild after internal fixation.[6] And the bird's ability to fly away does not guarantee that it can maintain itself in the wild. However, in spite of the frustration, the rewards warrant the effort.

Acknowledgments

Thanks are extended to Dr. D. Piermattei, Colorado State University; Dr. P. Redig, University of Minnesota; Dr. M. Bush, Smithsonian Institute; and Dr. G. Hayes, Boulder, Colorado for reviewing this manuscript.

REFERENCES

1. Wingfield WE, DeYoung DW: Anesthetic and surgical management of eagles with orthopedic difficulties. *VM SAC* 67:991-993, 1972.
2. Bush M, James AE: Some considerations of practice of orthopedics in exotic animals. *JAAHA* 11(4):587-594, 1975.
3. Bush M: External fixation of avian fractures. *JAVMA* 171(9):943-946, 1977.
4. Bush M, Hughes JL, Ensley PK, James AE: Fracture repair in exotics using internal fixation. *JAAHA* 12(6):746-753, 1976.
5. James AE, Montali RJ, Novak GR, Bush M: The use of xeroradiographic imaging to evaluate fracture repair in avian species. *Skeletal Radiol* 2:161-168, 1978.
6. Griffin CR, Redig PT: Successful rehabilitation and reintroduction of bald eagles. *Wildlife Soc Bull* 6(1):44-45, 1978.
7. Newton CD, Zeitlin S: Avian fracture healing. *JAVMA* 170(6):620-625, 1977.

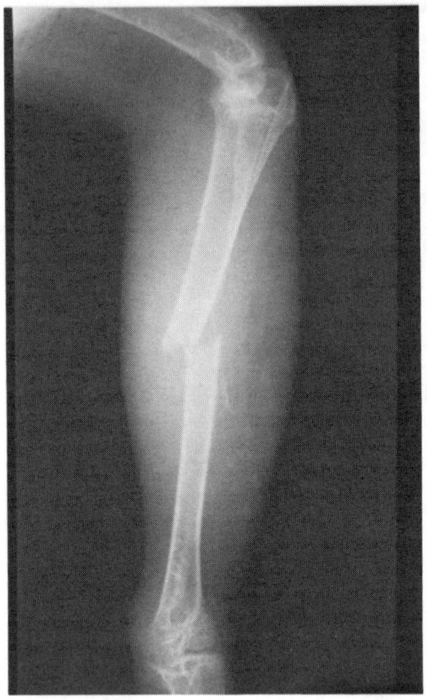

Figure 5A

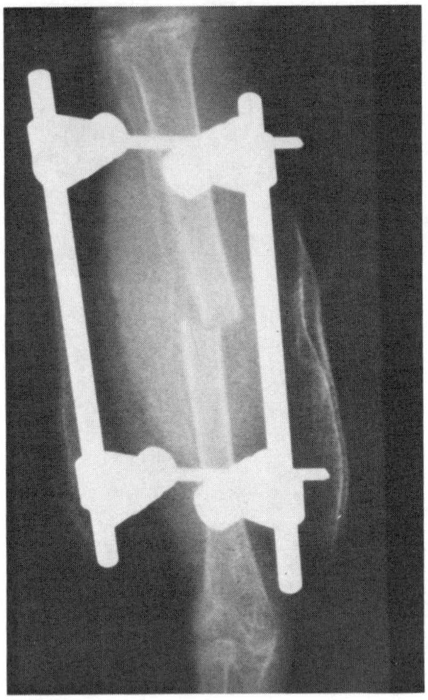

Figure 5B

Figure 5—**(A)** An almost transverse fracture of the tibia (tibiotarsus) in a red-tailed hawk. **(B)** Through-and-through external pin splint. Alignment is not perfect, but 50% cortical contact was considered adequate. **(C)** Postoperative view of pin splint on leg.

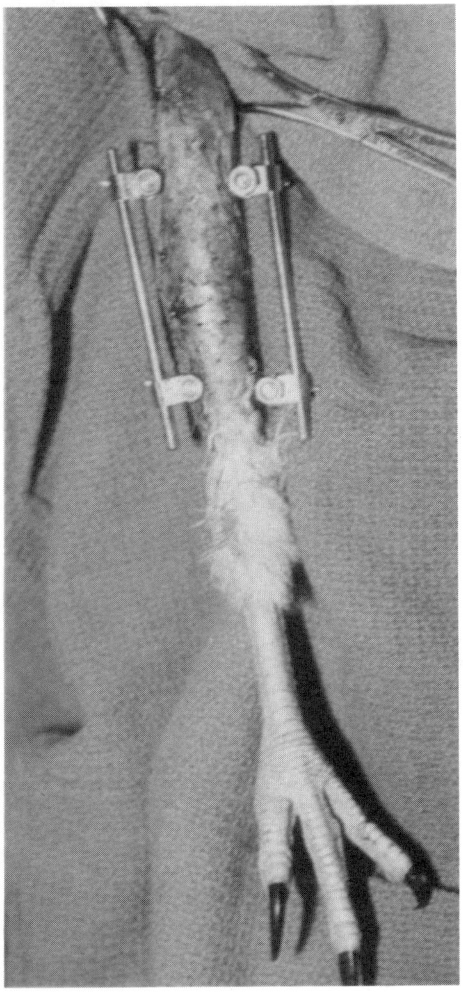

Figure 5C

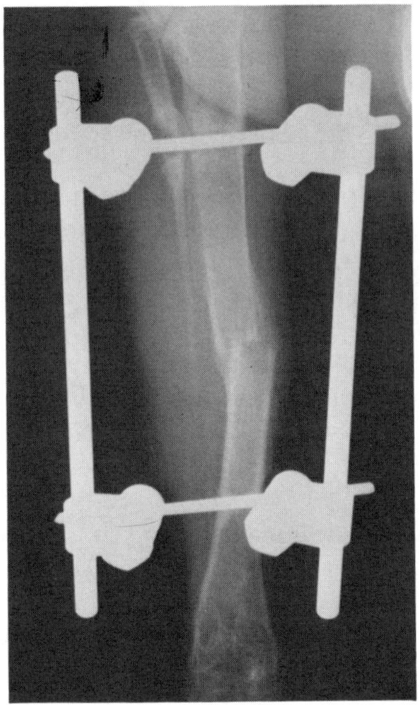

Figure 5D

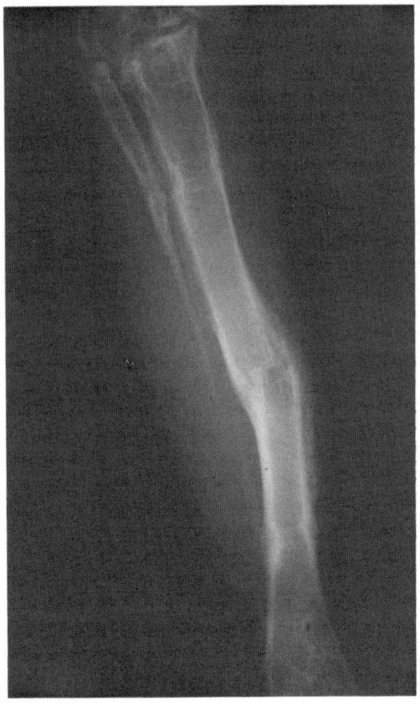

Figure 5E

Figure 5—**(D)** Four-week postoperative view of healed fracture. Slight valgus deformity exists, but leg is 100% functional. Note typical lysis around top pin hole. This is probably caused by slight motion. **(E)** Seven-week view just before release showing pin tract filled in and continued remodeling of fracture site.

8. Bush M, Montali RJ, Novak GR, James AE: The healing of avian fractures: A histologic xeroradiographic study. *JAAHA* 12(6):768-773, 1976.
9. Montali RJ, Bush M: Avian fracture repair, radiographic and histopathologic correlation. *Proc Am Assoc Zoo Vet*:150-154, 1975.
10. Redig P, Roush JC: Orthopedic and soft tissue surgery in raptorial birds, in Fowler ME (ed): *Zoo and Wild Animal Medicine*. Philadelphia, WB Saunders Co, 1978, pp 246-253.
11. Bush M, James AE: A new system of casting fractures in exotic animals. *VM SAC* 71:1288-1295, 1976.
12. Rickards DA, Hinko PJ, Morse EM: Orthopedic procedures for laboratory animals and exotic pets. *JAVMA* 161(6):728-732, 1972.
13. Roush JC: Avian orthopedics, in Kirk RW (ed): *Current Veterinary Therapy VII*. Philadelphia, WB Saunders Co, 1980, pp 663-673.
14. Galvin C: Care and treatment of captive wild birds, in Kirk RW (ed): *Current Veterinary Therapy VII*. Philadelphia, WB Saunders Co, 1980, pp 692-696.

Avian Gastrointestinal Radiography

Marjorie C. McMillan, DVM
Director of Radiology
Angell Memorial Animal Hospital
Boston, Massachusetts
The Windhover Bird Clinic
Walpole, Massachusetts

Contrast studies of the avian gastrointestinal tract may be necessary for a complete evaluation of gastrointestinal disturbances.

Medical Considerations and Indications for a Gastrointestinal Barium Examination

Since infectious diseases, parasites, toxins, and metabolic disturbances associated with kidney and liver diseases are common causes of gastrointestinal signs in birds, a complete history, thorough physical examination, survey radiographs, and laboratory data are indicated prior to contrast radiography. The primary indications for a gastrointestinal barium examination in birds are acute, chronic, or nonresponsive regurgitation, vomition, or diarrhea; palpation of an abnormal crop or abnormal abdomen; hemorrhagic diarrhea; or abnormal survey radiographic findings such as an obstructive pattern or organ displacement.

When clinically evaluating avian gastrointestinal problems, differentiation between physiologic and pathologic regurgitation and between diarrhea and polyuria is important. Physiologic regurgitation is associated with courtship feeding or affection toward an owner. These birds are healthy, and sexual display often precedes the regurgitation. The regurgitated material contains undigested food and does not have a foul odor. Pathologic regurgitation is not associated with sexual behavior and often has a foul or abnormal odor. These birds regurgitate undigested food or tenacious mucus, often have weight loss, and appear unhealthy.

Polyuria is a more common cause of loose droppings than diarrhea. The fecal portion of the dropping is well formed and surrounded by a clear or opaque, watery urate (Figure 1, A and B). Determination of renal function by uric acid levels and liver involvement by serum aspartate aminotransferase (SAST; SGOT) rather than barium examination is indicated. Change in color of the fecal portion is more common than change in consistency.

Lime green or mustard green feces are associated with hepatic disease and impaired excretion of biliverdin.[1] Brown or hemorrhagic feces usually indicate enteric problems. However, determining whether bloody droppings originate from gastrointestinal or renal problems can be difficult.

Infectious diseases such as psittacosis, colibacillosis, candidiasis, and Pacheco's viral hepatitis are frequent causes of alimentary tract distur-

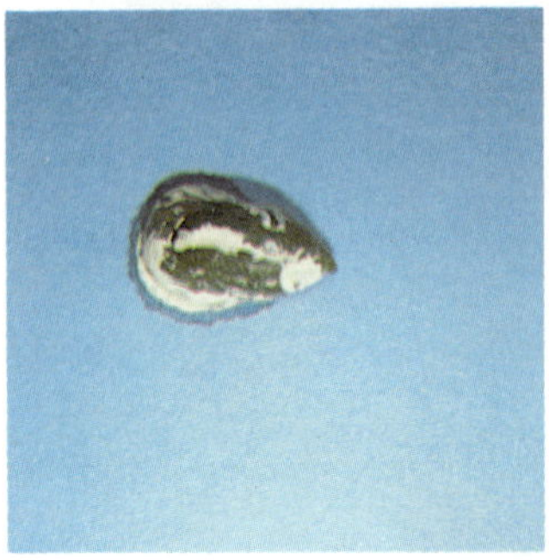

Figure 1A—Normal droppings from an Amazon parrot.

Figure 1A

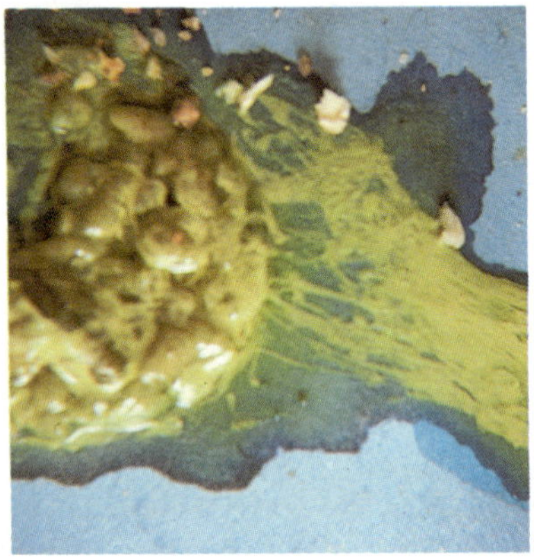

Figure 1B—Lime green droppings associated with abnormal liver and kidney functions.

Figure 1B

bances in newly acquired birds. A crop or cloacal culture helps to identify abnormal bacteria, yeast, and chlamydia. Survey radiographs in these instances show a distended, fluid-filled crop and intestines, hepatomegaly, and enlarged kidneys. Radiographs of an Amazon parrot showing enlarged kidneys and liver secondary to *Escherichia coli* infection are shown in Figure 2.

Ingestion of toxic materials such as heavy metal or plants may produce gastrointestinal signs as well as neurological signs. Lead poisoning due to ingesting paint chips from any source can cause regurgitation, diarrhea, and neurologic signs.[2] Plants, wood, and other foreign material causing local irritation can result in enteritis. Overeating grit, improper hand rearing techniques, or ingesting thread and wool from cage coverings can cause impacted crops.

Gastrointestinal parasites are uncommon in pet birds because many birds are wormed in quarantine stations or aviaries. However, since ascarids, tapeworms, and coccidia are occasionally seen, fecal examination is recommended in birds with gastrointestinal signs. Crop washings in birds with chronic regurgitation can demonstrate parasites as well as fungus and bacteria.

Kidney and liver diseases cause secondary gastrointestinal signs. Infections, neoplasia, and metabolic disorders (lipidosis[3] and hemochromatosis[4]) produce serious impairment of these organs.

Iodine deficiency resulting in thyroid enlargement, which impairs normal crop emptying, is a common cause of regurgitation in the budgerigar as a result of extrinsic crop compression (Figure 3).

Radiographic Technique

Prior to contrast examination, evaluation of survey radiographs for proper radiographic technique, location of the abdominal viscera, presence of gas and fluid, bowel distention, and foreign material is important. The presence of large amounts of gas and/or fluid in the crop often indicates gastrointestinal problems unless respiratory-induced aerophagia is present or the bird is being tube fed. Birds normally do not have gas in the intestinal tract, so that the presence of gas with or without distention is abnormal. Distended fluid-filled intestinal loops indicate gastrointestinal problems except in mynahs and toucans. Because of the high water content in their diet, these birds normally have slightly distended fluid-filled intestinal loops. Any abnormal location of the gastrointestinal tract is noted.

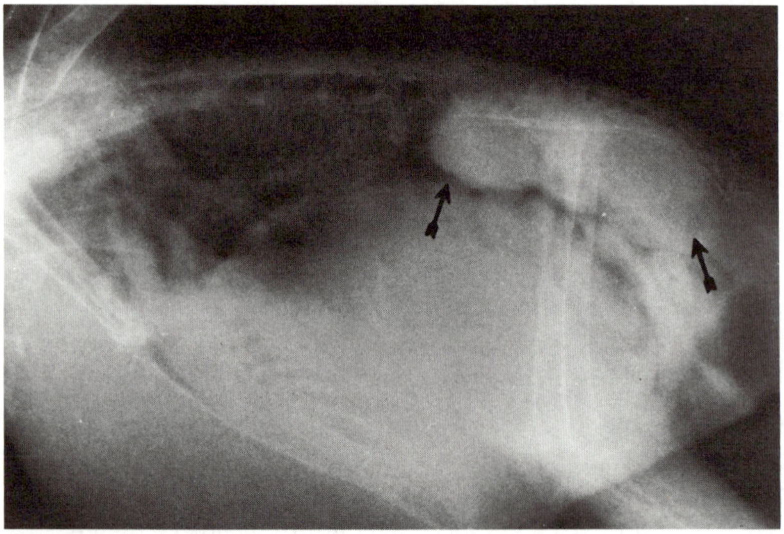

Figure 2A

Figure 2—(A) Lateral radiograph of an Amazon parrot showing enlarged kidneys *(arrows)* and liver secondary to *E. coli* infection. (B) Ventrodorsal view of the same parrot.

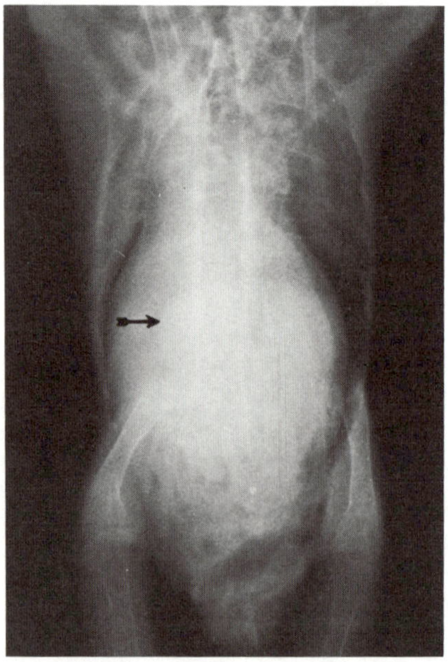

Figure 2B

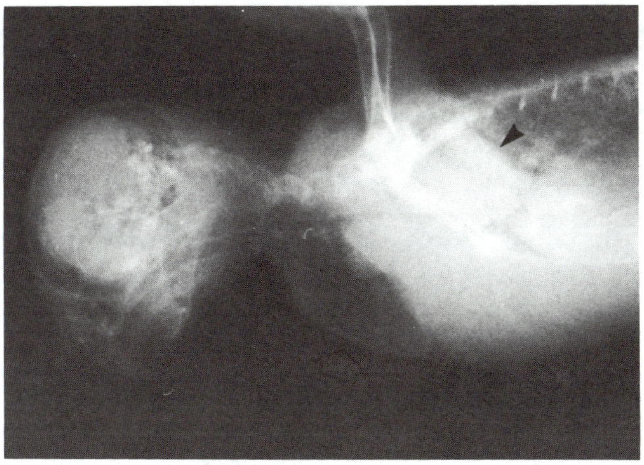

Figure 3—Lateral radiograph of the cranial thoracic area of a budgerigar showing an enlarged thyroid gland *(closed arrow)* and distended crop *(open arrow)*. The soft-tissue density visualized at the thoracic inlet extending into the crop may represent an enlarged thyroid or soft tissue displaced anteriorly by a larger caudal thyroid mass.

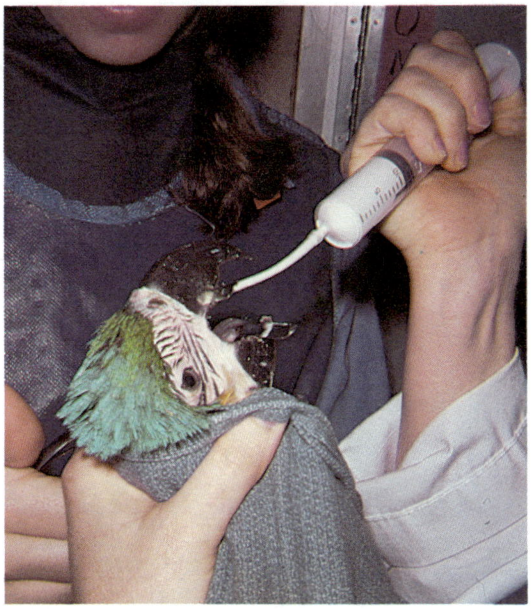

Figure 4—Administration of barium to a blue and gold macaw using a nasal speculum.

Displacement may be due to extrinsic masses or organ enlargement. Radiopaque material is normally present in the gizzard if the bird is receiving grit. Proper positioning[5] and at least two views, lateral and ventrodorsal, are necessary for evaluation. Because exposure factors vary with the size of the bird, film-screen combinations, and radiographic equipment, it is difficult to recommend a specific kilovolt peak, milliamperage, and time. For average parrots (weighing 350 to 500 g) a technique comparable to feline radiographic studies is appropriate. Parakeets require 5 to 10 kvp less and canaries and finches need a 15 kvp decrease. Larger parrots (macaws and large cockatoos) require about the same kilovolt peak setting as cats.[6] For par speed film-screen combinations, a tabletop technique at 100 mA for 1/60 second at 40 in. provides diagnostic radiographs.

Currently, a rare-earth ultradetailed film-screen[a] combination provides the most satisfactory avian radiographs. This film-screen combination requires a fivefold increase in the milliampere seconds over the par speed combination. Single-screen mammography packs with single-emulsion film can be substituted for the cassette system.

Tranquilizers and anesthetics are usually not necessary for radiographic procedures. Since the effects of these agents on gastrointestinal motility in birds is not thoroughly known, it is better not to use such agents when evaluating the gastrointestinal tract. A Plexiglas device[b] in combination with sandbags and tape provides adequate restraint and eliminates the need for personnel in the room during an exposure.

Procedure

The barium study is often tailored to the individual bird according to the history and clinical signs. If the crop is the area of concern, a double-contrast examination is indicated. Food and water are withheld for about four hours. Sometimes small amounts of seeds may remain in the crop or proventriculus. If the quantity is small, the study is still undertaken, though it is best to have the gastrointestinal tract empty. Barium sulfate suspension is administered orally into the crop[d] via a stomach tube (Figure 4). The size of the bird determines the volume of barium and whether an oral speculum is necessary (Table I). When the tube is palpated in the crop, a volume of barium is slowly given to gently distend the crop. If a double-contrast study of the crop is performed, half the amount of barium is given and the remainder of the volume is given as air.

Radiographs are made in the ventrodorsal and lateral planes immediately after administration of contrast medium and 30 minutes, 60 minutes, 2 hours, 4 hours, and 24 hours later. Timing of the radiographs may vary

[a]Kodak Lanex fine single or Kodak Ortho M-1, Eastman Kodak Co., Rochester, NY 14650.
[b]B.D. Creations, Lindenhurst, NY 11757.

[c]Liquid Polibar 55% W/W, E-Z-M Co., Inc., Westbury, NY 11590.
[d]In birds without crops, such as canaries, finches, and mynahs, the barium is given into the esophagus or proventriculus.

TABLE I

VOLUME OF BARIUM SULFATE IN AVIAN GASTROINTESTINAL RADIOGRAPHY[6]

Bird	*Volume (ml)*	*Tube (French)*	*Type of Speculum*
Canary, finch	0.25–0.5	5	None
Parakeet	1.0–3.0	5	None
Cockatiel, conure, lovebird	3.0–5.0	8	Hemostat
Smaller parrots	10.0	10	Nasal
Larger parrots	15.0	12	Nasal

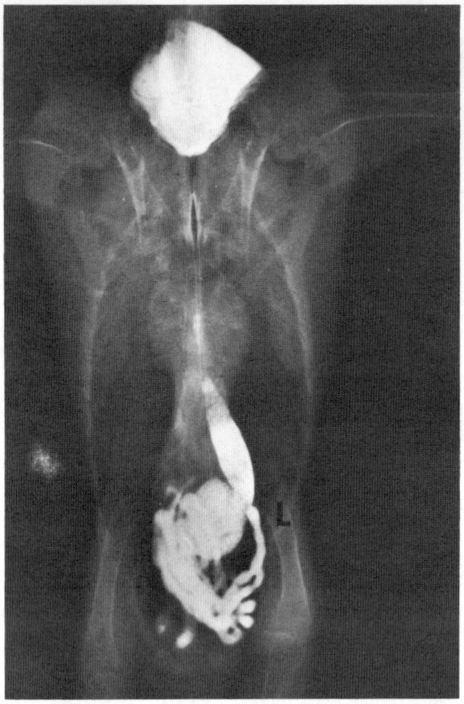

Figure 5A

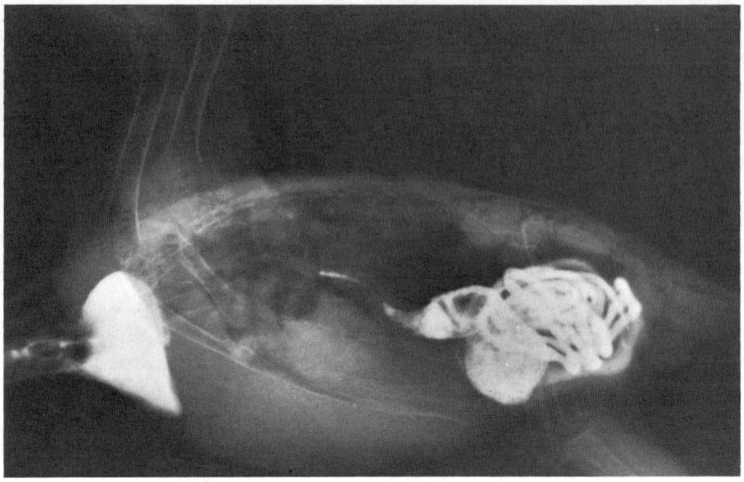

Figure 5B

Figure 5 (**A** and **B**)—A normal barium series. One-hour radiographs show filling of the crop, proventriculus, gizzard, and small intestines with barium. The radiolucent area in the proventriculus is a gas bubble.

depending on whether the upper gastrointestinal tract or lower region is of concern. Results of radiographs during the study may also alter the scheduling.

In normal studies in the immediate radiographs, the crop is filled with barium and a small amount of barium may be present in the esophagus and proventriculus (Figure 5). In 15 to 30 minutes, the proventriculus and gizzard and about half of the small intestines are filled. There is a decrease in the amount of contrast in the crop. By one hour the barium has filled the gastrointestinal tract. In four hours, the crop should be completely empty, although varying amounts of barium may remain in the proventriculus, gizzard, and intestines.

Radiographic Interpretation

Changes in transit time, thickening and/or irregularity of mucosal lining, distention, displacement of the gastrointestinal tract, and filling defects are radiographic signs associated with gastrointestinal disorders. When evaluating the significance of radiographic changes in contrast examinations, persistence of a lesion in subsequent radiographs is important. Motility in a dynamic system such as the gastrointestinal tract causes normal anatomic variation, which when visualized on only one radiograph leads to misinterpretation.

Delay in transit time results from functional or mechanical ileus. Mechanical ileus from extraluminal lesions or intraluminal masses such as foreign bodies is unusual in birds (Figure 6).

Functional ileus associated with severe gram-negative gastroenteritis is a more common cause of delayed transit of barium. Distention of the entire gastrointestinal tract is observed with severe gram-negative infections rather than obstruction (Figure 7). In addition to infection, lead toxicity, parasites, and egg peritonitis are associated with functional ileus. An increase in transit time has not been observed.

Thickening and irregularity of the crop and esophagus (Figure 8) are associated with candidiasis. Mucosal irregularity from neoplasia is difficult to distinguish from gastrointestinal fungal infections (Figures 9 and 10). Pathologic filling defects are unusual but do occur with neoplasia and fungal granuloma (Figure 11). Commonly, residual seed coated with barium is mistaken for filling defects. Thickening of the proventriculus, gizzard, and intestines has not been visualized radiographically.

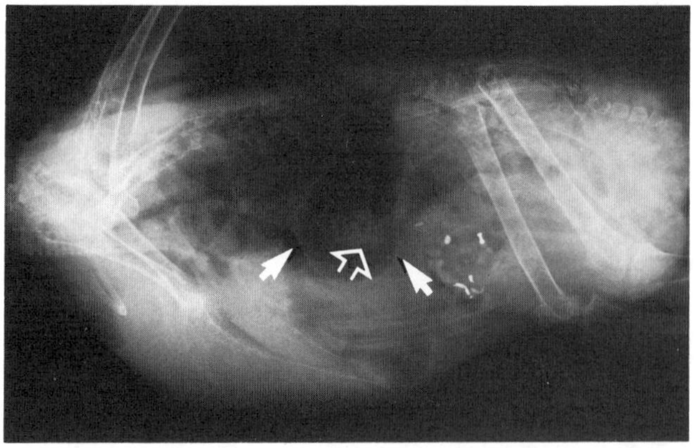

Figure 6—Distention of the proventriculus *(closed arrows)* with gas secondary to obstruction in a greater sulfur crested cockatoo. This parrot had ingested electric wire. If the type of heavy metal cannot be determined through historical information, the possibility of heavy-metal intoxication such as lead poisoning, in addition to obstruction, should also be considered. Foreign material *(open arrow)* is present in the lumen. Metallic foreign material is present in the gizzard.

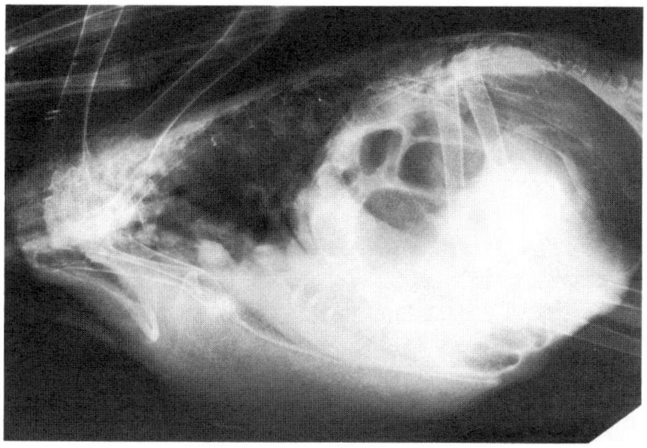

Figure 7A

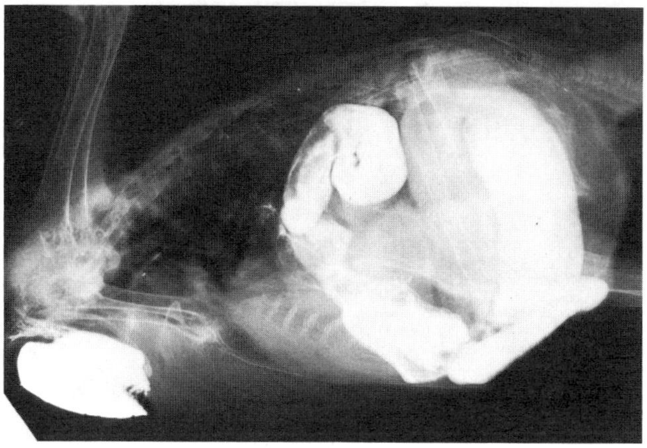

Figure 7B

Figure 7—**(A)** Survey radiographs of a blue and gold macaw showing marked distention of the gastrointestinal tract with gas. **(B)** In the one-hour radiograph, there is displacement of the duodenum and distention of the loops of intestines with barium. On autopsy, there was no evidence of obstruction. Serositis and associated gram-negative infection produced a functional ileus.

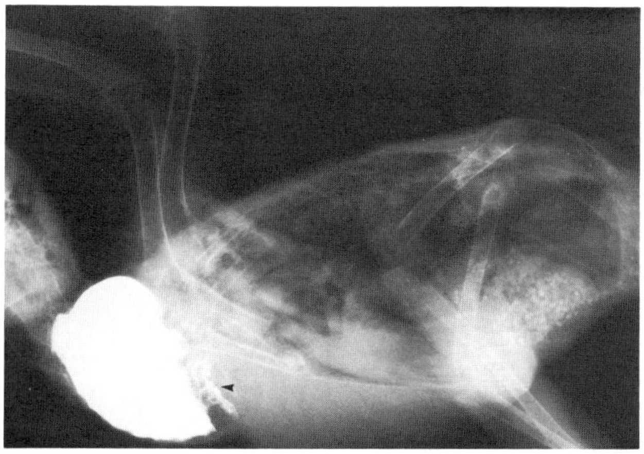

Figure 8A

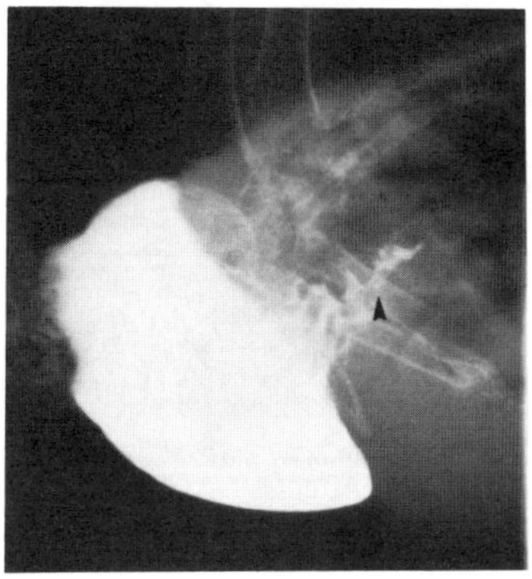

Figure 8B

Figure 8—**(A)** A double-contrast study of the crop showing thickening and irregularity of the crop wall due to candidiasis *(arrow)*. **(B)** Esophageal abnormality in same bird also due to candidiasis *(arrow)*.

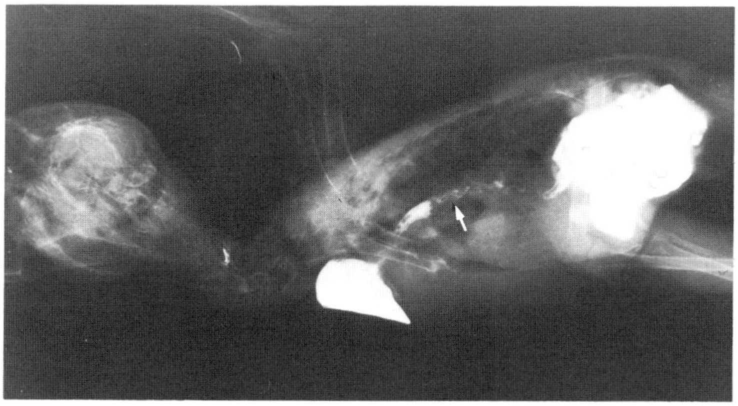

Figure 9—Squamous cell carcinoma causing a nodular mass *(large arrow)* and mucosal irregularity *(small arrow)* in the esophagus and proventriculus of a 47-year-old Amazon parrot.

Localized distention of the crop occurs secondary to enlarged thyroids, lead toxicity, and obstruction in the proventriculus, gizzard, or upper intestines. Distended atonic cloacae can occur secondary to spinal trauma and neoplastic involvement of sacral nerves.

Displacement of the gastrointestinal tract due to extrinsic mass or organ enlargement may be visualized by barium contrast examination. Viewing the direction

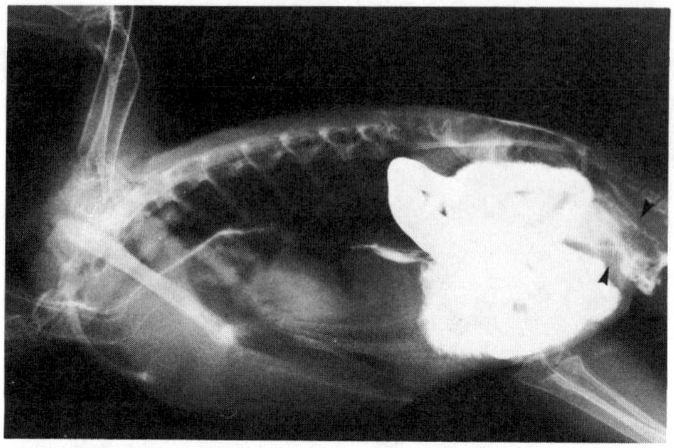

Figure 10—Filling defects and mucosal abnormality *(arrows)* in the rectum of a mynah with an adenocarcinoma.

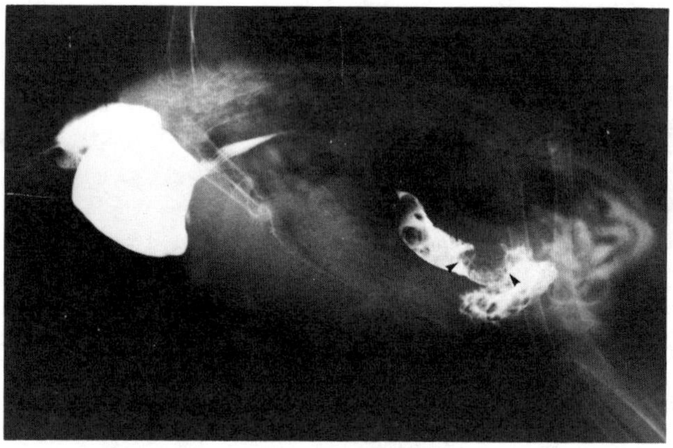

Figure 11—*Aspergillus* granuloma in an Amazon parrot *(arrows)* causing a large filling defect in the proventriculus.

in which the gastrointestinal tract is displaced will aid in determining which organ or organs may be involved (Figure 12).

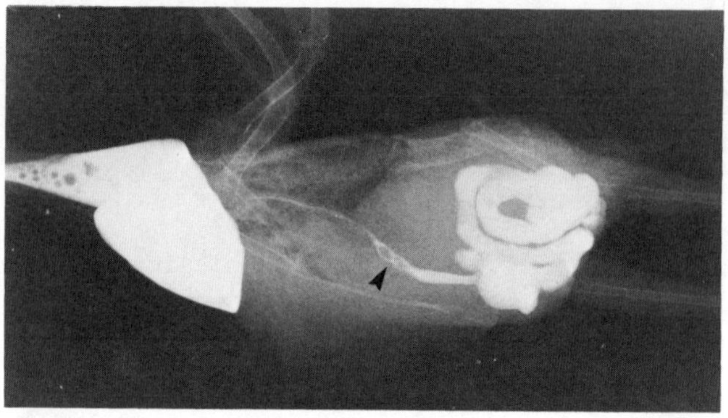

Figure 12—Ventral displacement of the esophagus and proventriculus *(arrow)* in a budgerigar from a renal tumor.

Summary

Barium contrast examination is indicated for thorough evaluation of avian gastrointestinal disturbances. An appropriate diagnostic workup should precede radiographic examination. Findings on survey radiographs suggest that gastrointestinal problems can be pursued with a barium study. In the author's experience, the most common finding on survey radiographs indicating a gastrointestinal abnormality is distention of the gastrointestinal tract with gas and fluid. Obstructive ileus causing this pattern is unusual, and other causes such as infection and toxicity should be considered. Delayed transit time, distention of intestines, and mucosal irregularities are common lesions observed during the barium series.

REFERENCES

1. McDonald SE, Bayer EV: Psittacosis in pet birds. *Calif Vet* 4:6-17, 1981.
2. Woerpel RW, Rosskopf WJ: Heavy-metal intoxication in caged birds. Part 1. *Compend Contin Educ Pract Vet* 4:729-738, 1982.
3. Leav I, et al: A naturally occupying lipidosis in shell parakeets, *Melopsittacus undulatus. Lab Invest* 18(4):433-437, 1968.
4. Lowestine LJ, Petrak ML: Iron pigment in the livers of birds, in Montali RJ, Migaki G (eds): *The Comparative Pathology of Zoo Animals.* Washington, DC, Smithsonian Institute Press, 1980, pp 127-135.
5. Evans SM: Avian radiographic diagnosis. *Compend Contin Educ Pract Vet* 3:660-666, 1981.
6. McMillan MC: Avian radiology, in Petrak ML (ed): *Diseases of Cage and Aviary Birds.* Philadelphia, Lea & Febiger, 1982, pp 329-360.

Radiographic Diagnosis of Avian Abdominal Disorders

Marjorie C. McMillan, DVM

School of Veterinary Medicine
Tufts University
North Grafton, Massachusetts

Angell Memorial Animal Hospital
Boston, Massachusetts

Windhover Bird Clinic
Walpole, Massachusetts

Many avian diseases create radiographic abnormalities, and failure to recognize them may lead to misdiagnoses and inappropriate treatment. Radiographic examination, however, must complement an accurate history, thorough physical examination, and clinical laboratory data. It is not a substitute for these procedures. The interpretation and significance of certain radiographic abnormalities vary with species, age, sex, and duration in captivity. In addition, the frequency of certain radiographic findings varies with the species of bird under consideration. For example, traumatic injury to the extremities and skull predominates in raptors, whereas infectious diseases and nutritional deficiencies are common in exotic birds.

The radiographic technique used for birds as well as the normal radiographic anatomy of birds are reported in the literature[1,2]; specifically, birds and mammals differ in that birds lack an omentum, well-developed mesenteric attachments, and a falciform ligament. Because of short mesenteric attachments, the abdominal organs of birds remain relatively fixed in position. Fat deposits between organs are minimal, and thus differentiation of specific organ margins is more difficult in birds than it is in dogs and cats. Because only a rudimentary, incomplete diaphragm is present, the cardiac silhouette and bilobed liver blend into a homogeneous soft tissue that has an hourglass appearance on ventrodorsal radiographs. The soft tissue density of abdominal viscera contrasts with the radiolucent surrounding air sacs.

Radiographic findings associated with abdominal disorders are:

1. Changes in the size, shape, position, and density of specific organs
2. Homogeneous abdominal density
3. Loss of abdominal air sac space
4. Visualization of a mass.

Radiographic Abnormalities

Hepatomegaly is a common radiographic finding in psittacines. In a lateral radiograph, the liver normally does not extend beyond the sternum. If the bird is positioned properly for a ventrodorsal view, the liver normally does not extend laterally beyond a line parallel to the sternum connecting the scapula and acetabulum (Figure 1).

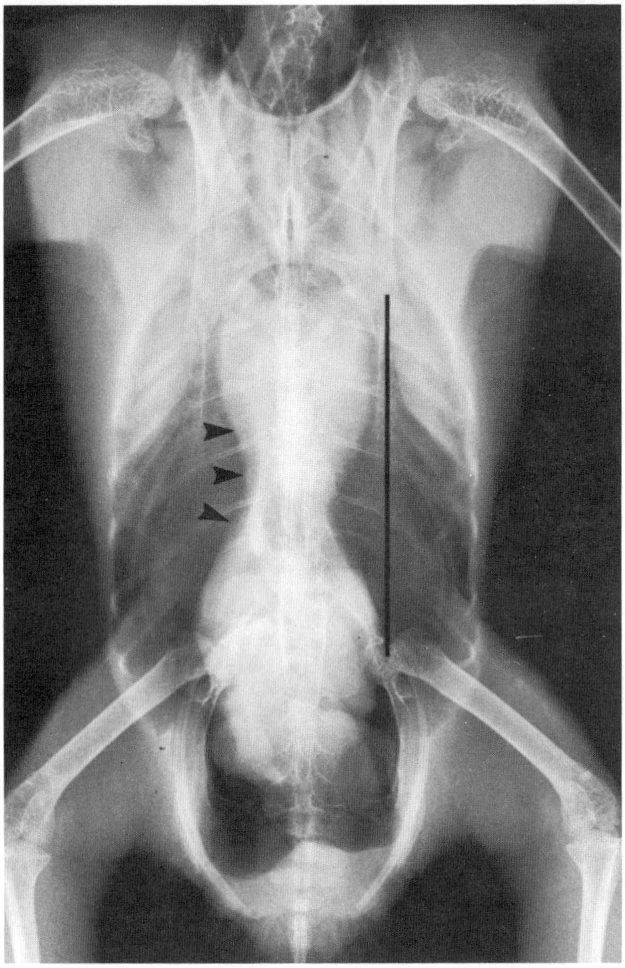

An enlarged liver may cause cranial displacement of the cardiac silhouette, dorsal displacement of the proventriculus, and caudodorsal displacement of the ventriculus. The hourglass configuration of the cardiohepatic silhouette is altered, and the liver is visualized as bulging into the abdominal air sacs. Many viral diseases[3-6] (such as Pacheco's disease, REO [respiratory enteric orphans] disease, Newcastle disease virus, and papovavirus) and bacterial infections (particularly gram-negative organisms, mycobacteria,[7,8] and chlamydia) may result in hepatomegaly (Table I). Often, splenomegaly also is present (Figure 2). Parasites are an uncommon cause of liver disease, although toxoplasmosis in mynahs (*Acridotheres* spp.)[9] and liver flukes in a sulphur-crested cockatoo (*Kakatoe galerita*)[10] have been reported. Such metabolic abnormalities as hemochromatosis in mynahs (*Gracula religiosa*),[11,12] lipidosis in parakeets (*Melopsittacus undulatus*),[13] fatty degeneration, and gout may involve the liver, spleen, kidneys, and heart. Primary and metastatic neoplasia occur most commonly in parakeets; while lymphoma[14,15] (Figure 3), biliary adenocarcinoma, hepatocellular carcinoma,[16] and meta-

Figure 1—Ventrodorsal radiograph of a normal Amazon parrot demonstrates the hourglass appearance of a cardiohepatic silhouette (*arrows*) and the lateral extent of liver (*solid line*). Loss of hourglass configuration or extension of liver lobes beyond the solid line indicates hepatomegaly.

Figure 2—Lateral radiograph of a blue and gold macaw shows splenomegaly (*large arrows*) and kidney enlargement (*curved arrows*) associated with psittacosis.

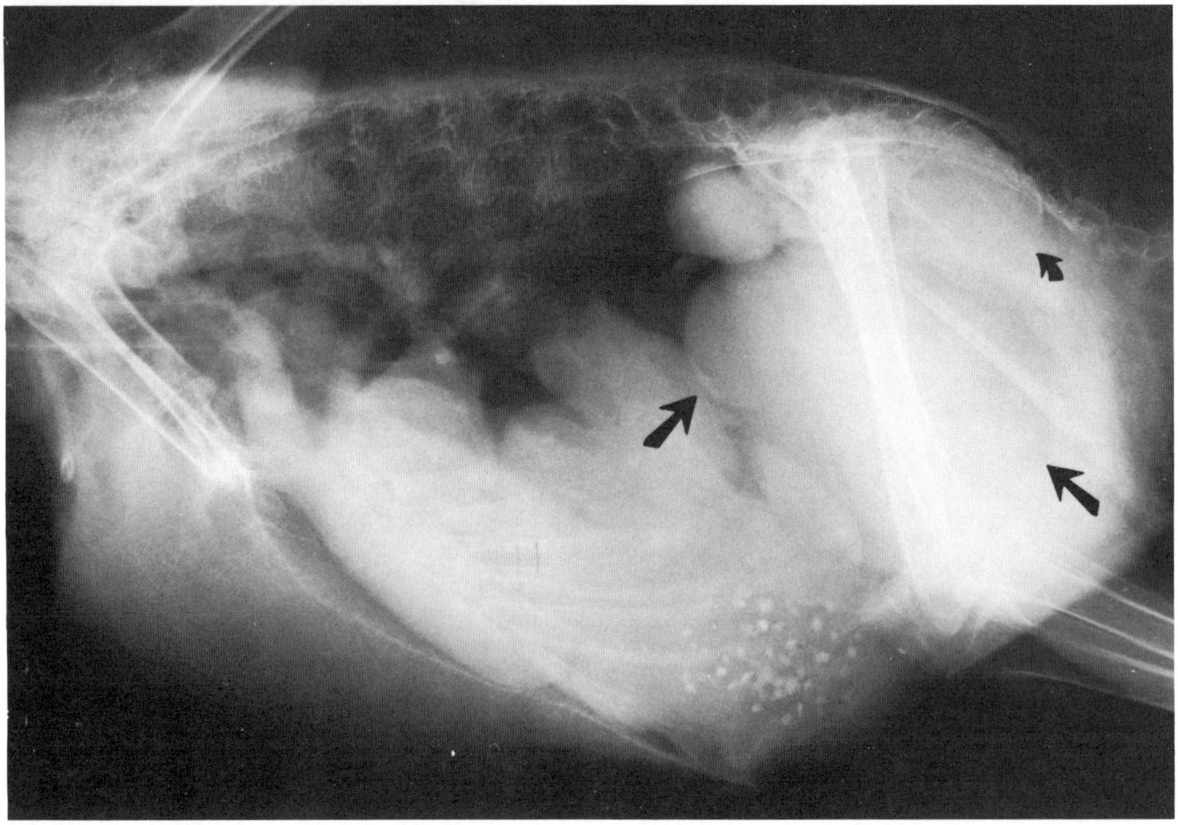

TABLE I
Causes of Hepatomegaly, Splenomegaly, and Nephromegaly

Hepatomegaly	*Splenomegaly*	*Nephromegaly*
Infectious	**Infectious**	**Infectious**
Viral	Viral	Bacterial
Bacterial	Bacterial	Chlamydial
Chlamydial	Chlamydial	
Mycobacterial	Mycobacterial	**Neoplastic**
Fungal		Adenocarcinoma
	Neoplastic	Embryonal nephroma
Neoplastic	Lymphoma	
Primary	Hemangiosarcoma	**Metabolic**
Hepatocellular carcinoma	Fibrosarcoma	Gout
Biliary adenocarcinoma	Leiomyosarcoma	Dehydration
Fibrosarcoma		Lipidosis
Hemangiosarcoma	**Metabolic**	
Hepatoma	Lipidosis	**Cystic**
Lymphoma	Hemochromatosis	
Metastatic		**Toxic**
Adenocarcinoma		Lead
Fibrosarcoma		
Melanoma		
Parasitic		
Toxoplasmosis		
Flukes (cestodes)		
Metabolic		
Hemochromatosis		
Lipidosis		
Fatty degeneration		
Gout		

static adenocarcinoma[16] have been reported in larger psittacines. In mynahs, hepatomas occur in association with hemochromatosis.[17]

The spleen usually is not apparent radiographically (Figure 4). Splenomegaly, often in combination with hepatomegaly, occurs in systemic infections, neoplasia, and such metabolic disorders as lipidosis and hemochromatosis (Table I).

The kidneys are firmly adherent to the synsacrum, have smoothly rounded cranial and caudal poles, are flattened dorsoventrally, and are surrounded by air. The kidneys are best visualized in a lateral radiograph. Obliteration of normal air density surrounding the renal silhouette indicates renal enlargement, dorsal displacement of abdominal viscera, or presence of abdominal fluid (Figure 5). Nephritis from gram-negative bacterial infection and chlamydiosis may cause renal enlargement (Table I).

Dehydration causes increased renal density and, sometimes, renal enlargement. Incomplete clearance and flushing of renal tubules lead to "renal constipation," with an accumulation of uric acid crystals in the kidneys.[18] Theoretically, any condition resulting in impaired renal clearance of uric acid crystals could result in nephromegaly and increased renal density. In addition, changes in kidney size and density are seen in psittacines in association with acute hemolysis caused by lead toxicity.[19] These changes probably are caused by hemoglobin blockage of kidney tubules, with resultant decreased renal tubular function. In contrast to generalized nephromegaly observed in the conditions mentioned, kidney tumors usually cause enlargement of only the cranial or caudal pole with ventral displacement of the ventriculum[2,20] (Figure 6).

Hormonal changes result in cyclic atrophy and recrudescence of the gonads. Hypertrophied testicles are visualized as symmetric enlargements in the ventrodorsal view and as superimposed circular soft tissue masses, cranial and ventral to the kidneys, in the lateral radiograph (Figure 6). An enlarged oviduct results in loss of air sac density below the kidneys and increased soft tissue density in the dorsal abdominal region (Figure 7). Pathologic enlargement of the testicles and ovaries occurs because of neoplasia.[21] In addition, increased medullary bone density occurs in females with ovarian tumors[22] and oviduct abnormalities.

Changes apparent on survey radiographs provide preliminary information for certain disease processes; however, abnormalities of the gastrointestinal tract are best evaluated by barium-contrast examination.[23] As an example, gas in the gastrointestinal tract of birds is abnormal. If an external source of gas (such as tube feeding or aerophagia) is eliminated, a gastrointestinal abnormality is the most likely cause.

Proventricular dilatation,[24] also called *blue and gold ma-*

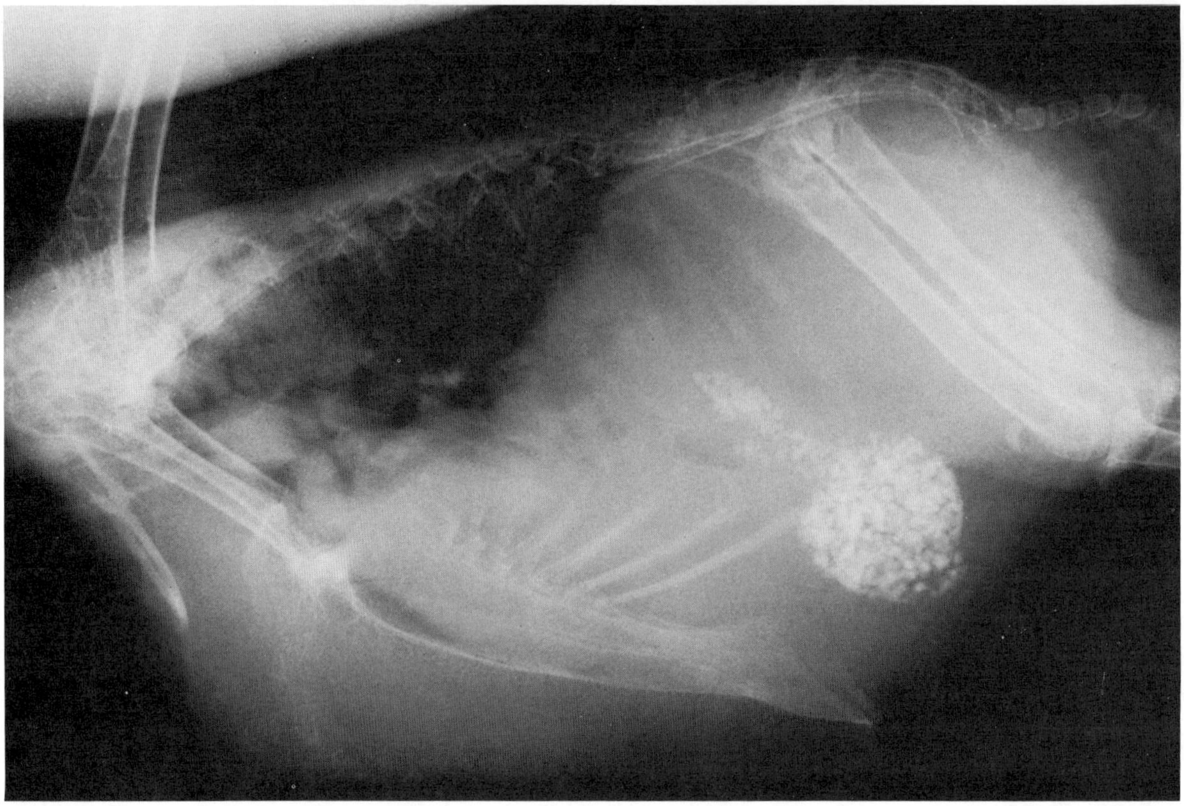

Figure 3A

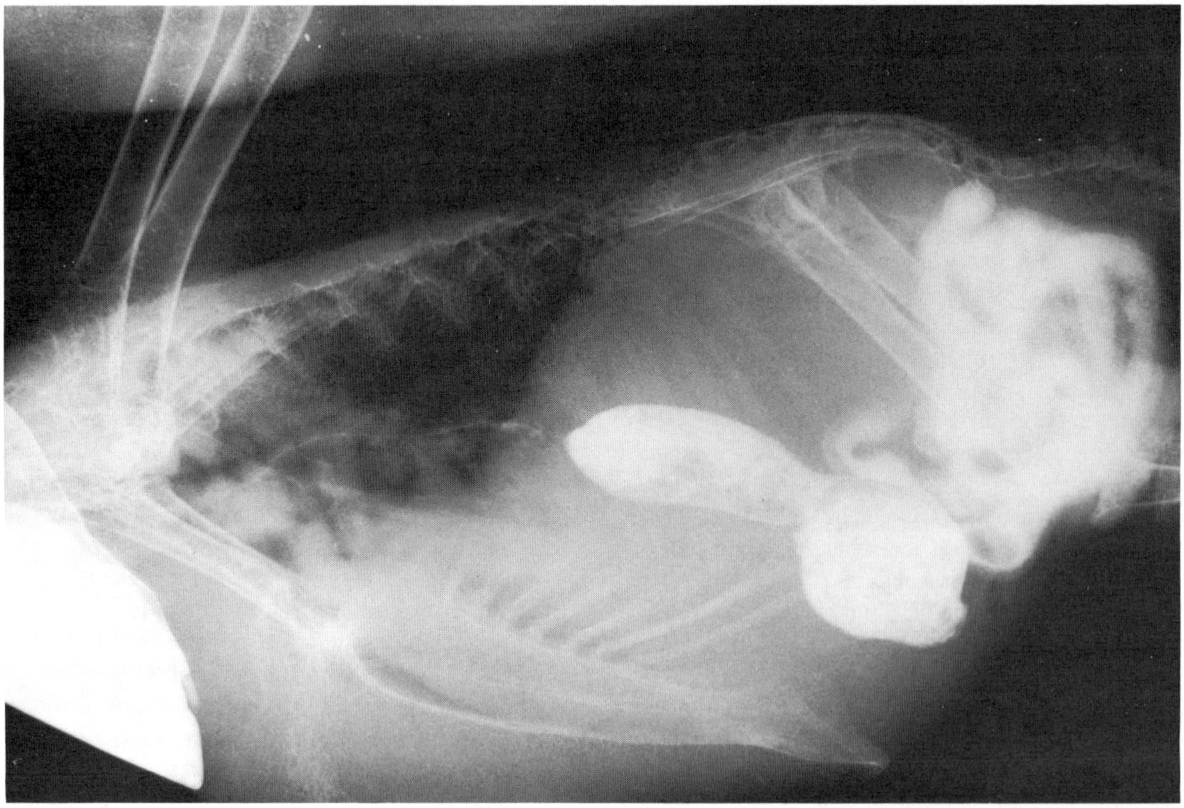

Figure 3B

Figure 3—(**A**) Survey lateral radiograph of an African gray parrot shows dorsal displacement of the proventriculus and caudodorsal displacement of the ventriculus by an enlarged liver. The homogeneous soft tissue mass in the dorsal abdomen obliterates the air sac space below the kidneys and between the lungs and viscera. (**B**) After one hour, the barium-contrast series indicated that the intestines were displaced caudally by a dorsal mass, which was an enlarged spleen. Hepatic and splenic enlargement were caused by lymphosarcoma.

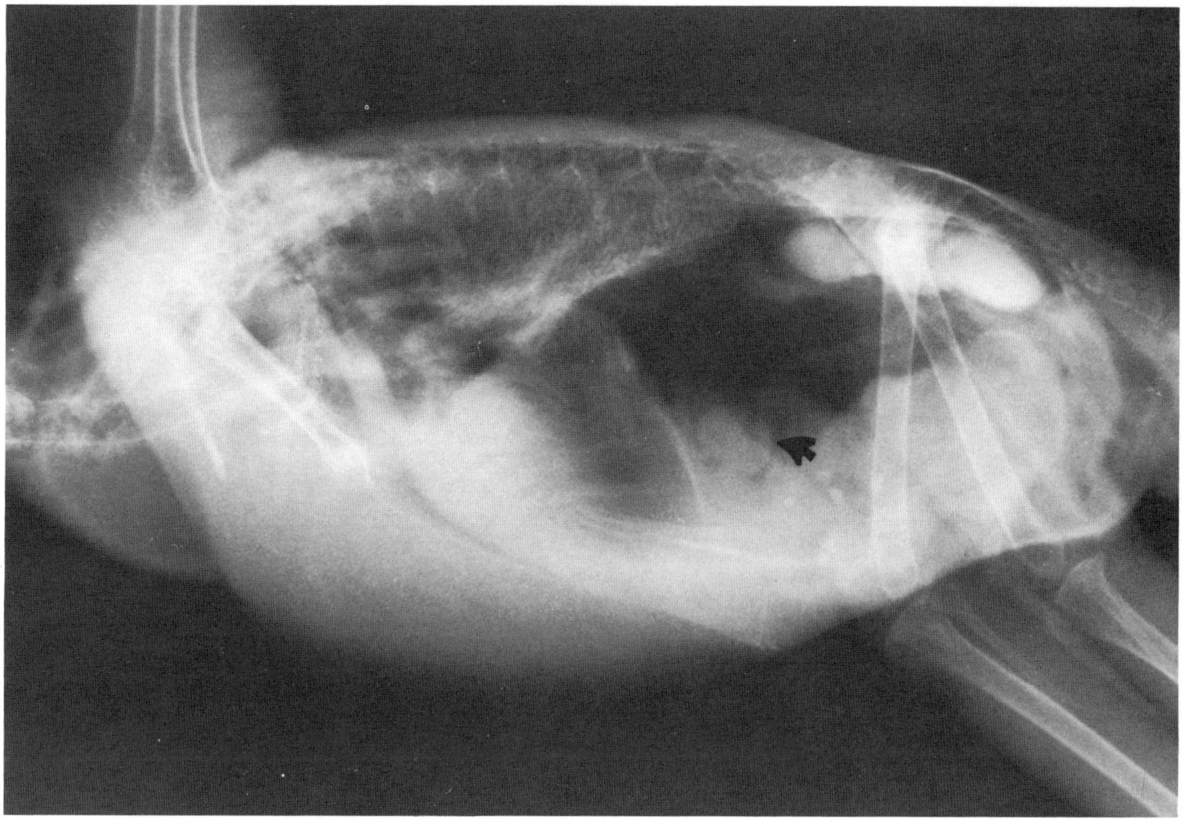

Figure 4—The normal size, shape, and location of the spleen (*arrow*) are apparent in this lateral radiograph of an African gray parrot. Peribronchial infiltrate is present in the hilar and mid region of the caudal lung.

caw syndrome[25] or *infiltrative splanchnic neuropathy*,[3] causes functional ileus resulting in marked gastrointestinal distention. Birds are presented with weight loss, uncontrollable regurgitation, history of passing undigested seeds, and dehydration. In all except a few cases, the disease is fatal. Radiographic changes range from slight distention of the proventriculus with gas to marked distention of the gastrointestinal tract (Figure 8). Barium may persist in the intestinal tract up to 72 hours after administration. The proventriculus is massively distended and may contain food or gas. The ventriculus also is distended and thin walled. The crop is usually distended with fluid. Histologically there is diffuse mononuclear cell infiltration of intrinsic and extrinsic splanchnic nerves supplying the crop, proventriculus, ventriculus, and duodenum. Although most commonly reported in the blue and gold macaw (*Ara ararauna*), the disease occurs in other macaws (e.g., the green-winged macaw [*Ara chloroptera*] and hyacinth macaw [*Hyacinthinus anodorhynchus*]) as well as in cockatoos, conures, and African gray parrots (*Psittacus erithacus*).

Functional ileus also occurs in association with inflammatory processes involving the abdomen. In birds with egg peritonitis, a generalized increased fluid density obscures abdominal detail and dilated gas-filled bowel loops may be apparent. Intestinal serosal adhesions associated with egg peritonitis also result in decreased intestinal motility (Figure 9). Gas-distended loops of intestine are also visualized in conjunction with the massive ascites commonly seen in mynahs with liver failure from hemochromatosis.

Gas and fluid distention of the intestinal tract caused by mechanical ileus can occur from a foreign body obstruction (Figure 10); stricture; neoplasia; and extrinsic masses involving the thyroid gland, oviduct, and spleen. Impaction of the ventriculus with grit results in upper gastrointestinal obstruction (Figure 11). Often these birds have been fed inappropriately sized grit, allowed to eat freely after being deprived of grit for a long period, or have a deprived appetite because of an underlying illness. Radiographs show an increased amount of grit firmly compressed in the ventriculus. Grit also may be visualized in the proventriculus and crop. Barium-contrast examination shows delayed emptying of the crop. Small amounts of barium may pass from the crop, through the ventriculus, and into the intestinal tract.

Atonic distention of the cloaca occurs with spinal trauma and infiltrative neoplastic processes involving the sacral nerves (Figure 12). Obstruction caused by cloacal polyps, papillomas, or adenocarcinoma also causes distention. Laying hens normally have a more dilated cloaca to facilitate passage of eggs; this should not be considered pathologic.

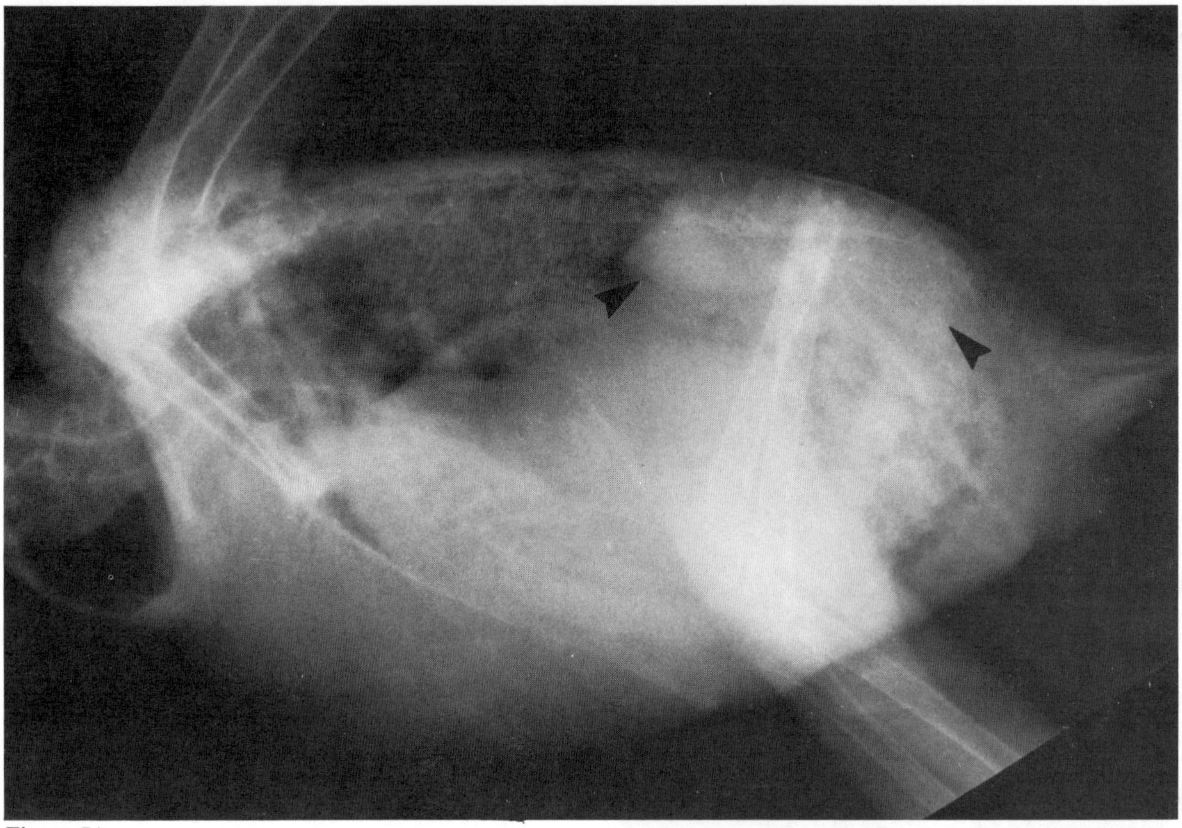

Figure 5A

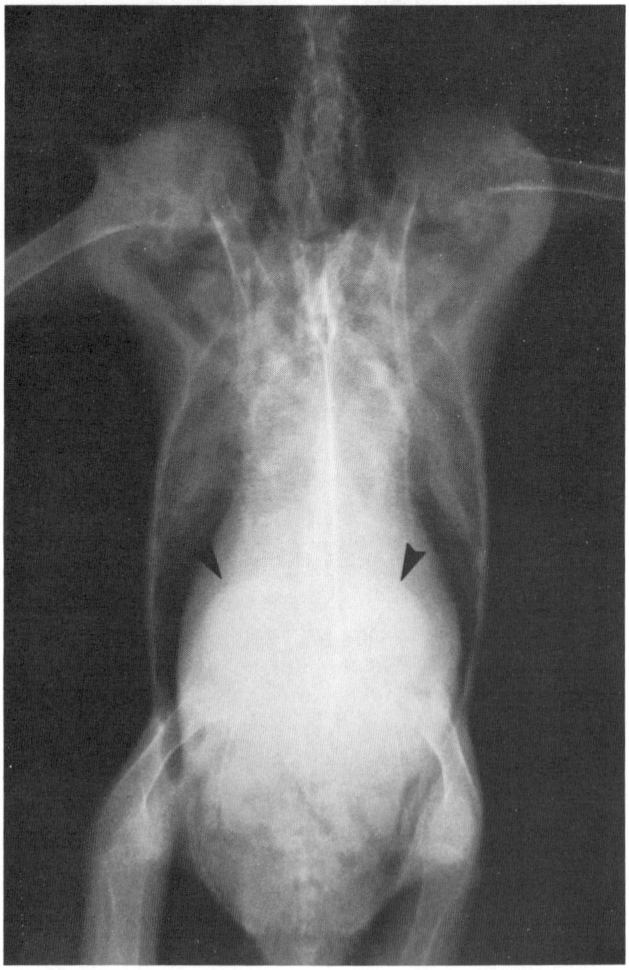

Figure 5B

Figure 5—(**A**) Kidney enlargement (*arrows*) with loss of air sac space ventral and cranial to kidneys is best demonstrated in a lateral radiograph. (**B**) Enlarged cranial kidney pole (*arrows*) is apparent in this ventrodorsal view. Nephromegaly in this Amazon parrot was caused by nephritis from *Escherichia coli* infection.

Additional Imaging Techniques

Urography,[2,26] ultrasonography,[27] and gastrointestinal barium-contrast studies[23] may aid in evaluating abdominal masses.

Urography outlines the kidneys, ureters, and cloaca. Radiographs taken at 10 seconds, 60 seconds, and 2 minutes after administration of contrast material provide the most useful information.[26] Irregularity of kidney size and shape and distention of the cloaca associated with renal neoplasia may be visualized by this means (Figures 6 and 12).

The presence of air sacs makes ultrasound examination difficult in birds. When abdominal fluid obliterates the air sacs, however, abdominal masses may be detected.

A gastrointestinal barium-contrast series helps the veterinarian localize abdominal masses and evaluate mechanical and functional ileus. Displacement of portions of the gastrointestinal tract by extrinsic masses, intraluminal masses, and hypomotility has been reported.

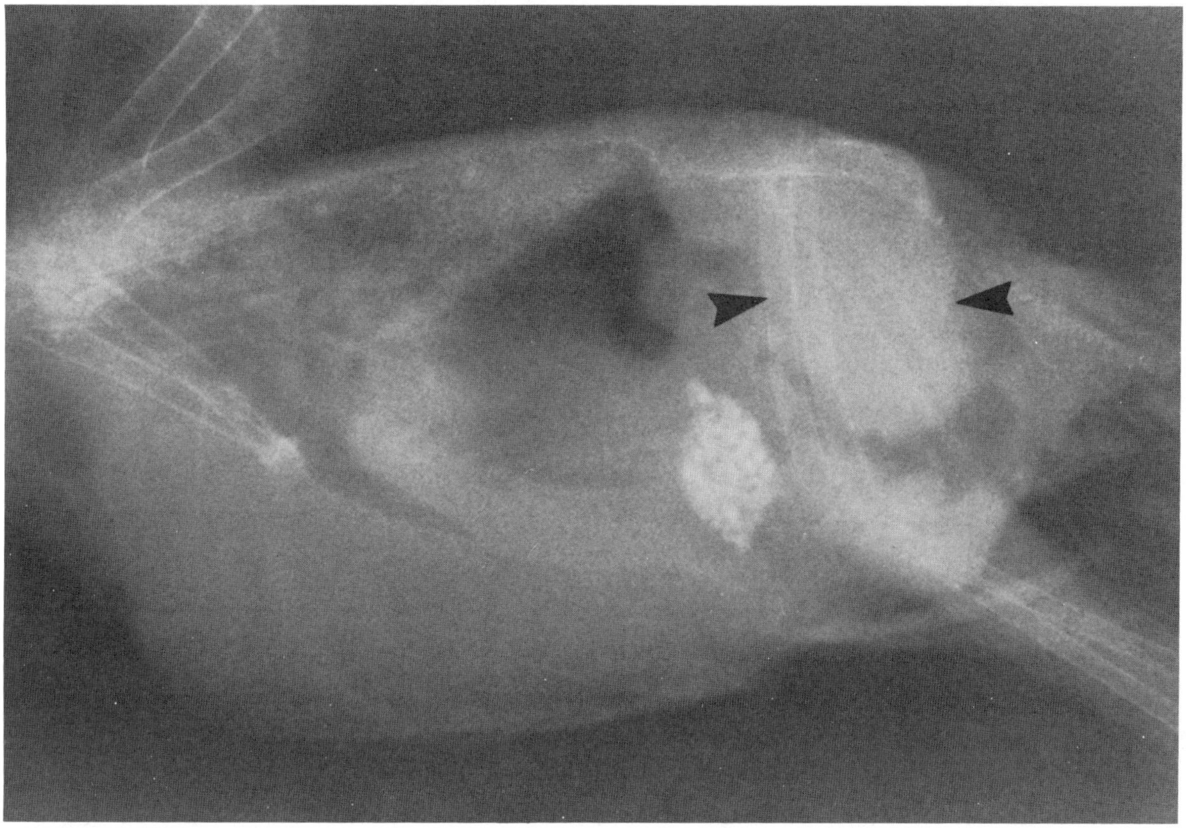

Figure 6A

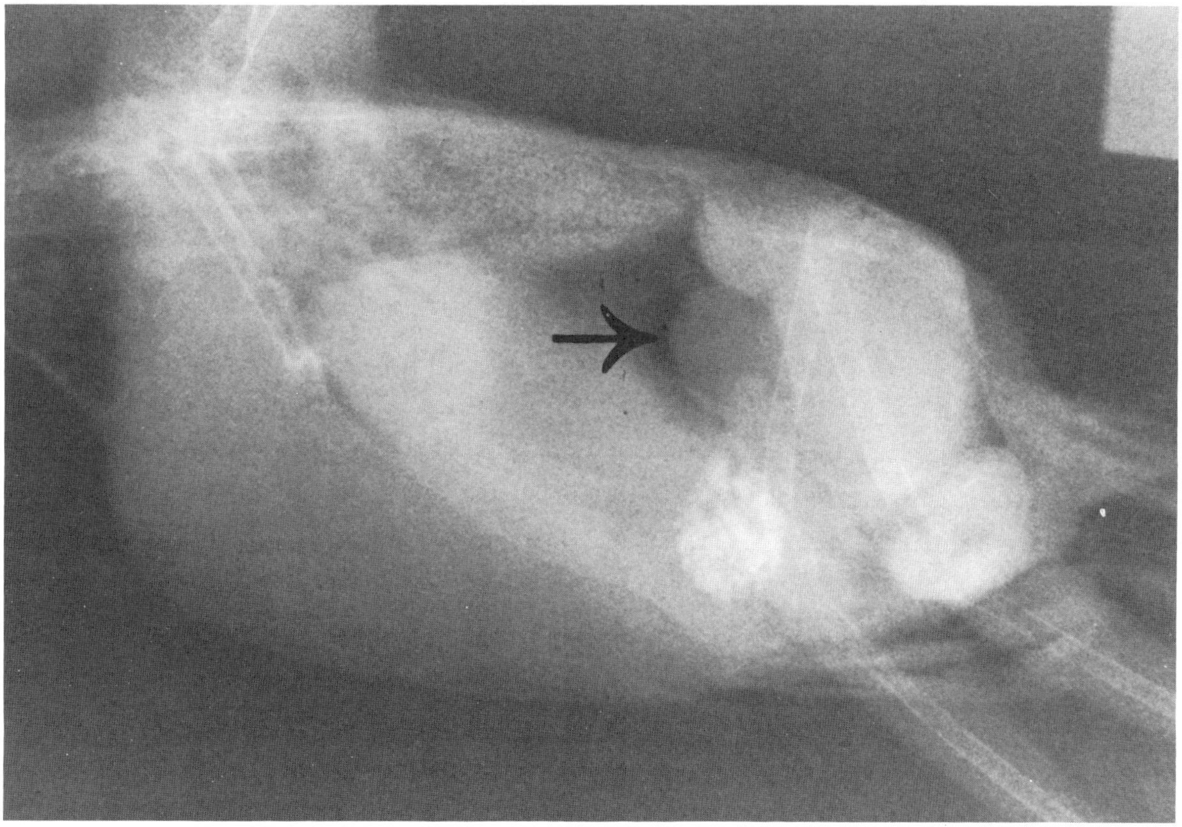

Figure 6B

Figure 6—(**A**) Renal adenocarcinoma (*arrows*) in this budgerigar is producing a large irregular mass from the caudal pole of a kidney. (**B**) The intravenous excretory urogram is enhancing the caudal pole renal adenocarcinoma in another budgerigar. The normal testicle (*arrow*) is ventral to the cranial kidney pole.

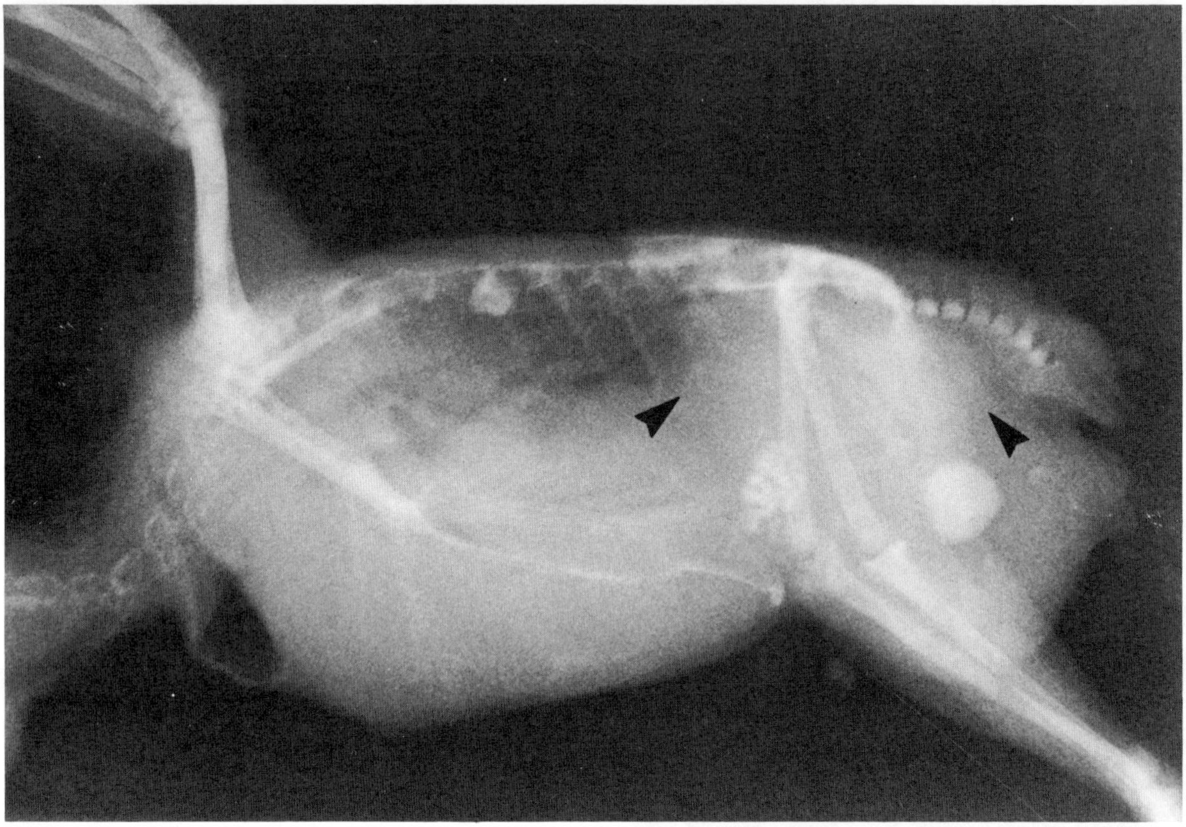

Figure 7A

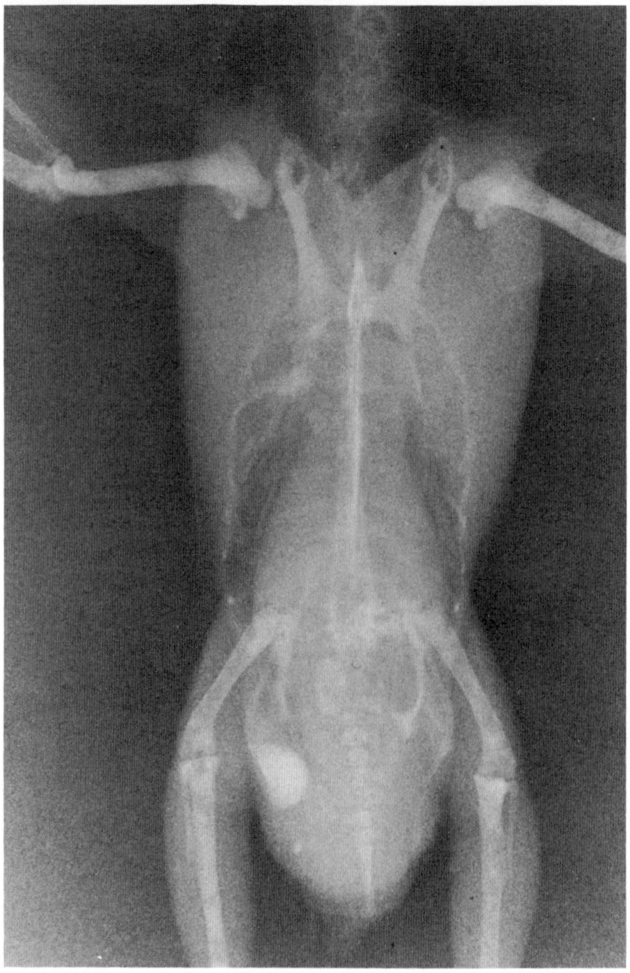

Figure 7B

Figure 7—(**A**) The soft tissue mass (*arrows*) in the dorsal abdomen obscuring visualization of the kidneys is an enlarged oviduct. The ventriculus is displaced cranially, and an abdominal hernia is apparent. (**B**) Mottled increased medullary bone density and well-defined circular regions of increased bone density involve the left pubis and ribs. These changes in budgerigars result from increased estrogen levels.

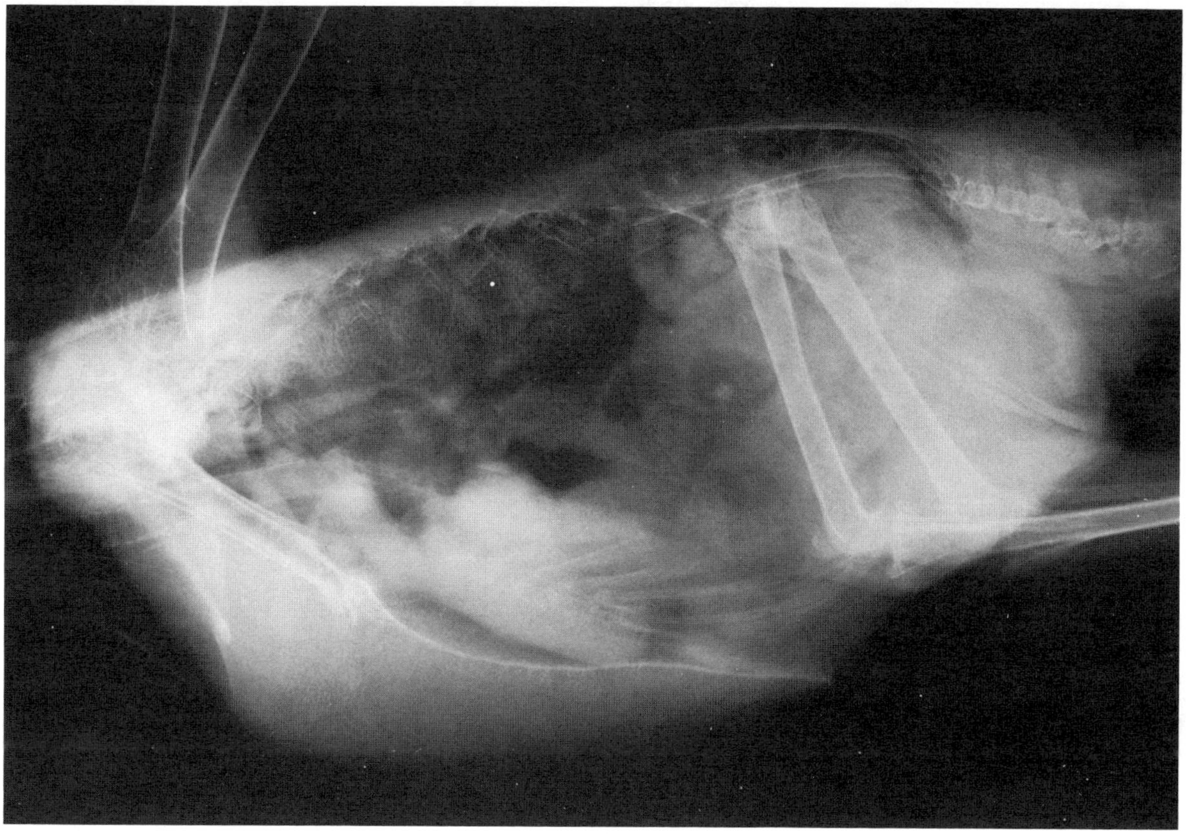

Figure 8A

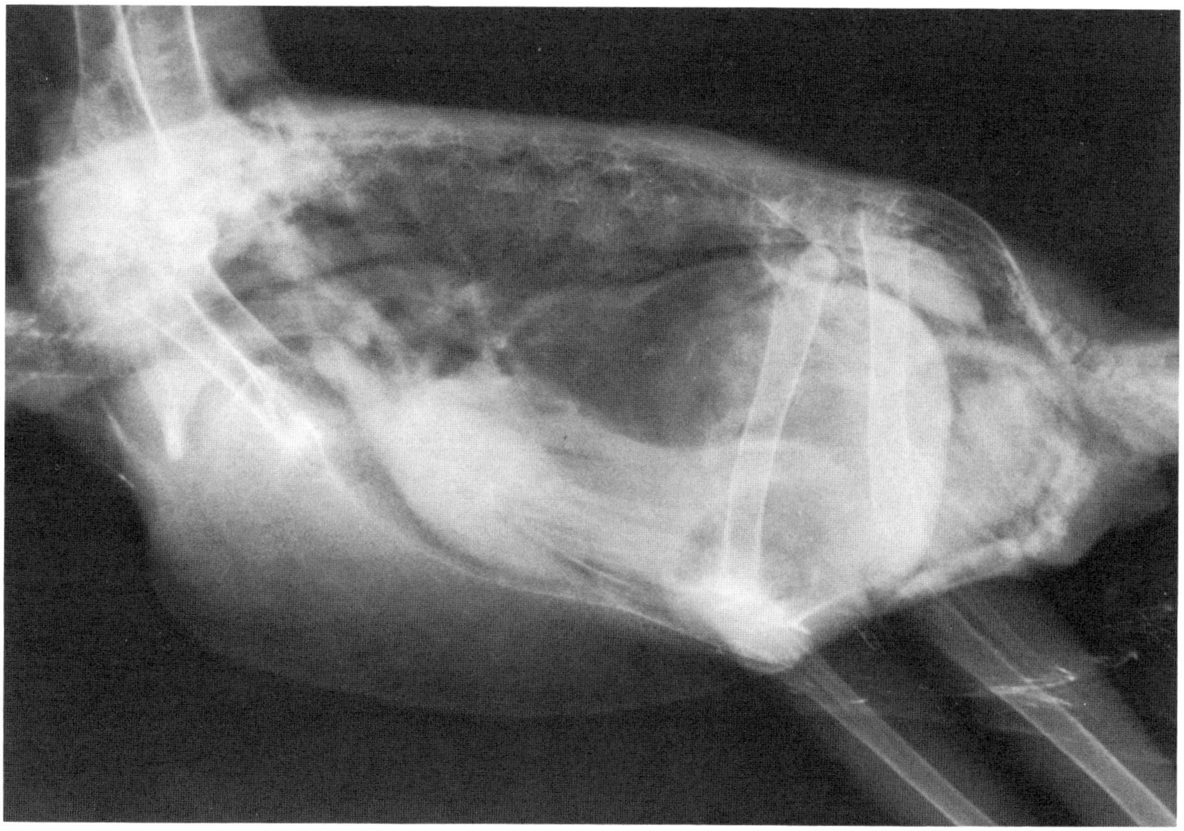

Figure 8B

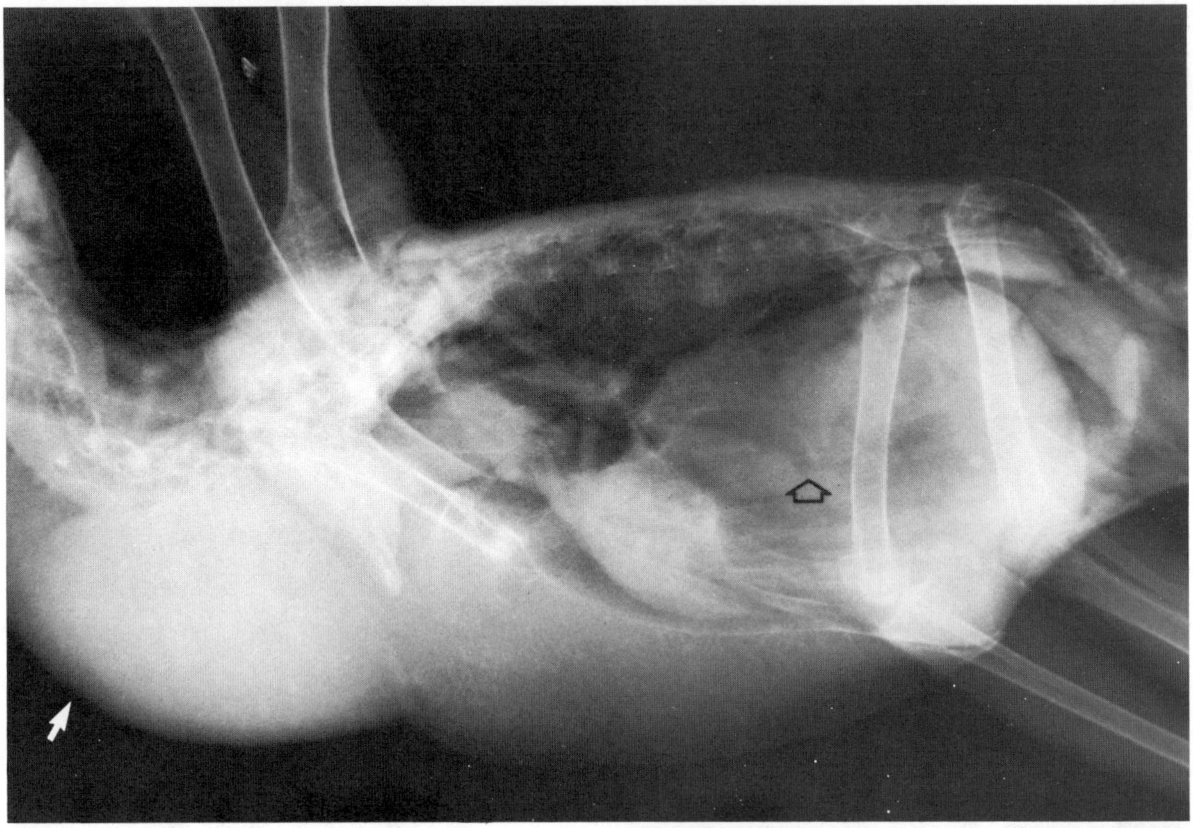

Figure 8C

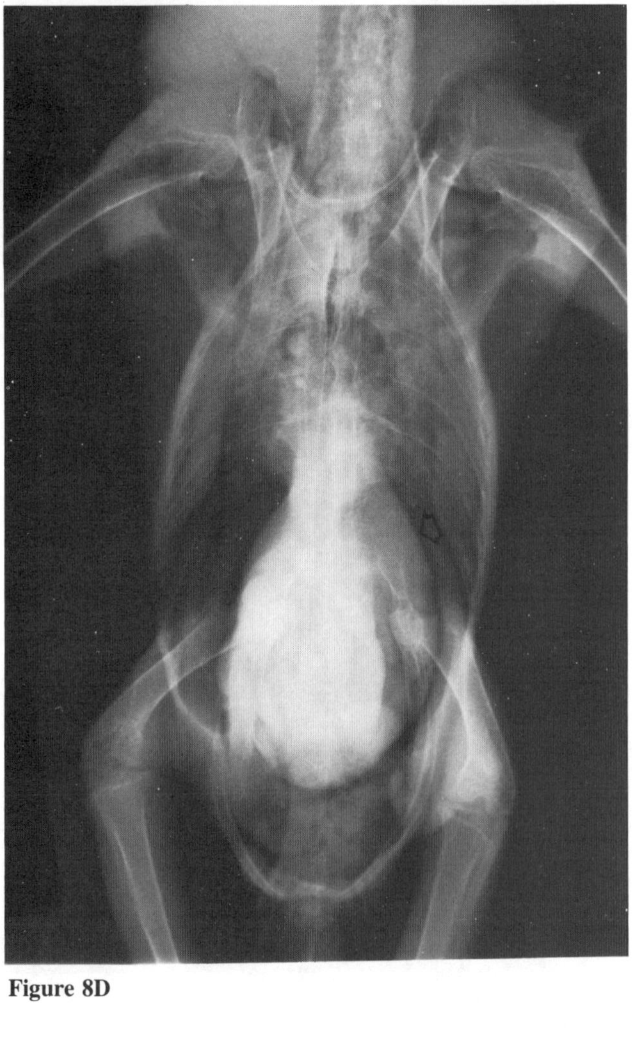

Figure 8D

Figure 8—(**A** through **F**) Radiographic changes associated with infiltrative splanchnic neuropathy. The radiographs are of blue and gold macaws. (**A**) Small amounts of gas and fluid are present in the proventriculus, ventriculus, and intestines. (**B**) Marked distention from the proventriculus and ventriculus being filled with gas and fluid. (**C**) Fluid-filled dilated proventriculus (*open arrow*) and ventriculus. The crop (*closed arrow*) is distended with fluid. (**D**) Ventrodorsal view of the parrot shown in **C**. The distended proventriculus (*open arrow*) could be mistaken for an enlarged liver lobe. (*Figure 8 continues next page*)

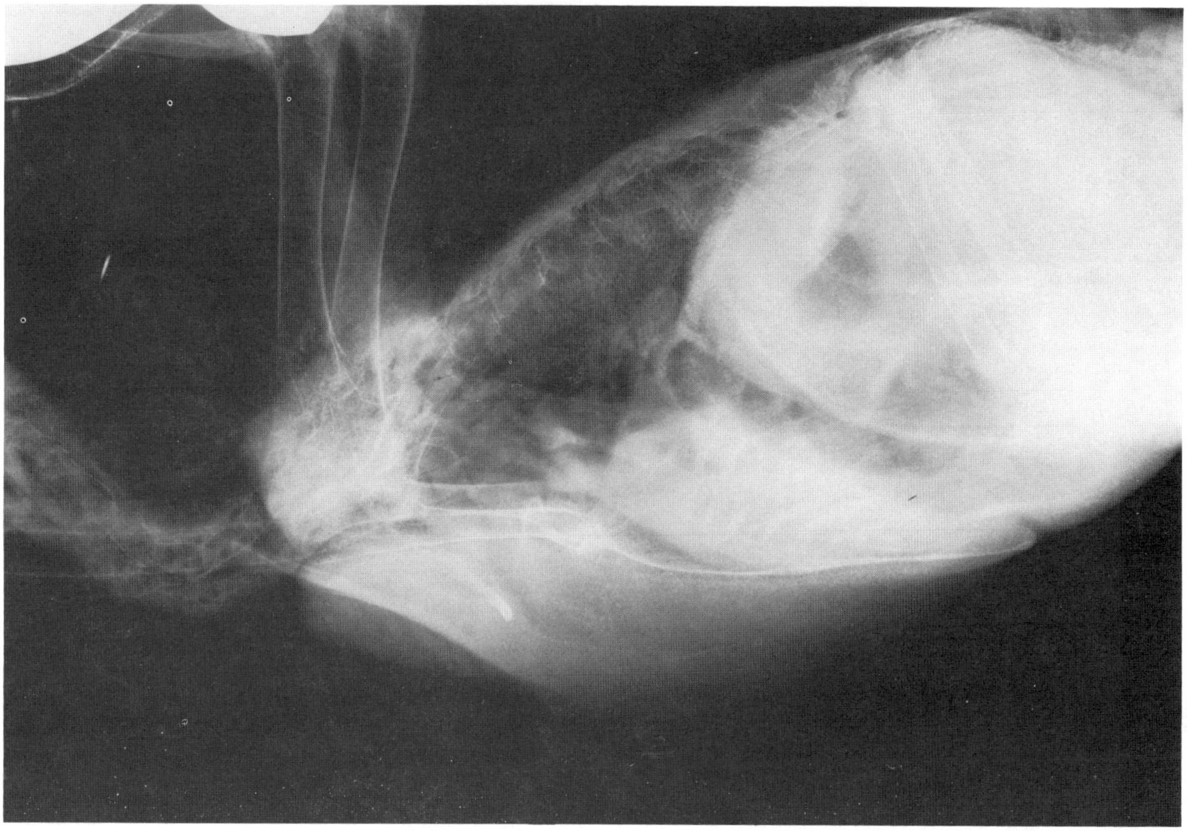

Figure 8E

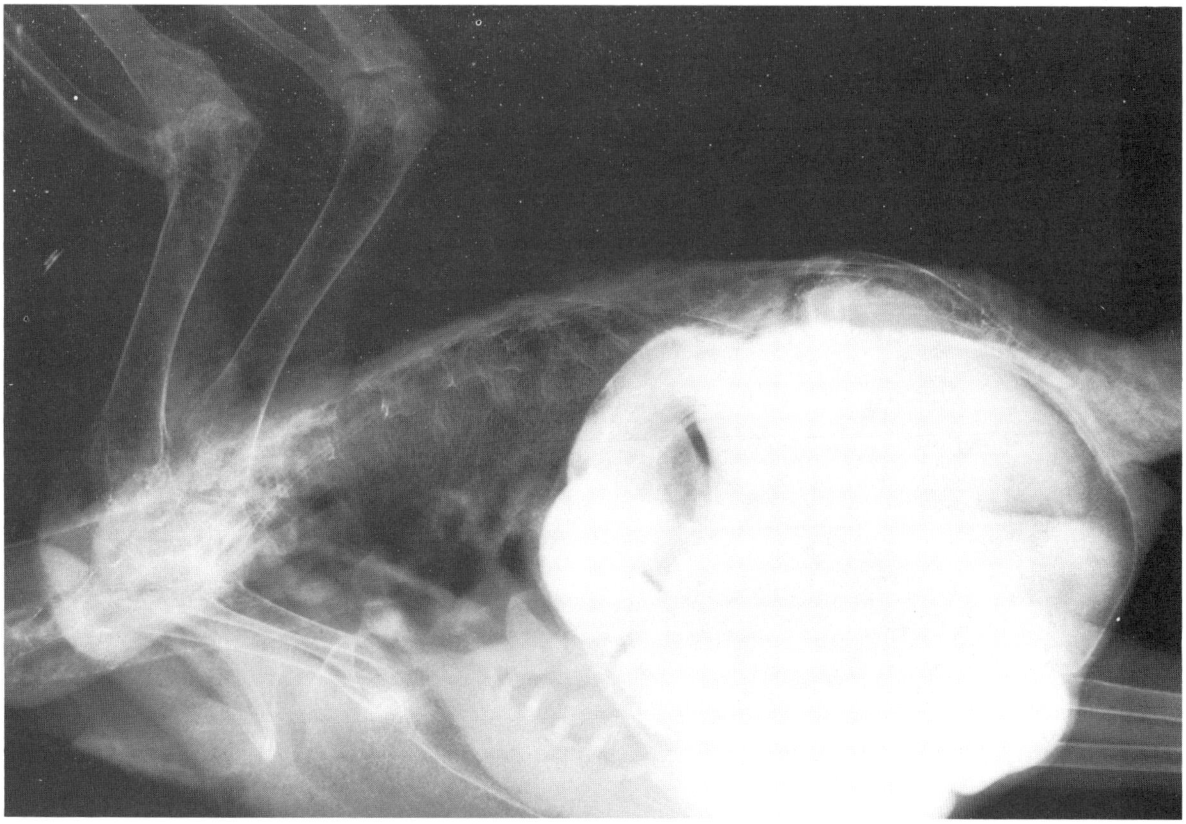

Figure 8F

Figure 8 continued—(**E**) Massive distention from the intestines being filled with gas and fluid because of functional ileus. (**F**) This radiograph shows retention of barium in dilated intestines eight hours after a barium-contrast series.

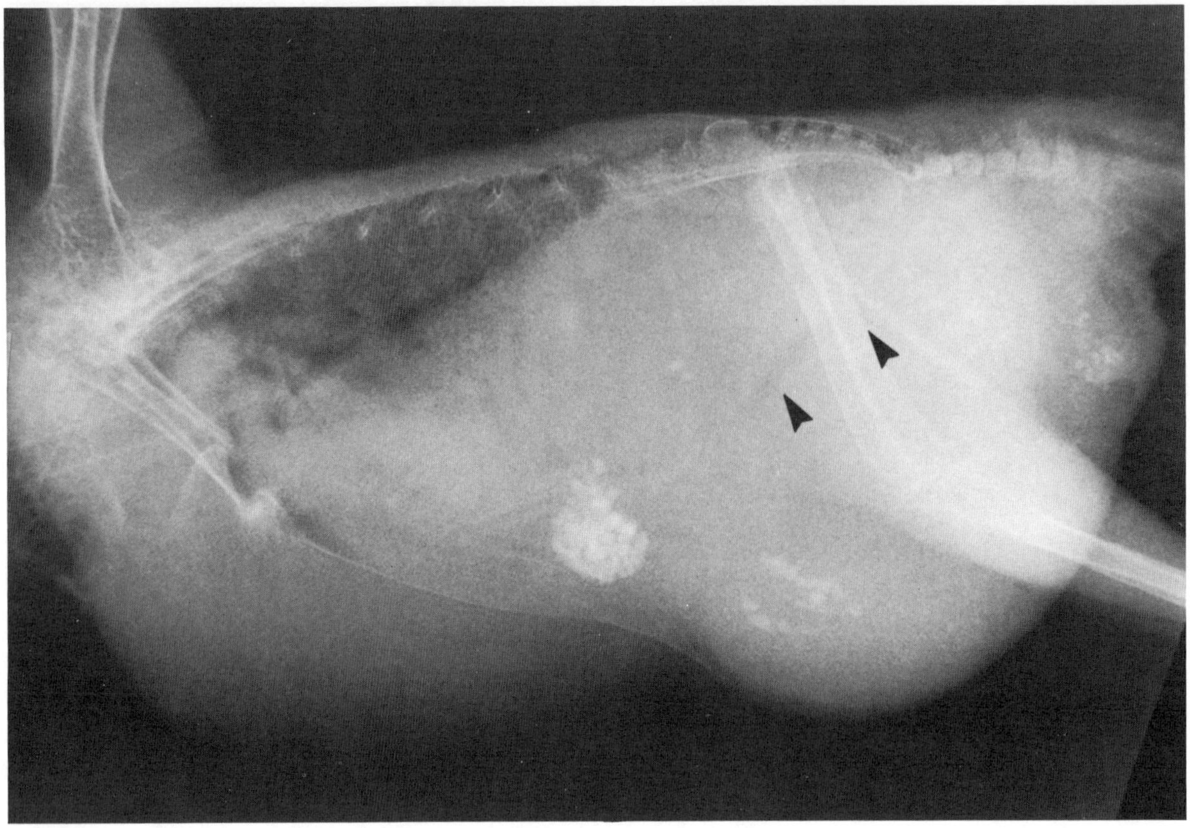

Figure 9A

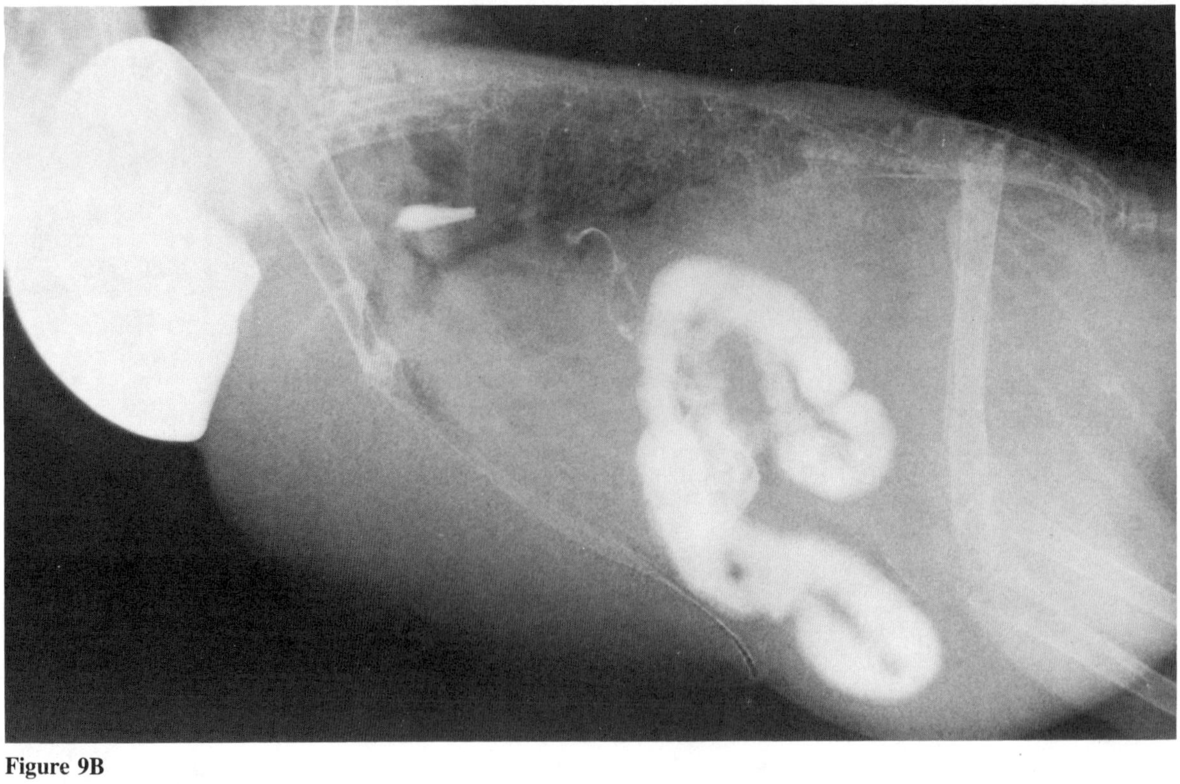

Figure 9B

Figure 9—(**A**) Distention of the abdomen, lack of contrast, and loss of air sac space are caused by abdominal fluid in this female cockatiel. A gas-filled intestinal loop (*arrows*) is present. The ventriculus is displaced cranially. (**B**) This radiograph shows abnormal positioning of the proventriculus, ventriculus, and intestines 30 minutes after a barium-contrast series. The intestines are dilated. Egg peritonitis with abdominal fluid and adhesions is present.

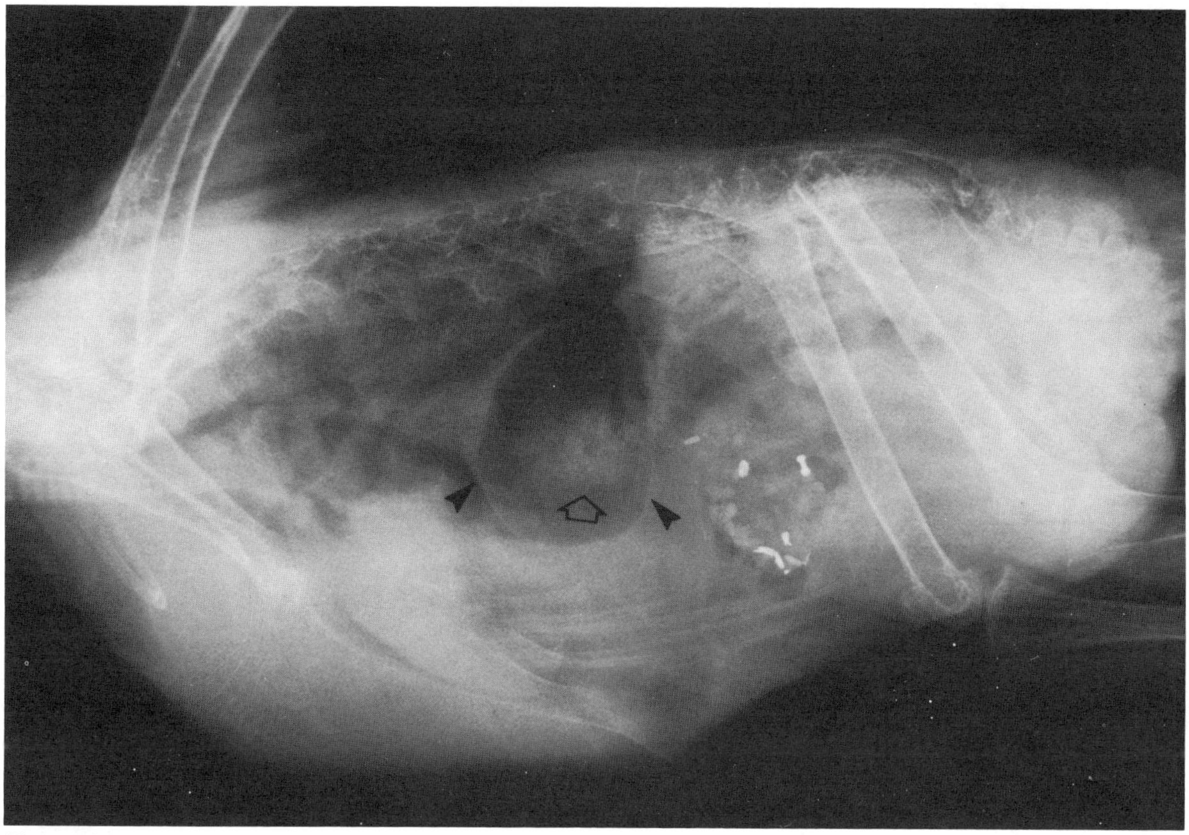

Figure 10A

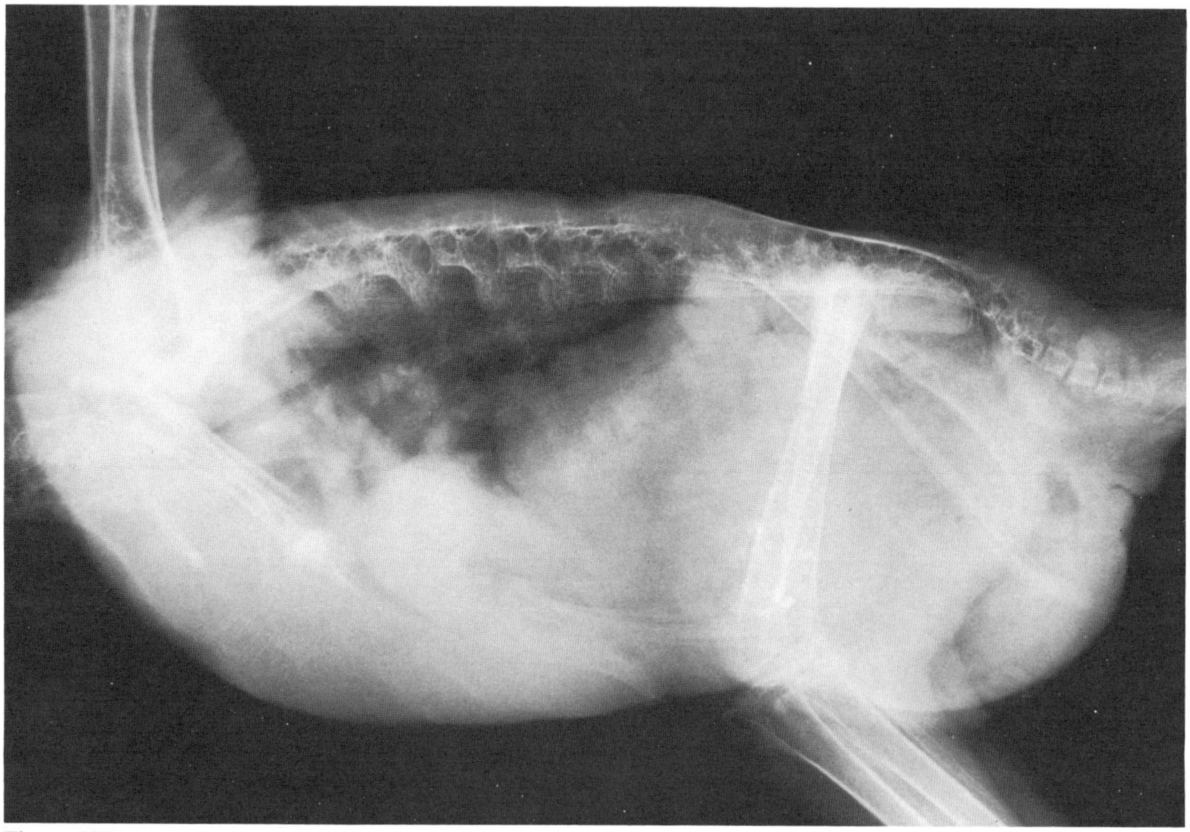

Figure 10B

Figure 10—(**A**) Gaseous distention of the proventriculus (*closed arrows*) and intraluminal foreign material (*open arrow*). Metallic foreign material is present in the ventriculus. (**B**) Radiograph taken 36 hours later shows that the foreign material still persists. Lack of abdominal contrast and mild abdominal distention are attributable to the presence of fluid. This cockatoo ingested a toy that perforated the gastrointestinal tract, causing peritonitis.

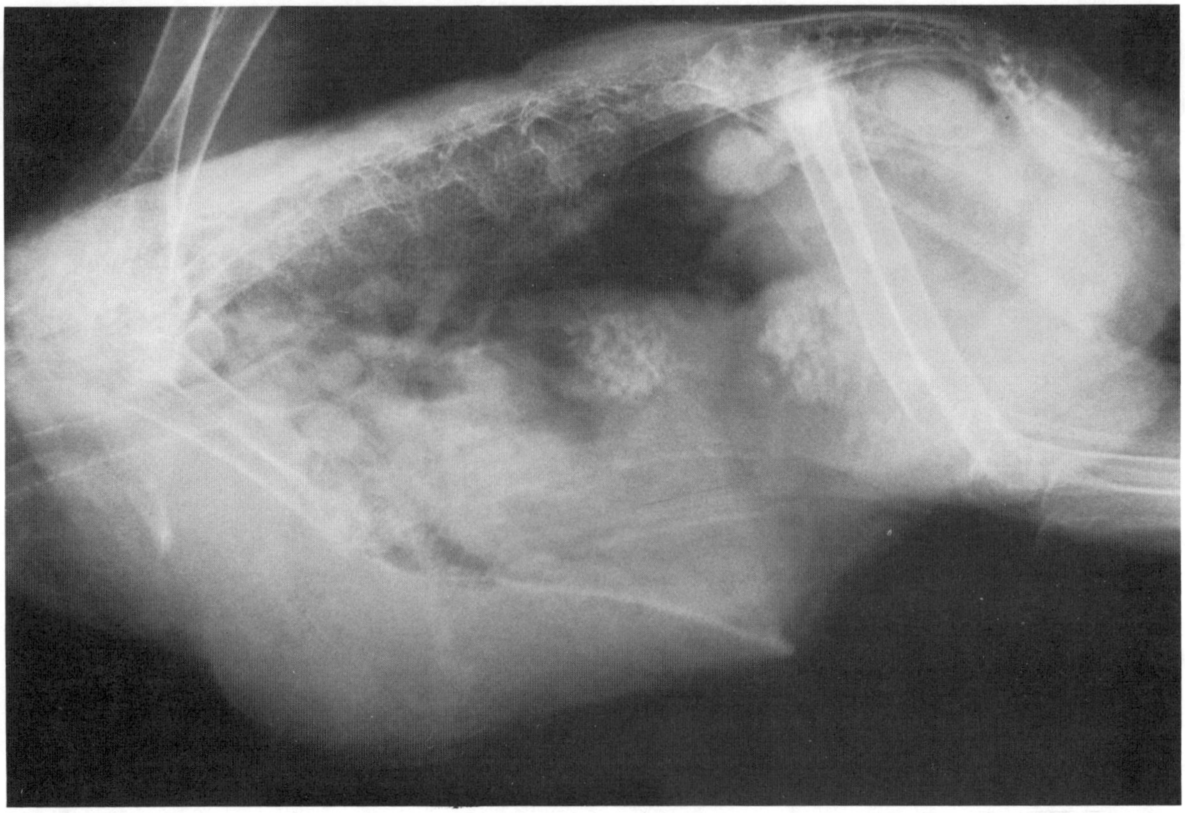

Figure 11A

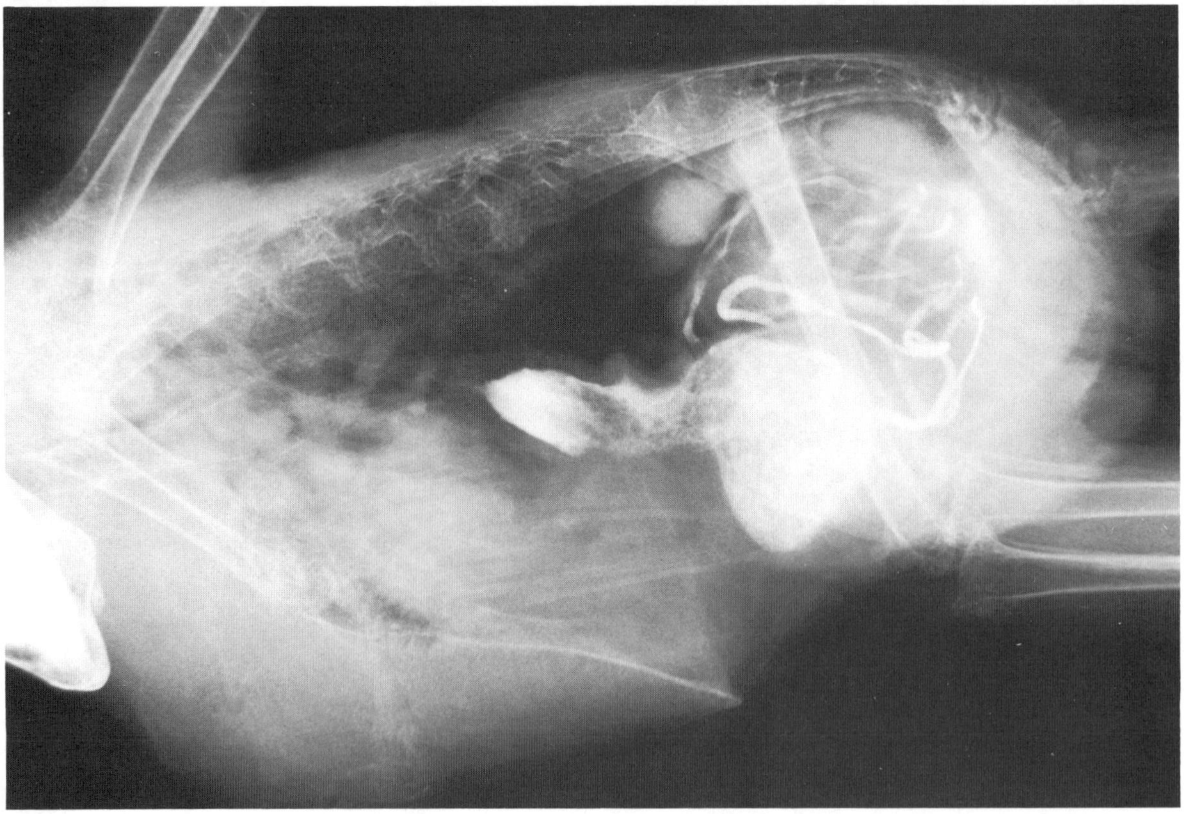

Figure 11B

Figure 11—(**A**) The presence of grit in the proventriculus is unusual. (**B**) A radiograph taken 36 hours after a barium-contrast series shows the barium still present in the crop, proventriculus, and ventriculus. Only small amounts of barium entered the intestines. This Amazon parrot was allowed to consume a large amount of grit after years of no access to grit. The impaction was removed surgically, and the parrot recovered uneventfully.

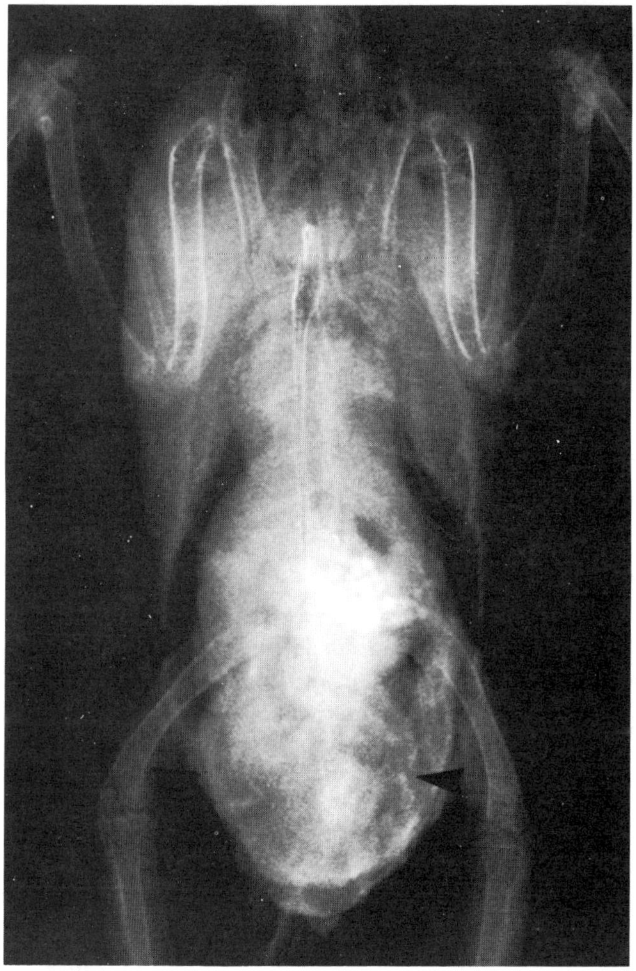

Figure 12—Intravenous excretory urogram shows irregularity in the kidney and distended cloaca (*closed arrows*). On autopsy, this budgerigar had a renal adenocarcinoma with involvement of sacral nerves.

REFERENCES

1. Evans SM: Avian radiographic diagnosis. *Compend Contin Educ Pract Vet* 3(7):660-666, 1981.
2. McMillan MC: Avian radiology, in Petrak ML (ed): *Diseases of Cage and Aviary Birds*. Philadelphia, Lea & Febiger, 1982, pp 329-360.
3. Graham DL: An update on selected pet bird virus infections. *Proc Annu Meet AAV*:267-280, 1984.
4. Gerlach H: Virus diseases in pet birds. *Proc Annu Meet AAV*:87-109, 1983.
5. Clubb SL: Infectious diseases. *Proc Annu Meet AAV*:91-101, 1982.
6. Simpson CF, Hanley JE: Pacheco's parrot disease in psittacine birds. *Avian Dis* 21(2):209-219, 1976.
7. Rosskopf WJ, Woerpel RW, Yanoff SR, et al: Tuberculosis in a parrot. *Mod Vet Pract* 62(10):777-778, 1981.
8. Dolphin RE, Olsen DE, Gallina AM: Tubercular infection in a sulfur-crested cockatoo. *VM SAC* 74(6):833-835, 1979.
9. Dhillon AS, Thacker HL, Winterfield RW: Toxoplasmosis in mynahs. *Avian Dis* 26(2):445-449, 1982.
10. Minsky L, Petrak ML: Diseases of the digestive system, in Petrak ML (ed): *Diseases of Cage and Aviary Birds*. Philadelphia, Lea & Febiger, 1982, pp 432-448.
11. Lowenstine LJ, Petrak ML: Iron pigment in the livers of birds, in Montali R, Migaki G (eds): *The Comparative Pathology of Zoo Animals*. Washington DC, Smithsonian Press, 1978, pp 127-135.
12. Randell MG, Patnaik AK, Gould WJ: Hepatopathy associated with excessive iron storage in mynah birds. *JAVMA* 179(11):1214-1217, 1981.
13. Leav I, Crocker AC, Petrak ML, et al: A naturally occurring lipidosis in shell parakeets, *Melopsittacus undulatus*. *Lab Invest* 18(4):433-437, 1968.
14. Palmer GH, Stauber E: Visceral lymphoblastic leukosis in an African gray parrot. *VM SAC* 26(9):1355-1356, 1981.
15. Petrak ML: Unpublished case material, Angell Memorial Animal Hospital, Boston, MA, 1983.
16. Petrak ML: Case presentations, AFA, Las Vegas, NV, 1980.
17. McMillan MC: Unpublished case material, Angell Memorial Animal Hospital, Boston, MA, 1978.
18. Knox DW: Gout in reptiles and birds, with observations on a comparable syndrome in man, in Montali R, Migaki G (eds): *The Comparative Pathology of Zoo Animals*. Washington DC, Smithsonian Press, 1978, pp 137-141.
19. Woerpel RW, Rosskopf WJ: Heavy metal intoxication in caged birds. Part I. *Compend Contin Educ Pract Vet* 4(10):729-738, 1982.
20. McMillan MC, Petrak ML: The clinical significance of abdominal enlargement in the budgerigar (*Melopsittacus undulatus*). *Compend Contin Educ Pract Vet* 3(10):898-904, 1981.
21. Petrak ML, Gilmore CE: Neoplasms, in Petrak ML (ed): *Diseases of Cage and Aviary Birds*. Philadelphia, Lea & Febiger, 1982, pp 606-637.
22. Schlumberger HG: Polyostotic hyperostosis in the female parakeet. *Am J Pathol* 35(1):1-23, 1959.
23. McMillan MC: Avian gastrointestinal radiography. *Compend Contin Educ Pract Vet* 4(5):273-284, 1983.
24. Ridgway RA, Gallerstein GA: Proventricular dilatation in psittacines. *Proc Annu Meet AAV*:228-230, 1983.
25. Woerpel RW, Rosskopf WJ, Hughes E: Proventricular dilatation and wasting syndrome: Mysenteric ganglioneuritis and encephalomyelitis of psittacines: An update. *Proc Annu Meet AAV*:25-28, 1984.
26. McNeel SV, Zenoble RD: Avian urography. *JAVMA* 178(4):366-368, 1981.
27. Peterson ME, Rantanen NW, Stauber E: Ultrasonic imaging in diagnosis of an abdominal mass in a pigeon. *Mod Vet Pract* 64(10):825-826, 1983.

Electrocardiography in the Parakeet and Parrot

R. D. Zenoble, DVM, MS
Diplomate, ACVIM
Department of Veterinary Clinical Sciences
College of Veterinary Medicine
Iowa State University
Ames, Iowa

Veterinarians are being asked to care for caged birds with the same degree of objectivity and sophistication used in the treatment of dogs and cats. Veterinarians must attempt to apply diagnostic procedures used in routine small animal practice to avian patients. Electrocardiography has become an accepted aspect of small animal practice and has potential value in avian medicine. However, the clinical use of electrocardiography in caged birds awaits establishment of normal values.

The electrocardiogram (ECG) of the chicken was first described in 1909. Electrocardiographic studies have been performed on the sea gull,[1] buzzard,[2] and quail.[3] The ECG has been best characterized in the turkey[4-6] and chicken.[7-9] ECG changes have been described in various natural diseases in turkeys, such as influenza infection,[10] round heart disease, and hypertension.[11,12] The effects of experimental factors such as potassium deficiency, thiamine deficiency, estrogen administration, various dietary deficiencies, and *Escherichia coli* infection on the chicken ECG have been reported.[13-17] Two cases of heart failure have been diagnosed antemortem in exotic birds. Congestive heart failure was diagnosed via clinical and radiologic evidence in a mynah bird and confirmed at necropsy.[18] Congestive heart failure and atrial fibrillation secondary to mitral valvular insufficiency were diagnosed in a Pukeko.[19]

In order to establish some normal values for ECGs in birds, some investigations were done on parrots and parakeets. Parrots (*Amazona* spp.) of mixed variety and parakeets (*Melopsittacus undulatus*) were studied. All birds were adults and believed to be free of disease. Each bird was given ketamine hydrochloride IM at approximately 15 to 20 mg/kg body weight. The birds then breathed halothane and oxygen via a face mask until the wing could be lifted without causing reflexive wing flapping. Needle electrodes were placed subcutaneously on the thorax just caudal and slightly ventral to the attachment of the wings and on the legs near the proximal attachment of the gastrocnemius muscle (Figure 1) according to the technique used by Szabuniewicz.[2,3,8]

The birds were positioned on their right sides with the legs held perpendicular to the torso. After a six-lead ECG was recorded, the birds were placed on their backs with the legs pulled caudally, and a second ECG was recorded. The paper speed was 50 mm/second, and 1 mV was standardized to 1 cm.

The tracings were analyzed under low magnification for heart rate and rhythm, P wave height and duration, P-R interval, QRS configura-

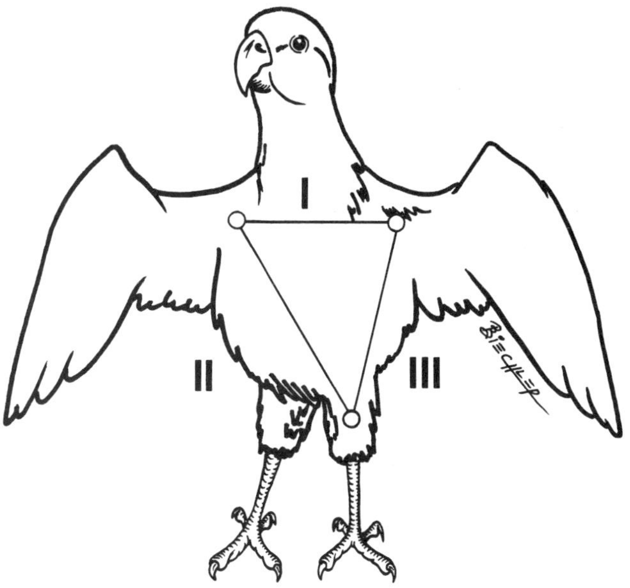

Figure 1—Proper lead placement on a parrot is shown.

tion and duration, T wave configuration, and arrhythmias. The ECG obtained in the lateral position was compared to the ECG obtained in the dorsoventral position.

The ventricular depolarization wave was described using standard terminology. The first downward deflection, when present, was designated *Q* and the second downward deflection was called *S*. The first positive deflection was designated *R*. If the QRS complex was a single negative deflection lasting for the usual QRS duration, it was described as a QS pattern. If the deflection magnitude was small, a lowercase letter was used.

Parakeet

The heart rate of the parakeets studied ranged from 600 to 750 beats/minute with a mean of 675 beats/minute. There was a normal sinus rhythm in 90% of the birds (Figures 2 and 3) and there were arrhythmias in 10% (Figures 4, 5, and 6). The arrhythmias disappeared after three to four minutes of monitoring (Figure 6).

The P wave was positive in leads I, II, III, and aVF (100%), negative in lead aVR (100%), and biphasic in lead aVL (80%). The P wave duration was 0.01 to 0.02 second. The P-R interval was 0.01 to 0.04 second.

The ventricular depolarization wave was a negative QS (60%) or rS (40%) in lead I with a range of −0.1 to −0.6 mV. In lead II the wave was QS or rS with a range of −0.2 to −1.1 mV. In lead III the wave was variable (RS [40%], QS [40%], and rS [20%]). In lead aVR the major deflection was positive, being either qR or R (80%) and QR (20%). In lead aVL the wave was either biphasic (QR [50%]) or positive (R [40%], qR [10%]). Lead aVF was negative or biphasic (rS or QS [90%], RS [10%]). The QRS complex duration was 0.01 to 0.03

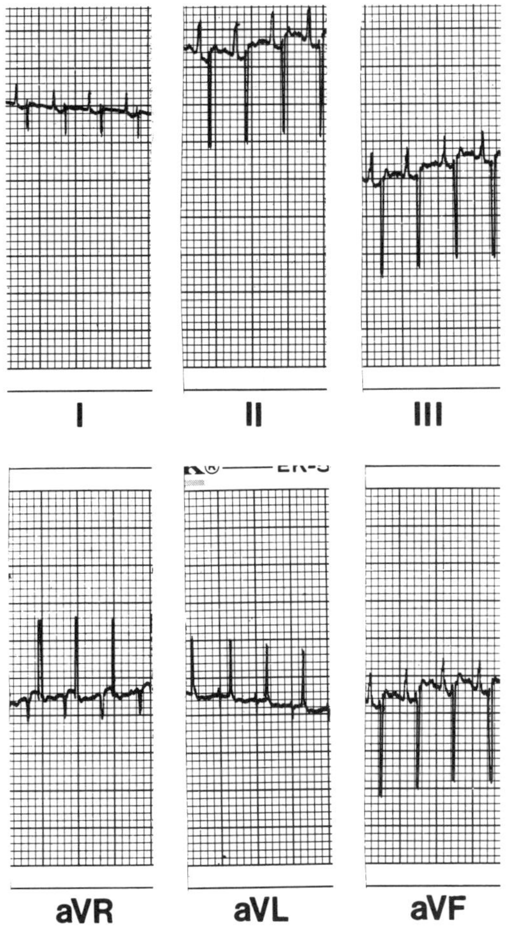

Figure 2—ECG from a normal anesthetized parakeet illustrating peaked positive P waves in leads I, II, and aVF; a notched P wave in lead III; and a negative P wave in lead aVR. The ventricular deflection is an rS wave in leads I, II, III, and aVF and a qR or R wave in leads aVR and aVL. The T waves are poorly illustrated in this example. (1 cm = 1 mV, 50 mm/second)

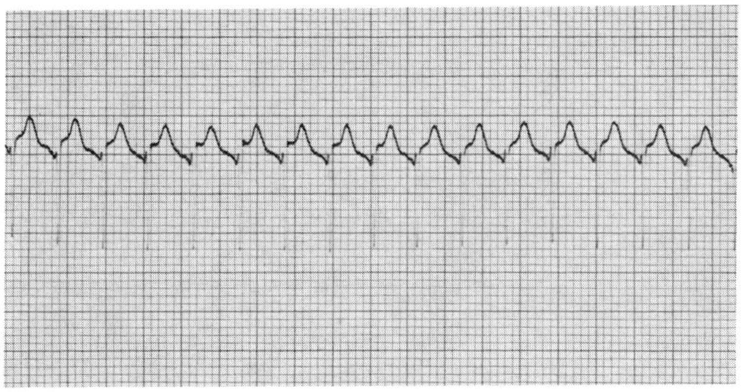

Figure 3—ECG from a parakeet showing overlapping of T and P waves during a rapid heart rate (lead II).

second. The T wave was small or unidentifiable in lead I, positive in leads II, III, and aVF, and negative in leads aVR and aVL. It was difficult to accurately measure the T wave because of the frequent overlap between the T wave and the next P wave.

A position change of the parakeet from right lateral recumbency to dorsoventral recumbency caused no change in 80% of the birds and a mild increase in the major ventricular deflection in 20%.

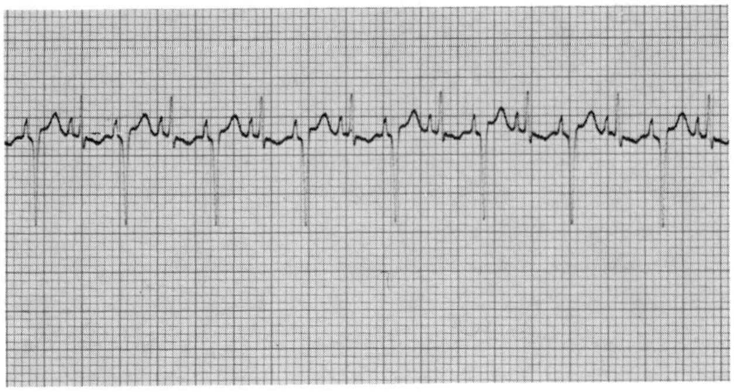

Figure 4—ECG from a parakeet showing a regular pattern of two different P-QRS-T complexes alternating with each heart beat (lead II).

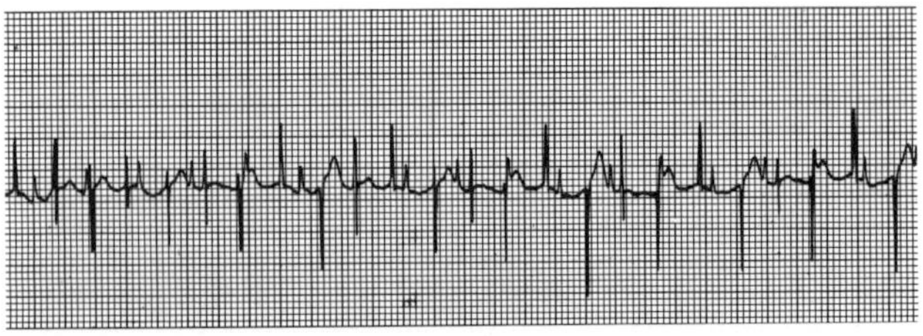

Figure 5—Transient arrhythmia from a parakeet showing QRS complexes that vary with each beat.

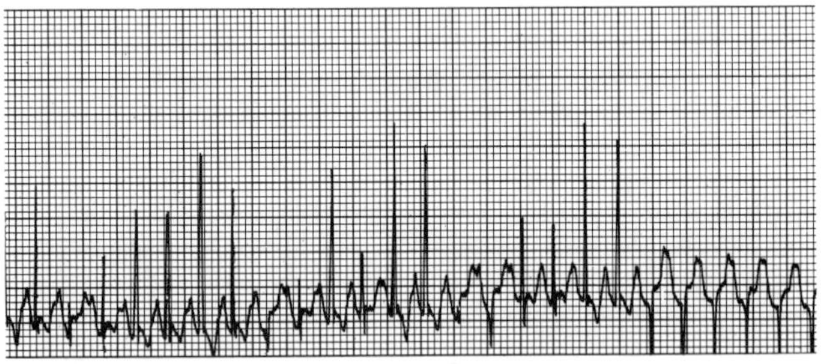

Figure 6—Transient arrhythmia similar to that in Figure 5 illustrating spontaneous conversion to a normal sinus rhythm.

Parrot

The parrots' heart rates ranged from 275 to 780 beats/minute with a mean of 390 beats/minute. There was a normal sinus rhythm in 75% of parrots (Figure 7) and there were arrhythmias in 25%. The arrhythmias were complex and difficult to characterize (Figure 8). In each case the arrhythmia disappeared within two to four minutes (Figure 8).

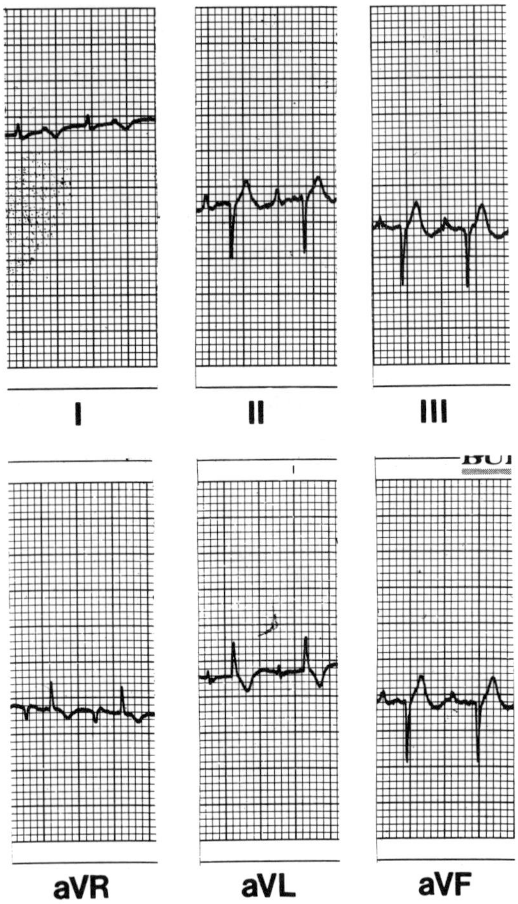

Figure 7—ECG from a normal anesthetized parrot. (1 cm = 1 mV, 50 mm/second)

The P wave was consistently positive in leads I, II, III, and aVF (100%), negative (80%) or biphasic (20%) in lead aVR, and slightly positive (20%) or biphasic (80%) in lead aVL. The P wave duration was 0.01 to 0.02 second and occasionally notched. The P-R interval was 0.03 to 0.07 second.

The QRS complex pattern was similar to the parakeet's QRS complex. In lead I, a small R wave (50%), QS (30%), and RS (20%) were found. In leads II, III, and aVF, a negative deflection was consistently present (QS or rS). Leads aVR and aVL had positive deflections (R or qR). The duration of the QRS complex was 0.01 to 0.02 second. The T wave was variable in lead I; it was positive, negative, or absent. A positive T wave was

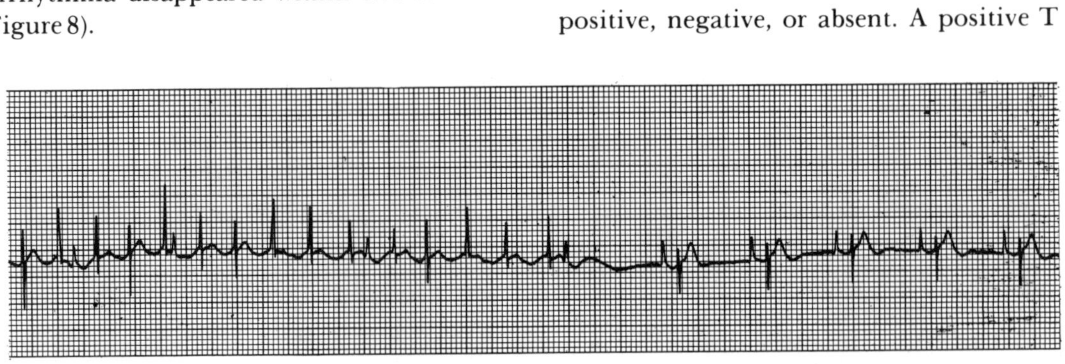

Figure 8—ECG from a parrot showing transient arrhythmia converting to normal sinus rhythm.

found in leads II, III, and aVF. A negative T wave was found in leads aVR and aVL.

Changing position of the parrot from lateral recumbency to dorsoventral recumbency caused no change in 90% of the birds and a marked increase in the amplitude of the ventricular deflection of 0.5 to 1.0 mV in the ECG in 10%.

Discussion

The ECG of birds is similar to that of mammals. In these investigations, there was a readily identifiable P wave representing atrial depolarization in all leads. The wave of atrial repolarization could not be found and was probably incorporated into the ventricular depolarization wave. The P wave was usually positive in leads I, II, III, and aVF. The P wave was usually negative or biphasic in leads aVR and positive or biphasic in lead aVL. Sometimes the P wave was notched. There was occasional overlapping of the P wave and the preceding T wave which made accurate measurements impossible at a paper speed of 50 mm/second. The duration of the P wave was 0.01 to 0.02 second.

The P-R interval was highly variable depending on the heart rate. The P-R interval range for the parakeet was 0.01 to 0.04 second, and for the parrot it was 0.04 to 0.08 second.

The wave of ventricular depolarization could be readily identified in all ECGs. The wave of ventricular depolarization (QRS) in lead I was usually negative in the parakeet but positive or isoelectric in the parrot. The QRS complex in leads II, III, and aVF was usually negative in both birds. The waves were usually a QS or rS wave with an occasional RS (isoelectric) wave. The QRS wave in leads aVR and aVL was usually positive (R, qR) with an occasional isoelectric wave (QR). The duration of the QRS complex was 0.01 to 0.03 second.

The T wave represents repolarization of the ventricles. Overlapping of the T and P waves was frequently found. In lead I, the T wave was either absent, positive, or negative. In leads II, III, and aVF it was either absent or positive, and in leads aVR and aVL it was absent or negative. The T wave configuration varied from tall and peaked, to a bump, to undetectable.

Arrhythmias were found in both groups of birds. The type of arrhythmia was difficult to identify because of the fast heart rate and impossibility of accurately measuring waves and intervals. One parakeet showed an arrhythmia that was complete A-V dissociation (Figure 5). The P-R interval varied from beat to beat, and occasionally the P wave followed the QRS wave. Arrhythmias were found in 25% of the birds during the initial ECG recording. The arrhythmias disappeared without an alteration of the anesthesia flow rate. It is believed that the cause of the transient arrhythmias was possibly the combination of the ketamine and halothane because a similar study using halothane alone on parrots showed no arrhythmias.[20]

Muscle-twitching artifacts were frequently seen when the legs were retracted away from the torso. If the legs were positioned and then allowed to relax, muscle-twitching artifacts were markedly reduced. Muscle twitching decreased as the depth of anesthesia was increased.

REFERENCES

1. Kisch B: Electrocardiographic studies in seagulls. *Exp Med Surg* 7:345-357, 1949.
2. Edjtchadi M, Rezakhani A, Szabuniewicz M: The electrocardiogram of the buzzard *(Buteo buteo)*. *Zbl Vet Med A* 24:597-600, 1977.
3. Szabuniewicz M, McCrady JD: The electrocardiogram of the Japanese *(Coturnix coturnix japonica)* and bobwhite *(Colinus virginianus)* quail. *Zbl Vet Med A* 21:198-207, 1974.
4. Hamlin RL, Pipers FS, Kondrich RM, et al: QRS component of the orthogonal lead, spatial magnitude and spatial velocity electrocardiograms, and vectorcardiograms of turkeys. *J Electrocardiol* 2(2):127-134, 1969.
5. Hunsaker WG, Robertson A, Magwood SE: The effect of round heart disease on the electrocardiogram and heart weight of turkey poults. *Poult Sci* 50:1712-1724, 1971.
6. McKenzie BE, Will JA, Hardie A: The electrocardiogram of the turkey. *Avian Dis* 15:737-744, 1971.
7. Kisch B: The electrocardiogram of birds (chicken, duck, pigeon). *Exp Med Surg* 9:103-124, 1951.
8. Szabuniewicz M, McCrady JD: The electrocardiogram of the chicken. *Southwest Vet* 20:287-294, 1967.
9. Sturkie PD: *Heart: Contraction, Conduction, and Electrocardiography in Avian Physiology*. New York, Springer-Verlag, Inc, 1976.
10. McKenzie BE, Will JA: Electrocardiographic changes following influenza infection in turkeys. *Avian Dis* 16:308-318, 1972.
11. Magwood SE, Bray DF: Disease condition of turkey poults characterized by enlarged and rounded hearts. *Can J Comp Med Vet Sci* 26:268-272, 1962.
12. Krista LM, Jankus EF, Waibel PE, et al: Comparison of electrocardiograms of hypertensive and hypotensive male turkeys. *Poult Sci* 49:700-703, 1970.
13. Sturkie PD: Further studies of potassium deficiency on the electrocardiogram of chicken. *Poult Sci* 31:648-650, 1952.
14. Sturkie PD: Effects of acute thiamine deficiency on the electrocardiogram of the chick. *Poult Sci* 33:508-510, 1954.
15. Sturkie PD, Singsen EP, Matterson LD, et al: The effects of dietary deficiencies of vitamin E and the B complex vitamins on the electrocardiogram of chickens. *Am J Vet Res* 15:457-462, 1954.
16. Sturkie PD: Role of estrogen on sex differences of the electrocardiogram of the chicken. *Proc Soc Exp Biol Med* 94:731-733, 1957.
17. Gross WB: Electrocardiographic changes of *Escherichia coli* infected birds. *Am J Vet Res* 27:1427-1436, 1966.
18. Ensley PK, Hatkin J, Silverman S: Congestive heart failure in a greater hill mynah. *JAVMA* 175:1010-1013, 1979.
19. Beehler BA, Montali RJ, Bush M: Mitral valve insufficiency with congestive heart failure in a Pukeko. *JAVMA* 177:934-937, 1980.
20. Altman RB: Effect of halothane and ketamine anesthesia on body temperature and electrocardiographic changes. Paper presented at the AAZA meeting, Denver, CO, Oct 1979.

Avian Radiographic Diagnosis

Sydney M. Evans, VMD
Resident, Section of Radiology
School of Veterinary Medicine
University of Pennsylvania
Philadelphia, Pennsylvania

Radiology can play an important role in diagnostic avian medicine. Birds are well suited for radiography because their air sacs provide intrinsic contrast. However, some birds' small size, fragile appearance, and rapid respiratory rate have discouraged practitioners from taking radiographs of them. Technically excellent diagnostic radiographs can be taken with minimal stress to these patients. Special studies such as upper gastrointestinal barium studies can be performed. These radiographic evaluations provide diagnostic and prognostic information which may otherwise be difficult to obtain.

Several articles have been published on avian radiology describing normal radiographic anatomy and some disease states.[1,2] This article will review the technical aspects of avian radiography and the pertinent gross and radiographic anatomy and physiology of the normal and abnormal caged bird.

Radiographic Technique

Before removing the patient from the cage, windows and doors should be closed and the x-ray panel set with the proper technique; several film-screen combination techniques are outlined in Table I. Most veterinary practices routinely use par speed screens and film, and this combination provides fine-quality avian radiographs. However, for better radiographic detail or if the highest milliamperage available is 200 mA, high-detail screens with par speed film are recommended (Table I). Single-screen cassettes are another option; however, this requires purchasing single-emulsion film (Table I).

When restraining the bird to remove it from the cage, the mandible is held between the thumb and forefinger. The body is supported in the palm of one hand and the feet can be controlled with the free hand. The bird should not be restrained by completely encircling the body; birds have no diaphragm and this interferes with sternum and rib motion and, therefore, with respiration. Larger birds can be caught using a towel or gloves. If clinically indicated, larger birds can be sedated with ketamine hydrochloride[a] 10 to 20 mg/kg intramuscularly. The duration of

[a]Ketaset®, Bristol Laboratories, Syracuse, NY 13201.

TABLE I

TECHNIQUES FOR AVIAN RADIOGRAPHY

Screen	*Film*	*Body Part*	*mA*	*kVp*	*Time (seconds)*	*Other*
Par speed*	Par speed†	Whole body	300	lateral = 42 ventrodorsal = 50	$\frac{1}{60}$	–
Par speed*	Par speed†	Extremity	100	42	$\frac{1}{20}$	–
High detail‡	Par speed†	Whole body	200	40 kVp for first 2 cm; add 2 kVp for each additional 1 cm	$\frac{1}{30}$	36-inch film-tube distance; Remove filter
Single screen§	Single emulsion‖	Whole body	200	lateral = 47 ventrodorsal = 50	$\frac{1}{30}$	36-inch film-tube distance Remove filter

*Par speed screens, E.I. Dupont DeNemours & Co., Wilmington, DE 19899.
†Kodak XRP–1 par speed film, Eastman Kodak Co., Rochester, NY 14650.
‡Kodak x-omatic fine intensifying screen in x-omatic cassette, Eastman Kodak Co., Rochester, NY 14650.
§Kodak Lanex fine screen in Kodak x-omatic cassette (extremity system), Eastman Kodak Co., Rochester, NY 14650.
‖Kodak NMB-1 film, Eastman Kodak Co., Rochester, NY 14650.

effect is approximately 45 minutes.[2] Patients can be taped to the cassette with masking tape[3] or, in larger species, held in place by assistants whose hands are shielded from the x-ray beam.

The keel and vertebrae are superimposed in a satisfactorily positioned ventrodorsal radiograph. The legs and wings are extended to preclude superimposition of extremity musculature over the abdominal and thoracic areas.[b] The right and left acetabula should be superimposed in a symmetrical lateral radiograph. In the left lateral recumbent position, the left wing and left hindlimb should be positioned caudal to the right wing and right hindlimb. The opposite is true for the right lateral recumbent position.

[b]Birds have no true diaphragm, and the body cavity is a coelom. The coelom is divided into the abdominal and thoracic areas.

Gastrointestinal Tract

In radiographs of normal birds (Figures 1A and 1B) the crop, a diverticulum of the esophagus, is proximal to the thoracic inlet. In the ventrodorsal radiograph, it may be right sided, left sided, or bilateral. The crop varies in size according to species. In many birds, the crop is empty and radiographically invisible. The esophagus and crop can be evaluated with 0.5 to 3 ml of air or barium administered via a stomach tube. One-half milliliter of barium was administered via a stomach tube to the budgerigar in Figure 2. After 15 minutes, barium is seen in a dilated esophagus as well as in

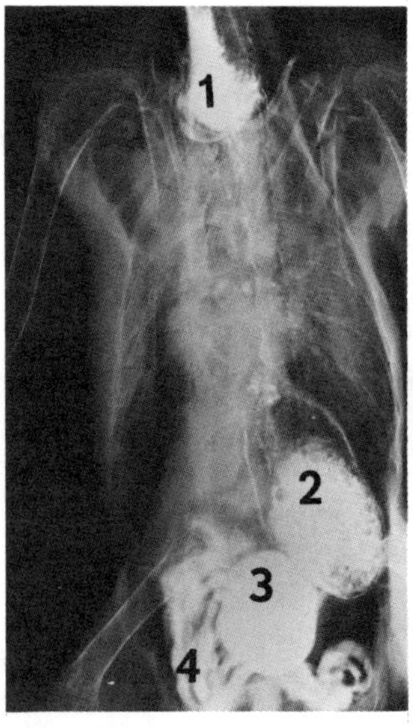

Figure 1A

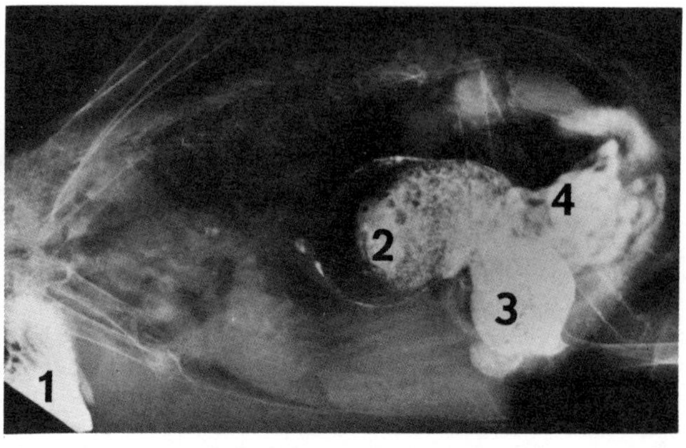

Figure 1B

Figure 1—Upper gastrointestinal series in a parrot. **A**, Ventrodorsal radiograph. Five milliliters of barium were administered via an orogastric tube. Barium is outlining the crop (*1*), proventriculus (*2*), gizzard (*3*), and small intestine (*4*). **B**, In the lateral radiograph, barium is seen in the crop (*1*), proventriculus (*2*), gizzard (*3*), and small intestine (**4**).

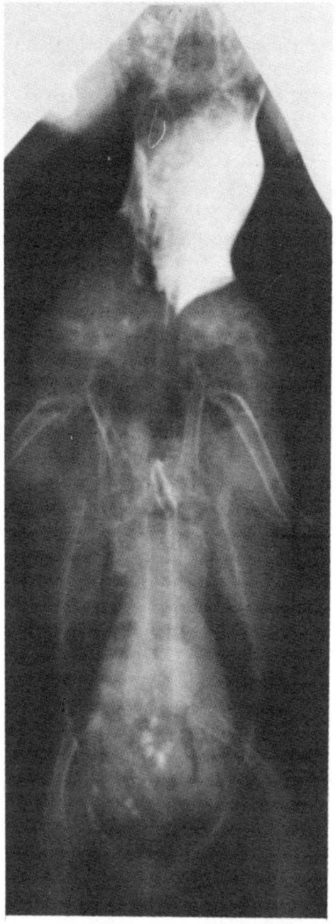

Figure 2—Esophagram in a budgerigar. One-half milliliter of barium was administered via orogastric tube. After 15 minutes, barium is seen in a dilated esophagus and in the soft tissues of the neck. At necropsy, the patient had a ruptured esophagus.

the soft tissues of the neck. At postmortem examination, the patient had a necrotic, ruptured esophagus.

The proventriculus (true stomach) usually cannot be identified in survey radiographs. Its location can be ascertained by the position of the gizzard, which is frequently filled with radiopaque grit. In the ventrodorsal radiograph, the normal gizzard is usually circular and lies to the left of the midline, with its cranial border at the level of the acetabula. In the lateral radiograph, the gizzard may be circular or elongated. Its most dorsal surface is one-half to three-quarters of the distance between the spine and the keel. The small intestine, cecum, and large intestine (rectum) are not seen radiographically unless they contain gas (Figures 3A and 3B). The liver and heart shadows merge, and the cardiac-hepatic shadow has an hourglass shape in the ventrodorsal radiograph. Unless the hind legs are fully extended and parallel, this normal hourglass shape may be altered. In the lateral radiograph, the liver lies caudal to the heart (Figure 3B). The spleen may be seen as a small, spherical, soft-tissue density cranial to the intestines and dorsal to the liver (Figure 4). In Figure 5, there is loss of the normal cardiohepatic hourglass shape. This change is characteristic of hepatomegaly. In this bird, the gizzard is in a normal position; however, in severe hepatomegaly, the gizzard is displaced caudally.

Radiographic changes in the small intestine may be similar to those seen in the dog and cat. Figure 6A shows gas distention of a single loop of small intestine, representing mechanical small bowel obstruction. There is loss of the normal cardiohepatic hourglass shape (Figure 6B). At necropsy, hepatomegaly, small intestinal adhesions, distention of a loop of small intestine, and air sacculitis were found. A paralytic ileus may also be

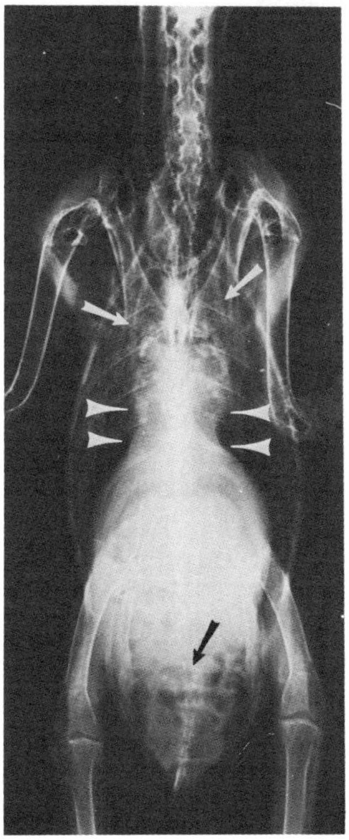

Figure 3A

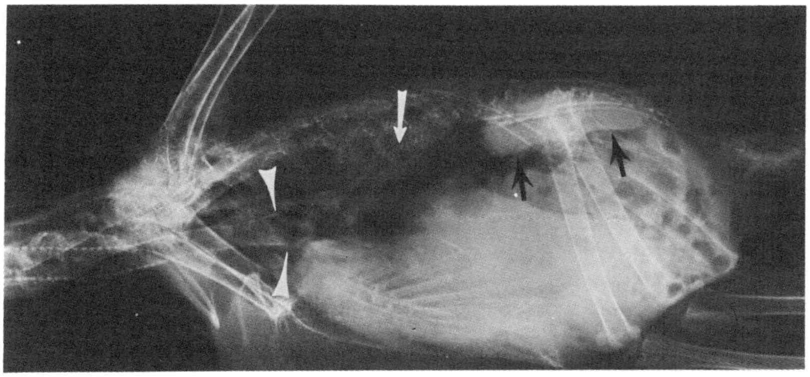

Figure 3B

Figure 3—(**A**) Ventrodorsal radiograph of a normal cockatiel. The fine reticular pattern of the lung is seen (*white arrows*), and the air sacs have a radiographic density similar to that of the surrounding air. There is an hourglass shape to the cardiohepatic shadow (*white arrowheads*). The small intestine contains gas (*black arrow*). The gizzard cannot be seen because it does not contain radiopaque grit. (**B**) Lateral radiograph of a normal cockatiel. The fine reticular lung pattern is seen (*white arrow*). The radiographic density of the air sacs is similar to that of the surrounding air. The syrinx is a slightly dilated portion of the distal trachea (*white arrowheads*). The kidneys are seen as elongated soft-tissue densities within the pelvic girdle (*black arrows*). Air-filled small intestine is seen ventral to the kidneys. The cardiac and hepatic shadows merge in the midventral coelom. The gizzard cannot be seen because it does not contain radiopaque grit.

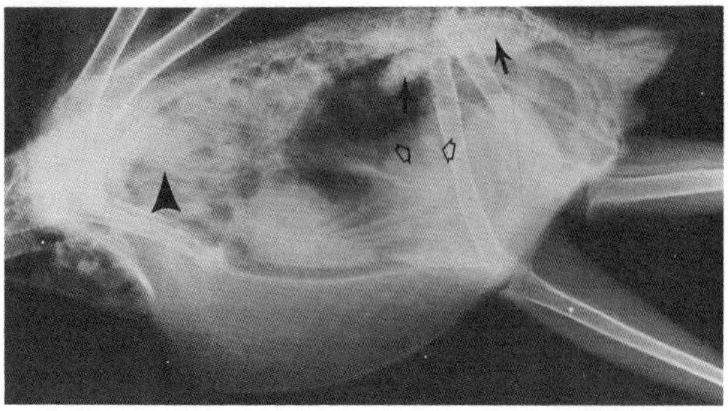

Figure 4—Lateral radiograph of a cockatoo. The fine reticular pattern of the lungs is mottled, especially in the cranial thoracic area of the coelom (*black arrowhead*). In addition, there is a calcium density in the area of the kidneys (*black arrows*). *Aspergillus fumigatus* was isolated from the pneumonia. The mineralization of the kidneys is thought to be due to calcium and/or urate crystals deposited in the kidney in the dehydrated bird. Note that the spleen can be identified on this radiograph (*open arrows*).

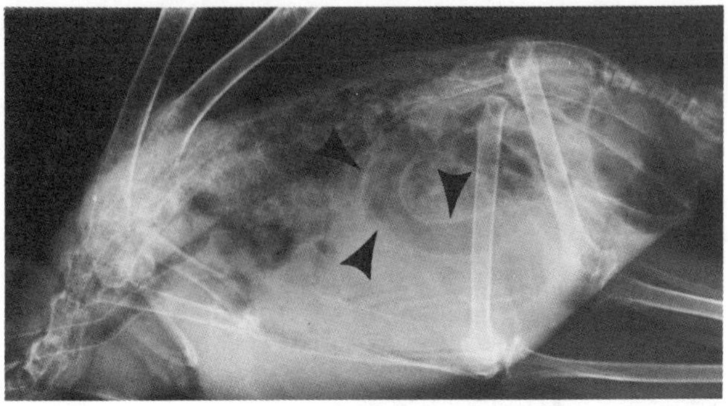

Figure 6A—Lateral radiograph of a cockatiel. A very large gas-distended loop of small intestine is seen (*arrowheads*).

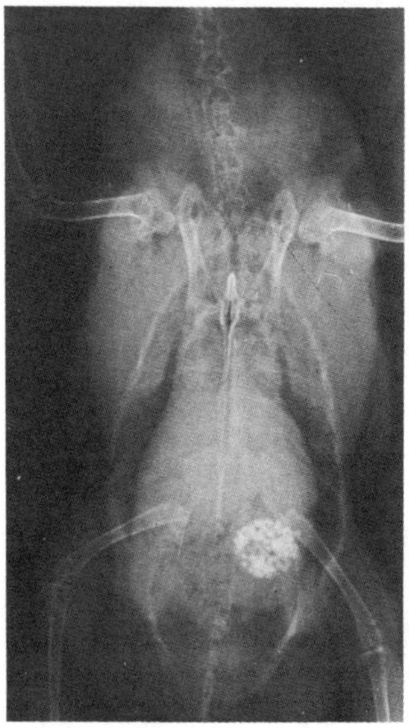

Figure 5—Ventrodorsal radiograph of a parakeet with hepatomegaly. There is loss of the normal cardiohepatic hourglass shape. The gizzard, filled with grit, is in a normal position to the left of the midline, at the level of the acetabula.

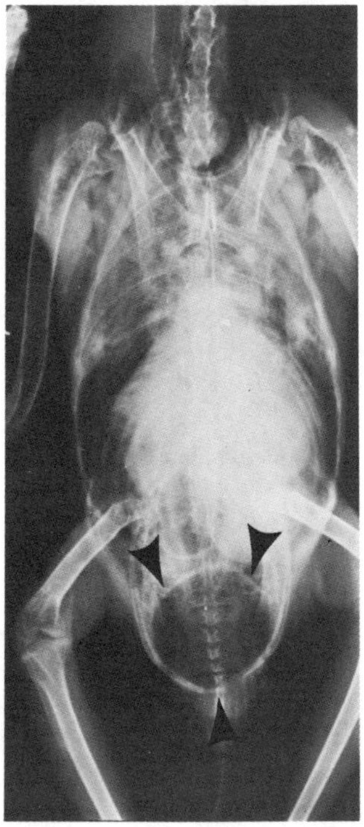

Figure 6B—Ventrodorsal radiograph of a cockatiel. There is an apparent loss of a normal cardiohepatic silhouette. An air-filled cloaca is seen (*arrow*). At necropsy, hepatomegaly, small intestinal adhesions, distended loop of small intestine, and air sacculitis were found.

seen in birds; it is characterized by multiple, equal-sized loops of gas-distended small intestine.

Lead poisoning can occur in birds, particularly in those that are allowed out of their cages. Birds presenting with neurologic and/or gastrointestinal signs should be radiographed for the presence of metallic material in their gastrointestinal tracts.[4,5]

A barium study may be performed to evaluate the gastrointestinal tract or its position with respect to other organs or masses. One-quarter to 10 ml of barium (the amount depending on the size of the patient[3]) is given via a stomach tube (Figures 1A and 1B). Gastrointestinal transit time is approximately two to three hours.

Urogenital Tract

The kidneys, adrenals, and gonads are located along each side of the vertebral column within the pelvic girdle. The kidneys are seen best on the lateral radiograph—they are bilobed and rectangular (Figure 3B). The ureters empty directly into the cloaca; there is no urinary bladder. The gonads and adrenals are located at the cranial aspect of the kidneys. The gonads are seen best in the lateral radiograph where they are cranial to the kidney and superimposed on the caudal thoracic air sac. With seasonal variation in mating behavior, the size of the gonads and thus their radiographic visibility vary. Seasonal enlargement of the gonads should be differentiated from pathologic enlargement, according to the clinical signs and physical examination. The kidneys and gonads lie adjacent to the roots of the lumbosacral plexus, and enlargements of these organs may result in impingement on the sciatic nerve. Figure 7 shows a mass lesion in the dorsolumbar area in a male budgerigar with signs of right leg lameness. At necropsy, a cystic right renal mass was found. In this patient, the position

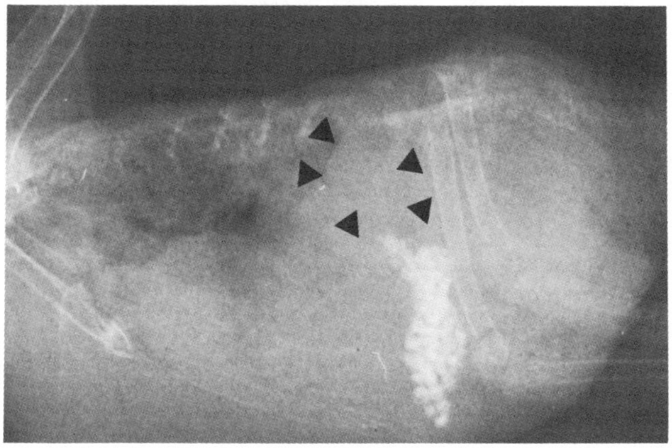

Figure 7—Lateral radiograph of a male parakeet with a history of right leg lameness. A soft-tissue mass (*arrowheads*) is seen cranial to the kidneys. The gizzard is normal in shape and position. It is elongated and its dorsal aspect is one-half the distance between the sternum and the keel. At necropsy, a cystic right renal mass was seen.

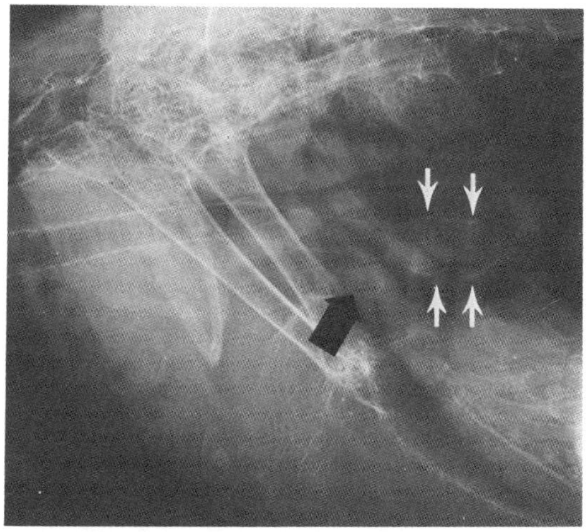

Figure 8—Lateral radiograph of the cranial thoracic area of the coelom. The apparent soft-tissue mass is an end-on view of a great vessel (*black arrow*). The fine reticular pattern of the normal lung is seen. The slightly dilated area in the distal trachea is the syrinx (*white arrows*).

of the gizzard was normal; however, renal enlargement may result in cranial, caudal, or ventral gizzard displacement.

The cloaca may be seen in the most caudal abdominal area if it contains air (Figures 6A and 6B) or an egg. An egg-bound bird is radiographically diagnosed by the presence of an egg in the cloaca and clinical signs of egg retention or an egg obviously too large to pass through the pelvic girdle. A soft-tissue mass in the caudal abdomen in a female bird may represent a noncalcified retained egg. These patients usually have insufficient vitamin D and/or calcium in their diets.

Respiratory and Cardiovascular Systems

The avian respiratory system is comprised of the trachea, syrinx (voice box), five sets of air sacs, and the lungs. The syrinx in most caged birds is a slightly dilated portion of the caudal trachea (Figures 3B and 8); however, in some species, the syrinx is a bizarre *osseous bulla* of the distal trachea[6] (Figures 9A and 9B). In the lateral radiograph, the lungs in the cranial-dorsal thorax have a fine, reticular pattern which represents end-on views of terminal bronchioles (Figure 9A). The most rostral air sac is the interclavicular sac, which communicates with the pneumatic humeri. The remaining air sacs extend caudally, and the abdominal air sacs are located dorsolateral to the gastrointestinal tract. The air sacs should have the same radiographic density as the background air (Figures 2A and 2B). There is no diaphragm and respiration depends on a bellows action which involves the ribs and sternum.

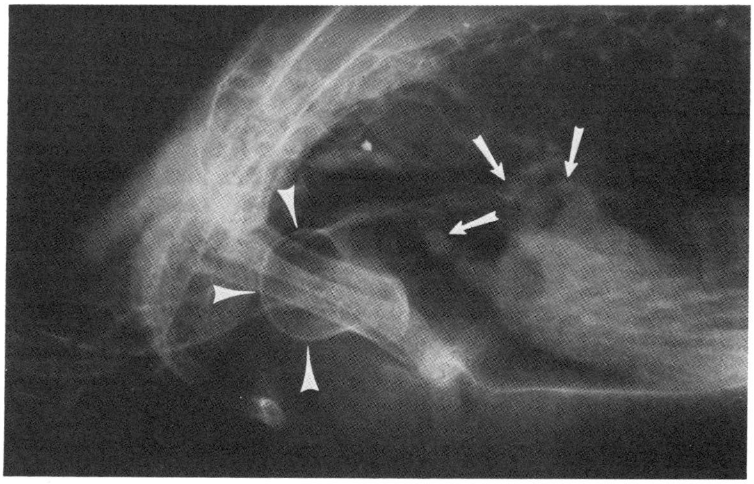

Figure 9A

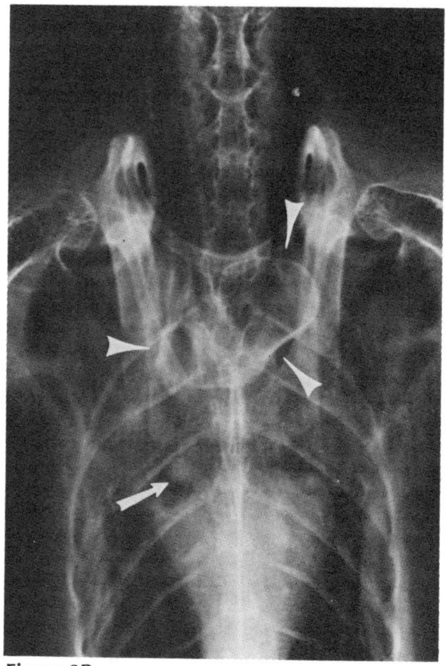

Figure 9B

Figures 9A and 9B—Lateral and ventrodorsal radiographs of the thoracic area of the coelom of a duck. The syrinx is a bizarre *osseous bulla* of the distal trachea (*arrowheads*). The soft-tissue masses seen (*arrows*) cranial to the heart are end-on views of the great vessels.

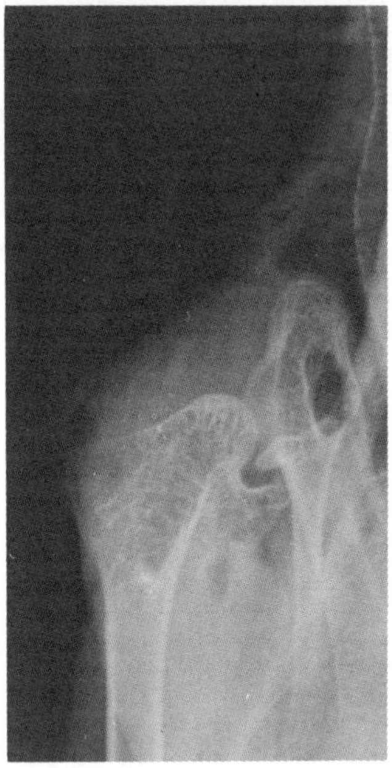

Figure 10—Normal scapulohumeral joint of the macaw. The bones appear osteoporotic, lytic, and expansile because they are pneumatic.

Air sacculitis results in the normally radiolucent air sacs having a soft-tissue density. In Figure 4, the caudal air sacs are as radiolucent as in a normal bird; however, the reticular pattern of the lungs is obliterated. *Aspergillus fumigatus* was identified as the causative agent in this pneumonia. This patient also had *Aspergillus* granulomas in the soft tissues, and the fungal hyphae were identified on a soft-tissue biopsy. Fungal disease may involve bone, soft tissue, air sacs, and lungs simultaneously.

Cardiac disease in birds is rare. Radiographic signs include cardiomegaly and ascites.[7,8] In the lateral radiograph of the thoracic area, the major cardiac vessels are prominent cranial to the heart (Figure 8); they should not be confused with lung or air sac masses.

Skeletal System

Most avian long bones are pneumatic and, as a result, the normal proximal and distal portions appear expanded, lytic, and osteoporotic. The proximal humerus, in particular, may look abnormal because it communicates with the interclavicular air sac (Figure 10). The avian ulna is larger than the radius, and the carpal and metacarpal bones are fused to form the carpometacarpus. In the hindlimb, the tibia and proximal row of tarsal bones are fused to form the tibiotarsus, and the distal tarsal bones and second through fourth metatarsal bones are fused to form the tarsometatarsus.

In caged birds on improper diets, pathologic fractures of long bones occur. Survey radiographs must be examined for poor bone quality, characterized by decreased contrast between bone and soft tissue. Open fractures of the long bones of the wing and leg may result in complications. Especially in the humerus, secondary bacterial air sacculitis can result from the intercommunication between the humeral medullary cavity and the interclavicular air sacs.

Radiographs of a cockatoo with a history of hindlimb weakness show a mottled soft-tissue density in the medullary cavity of the left femur (Figures 11A and 11B). In addition, several soft-tissue masses were seen in the neck. At postmortem examination, soft-tissue masses were found in the soft tissues of the neck, in the liver, and in the medullary cavity of the left femur and tibiotarsus. The histologic diagnosis was acid-fast-positive granulomatous disease.

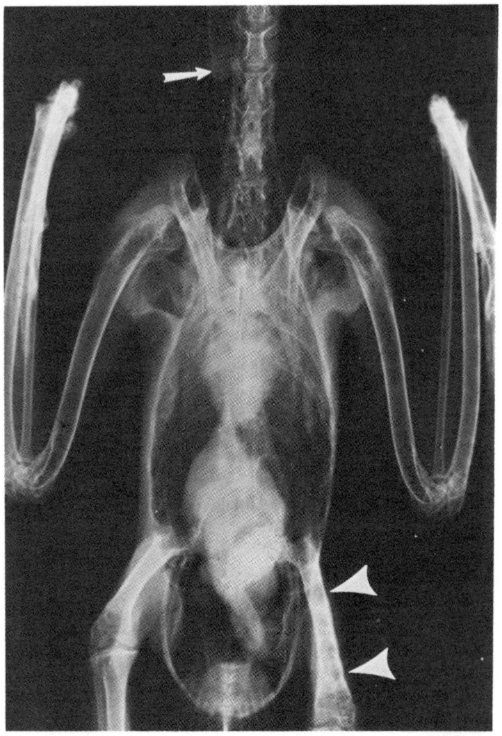

Figure 11A

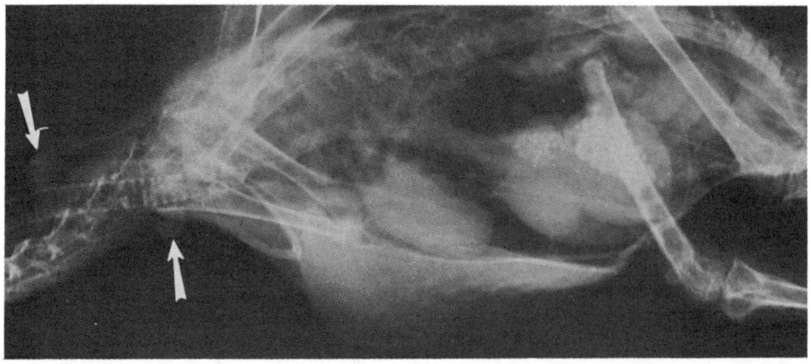

Figure 11B

Figure 11—(**A**) Ventrodorsal radiograph of a cockatoo with left hindleg lameness. Radiographs show a mottled soft-tissue density in the left femoral medullary cavity (*arrowheads*). In addition, a soft-tissue nodule is seen in the neck (*arrow*). The liver is smaller than normal. (**B**) Lateral radiograph of the same patient as in Figure 11A. Soft-tissue nodules are again seen in the neck (*arrows*). Granulomas in the neck, liver, and the left femoral medullary cavity were found at necropsy. The histologic diagnosis was acid-fast-positive granulomatous disease.

REFERENCES

1. Altman RB: Radiology. *Vet Clin North Am* 3:165-173, 1973.
2. Silverman S: Avian radiographic technique and interpretation, in Kirk RW: *Current Veterinary Therapy VI*. Philadelphia, WB Saunders Co, 1977, pp 671-674.
3. Morgan JP, Silverman D, Zontine WJ: *Techniques of Veterinary Radiography*, ed 2. Davis, CA, Veterinary Radiology Assoc, 1977, pp 284-292.
4. Jansen DL, Robinson PT, Ensley PK: Lead poisoning in birds. *Am Assoc Zoo Vet Annu Proc:* 40-41, 1979.
5. Redig PT, Stone CM, Barnes DM, Arent TD: Lead toxicosis in raptors. *JAVMA* 177(9):941-943, 1980.
6. Evans HE: Anatomy of the budgerigar, in Petrak ME (ed): *Diseases of Cage and Aviary Birds*. Philadelphia, Lea & Febiger, 1969, pp 45-112.
7. Ensley PK, Hatkins J, Silverman S: Congestive heart failure in a greater hill mynah. *JAVMA* 175(9):1011-1013, 1979.
8. Beehler BA, Montale RJ, Bush M: Mitral valve insufficiency with congestive heart failure in a puteko. *JAVMA* 177(9):934-937, 1980.

Radiology of Avian Respiratory Diseases

Marjorie C. McMillan, DVM
School of Veterinary Medicine
Tufts University
North Grafton, Massachusetts

Angell Memorial Animal Hospital
Boston, Massachusetts

Windhover Bird Clinic
Walpole, Massachusetts

The anatomy and physiology of the avian respiratory system result in changes in radiographic patterns that are different from the interstitial, alveolar, peribronchial, and vascular patterns described in mammals. Because birds lack a true pleural space, pneumothorax and pleural effusion do not occur. Pleural fluid is usually attributed to extension from abdominal disease. Avian lungs are firmly attached to the thoracic wall, and thus atelectasis is not associated with thoracic problems. Lung volume remains constant during the respiratory cycle. Because the bronchial tree consists of an interconnecting network of tubules, air bronchograms are not a feature of consolidating pulmonary change. The interstitium is poorly developed so that marked interstitial patterns do not occur radiographically.

Indications

Birds with signs of upper respiratory disease (e.g., sneezing, nasal discharge, and/or infraorbital and periorbital swelling) but that otherwise are healthy may not require radiographic examination on initial presentation. If signs persist or recur after proper medical management, radiographs are indicated. Dyspnea, open-mouthed breathing, wheezing, tail bobbing, coughing, oral abscesses, loss of vocalization, exercise intolerance, abdominal distention, weight loss, and auscultatory abnormalities are indications for radiographic examination.

Preradiographic Considerations

Birds with severe respiratory problems may tolerate only a cursory examination. If respiratory distress is severe or the patient is debilitated, supportive treatment with oxygen and fluids is necessary before physical or radiographic examination. Rapid intramuscular injection of fluids and stabilization in an atmosphere of 40% oxygen before beginning diagnostic procedures may be indicated. In stable patients, an oral speculum allows visualization of the choanal slit, pharynx, glottis, and tongue. Auscultation in a quiet area with a pediatric stethoscope placed over the pectoral region, back, and trachea may reveal abnormal clicks, wheezes, and fluid sounds as well as cardiac murmurs and arrhythmia. Differences in air flow, harshness of sounds, or lack of air flow may be detected if the nostrils are auscultated.

Because abdominal masses or fluid can compromise the respiratory system by extending into the lung or air sacs or by cranial displacement of viscera, abdominal palpation may suggest a cause of respiratory distress.

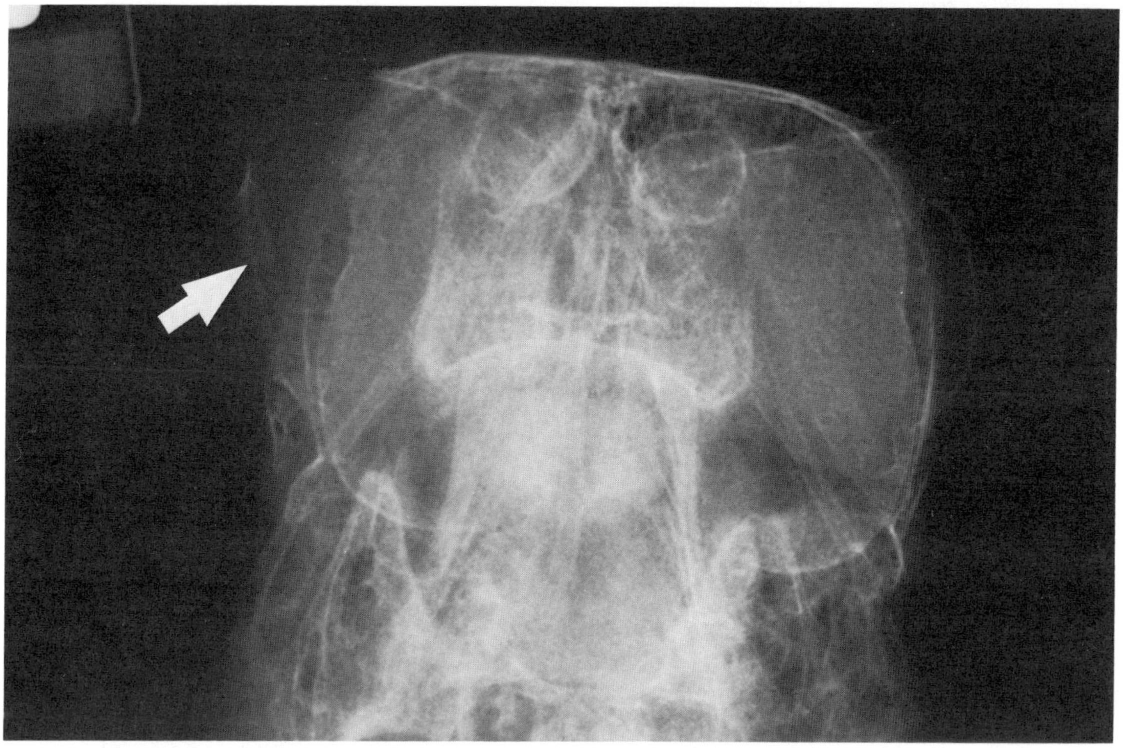

Figure 1—Rostrocaudal view of an Amazon parrot's skull shows a supraorbital abscess displacing scleral ossicle (*arrow*) with no bone erosion.

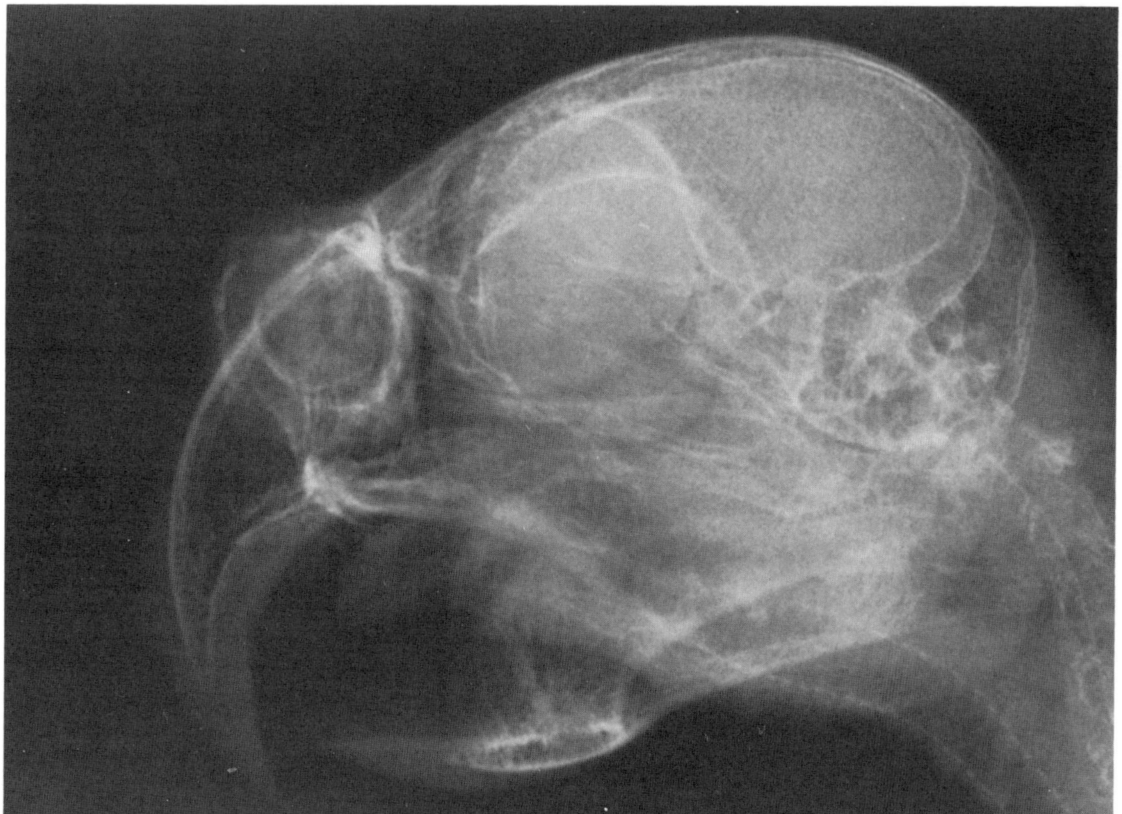

Figure 2—Lateral view of a Senegal parrot's skull demonstrates mineralization within a mass that involved the right nostril. Aspergillosis was diagnosed by biopsy and culture.

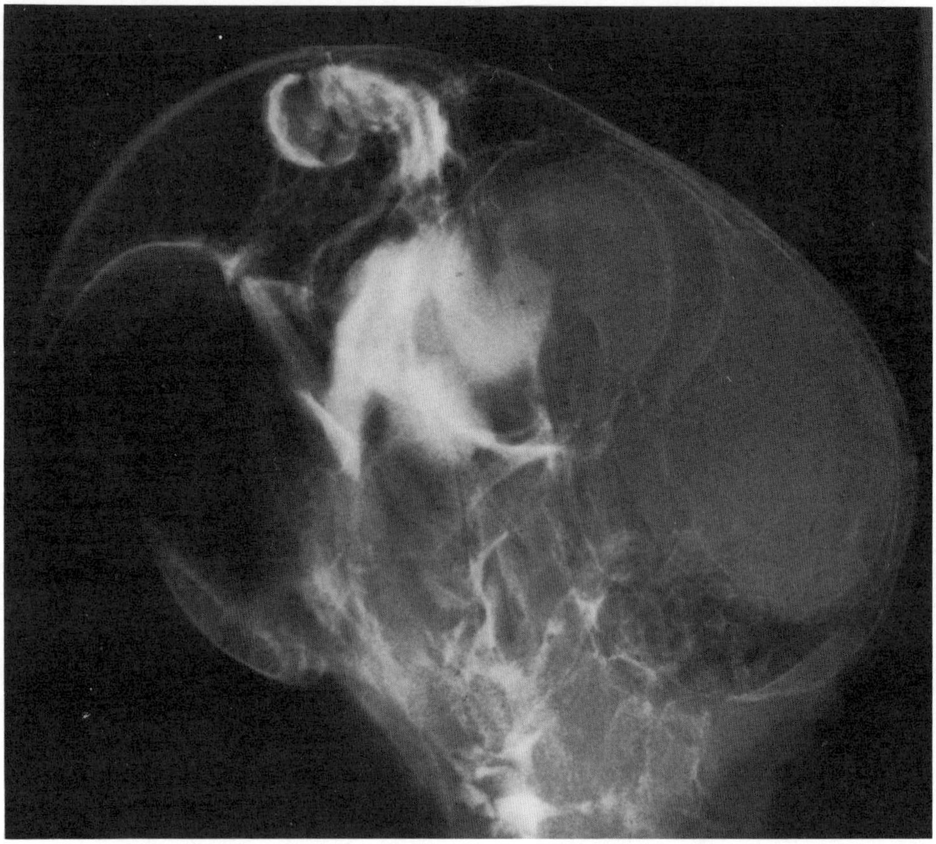

Figure 3A

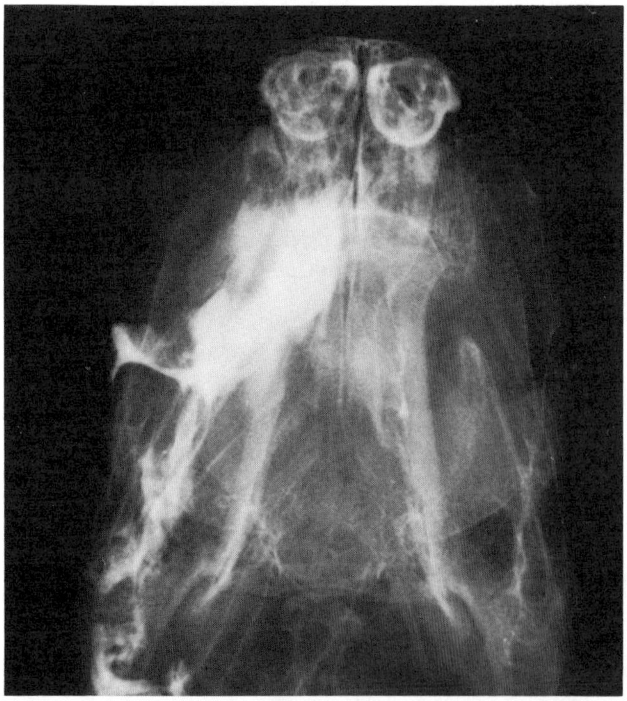

Figure 3B

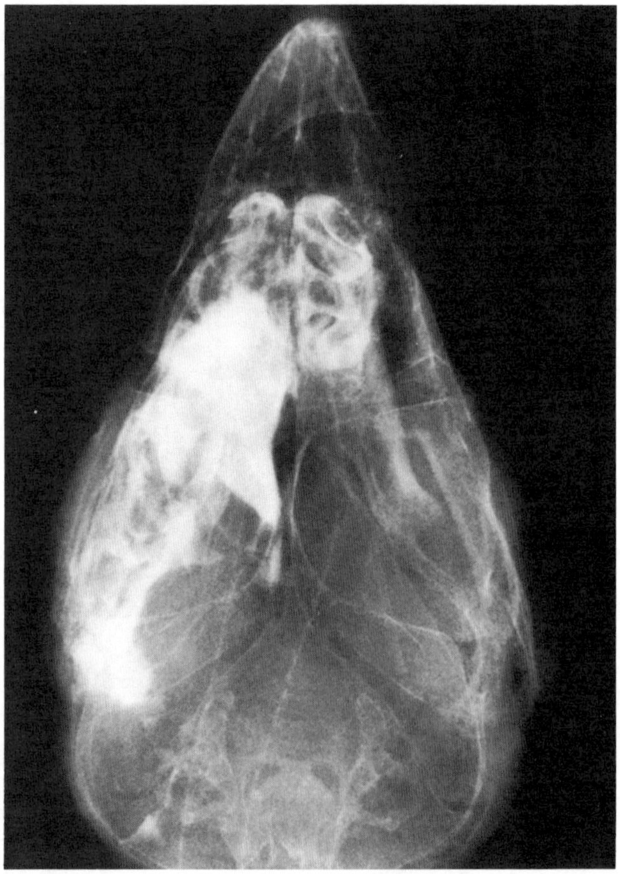

Figure 3C

Figure 3—Positive-contrast sinography of a normal parrot demonstrates the flow of contrast material into the contralateral sinus, nasal cavity, and periorbital and auricular regions. Contrast agent was injected into the right infraorbital sinus. (**A**) Right lateral, (**B**) rostrocaudal, and (**C**) ventrodorsal views.

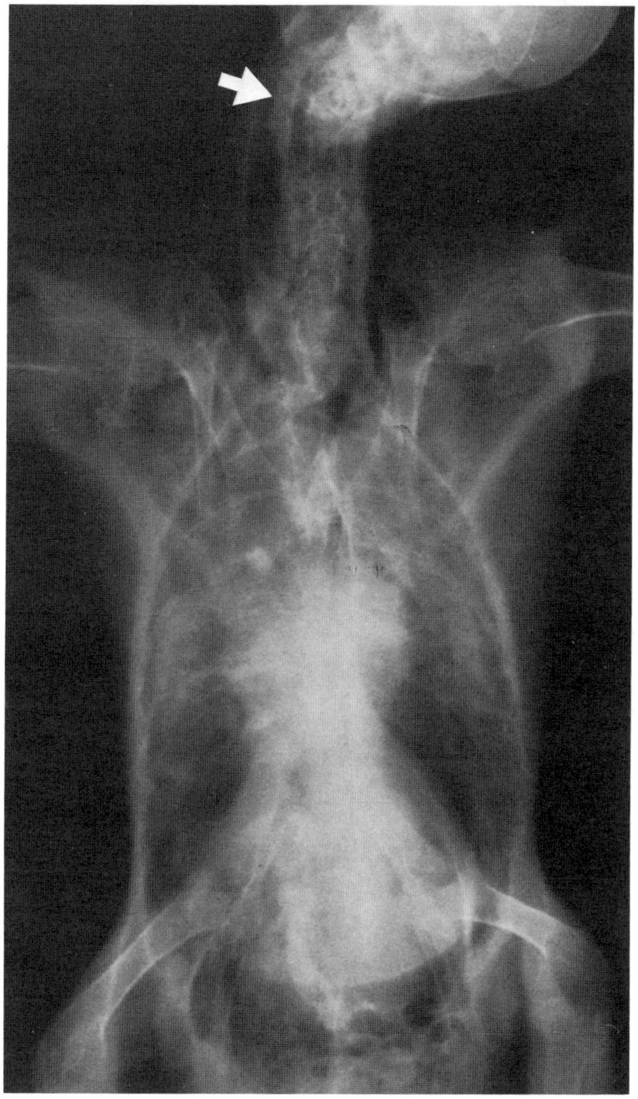

Figure 4—Increased parabronchial pulmonary density is present in the mid portion of both lungs of this parrot. The *arrow* points to a tracheal mass. Aerophagia is apparent. Pneumonia and tracheal abscess were secondary to hypovitaminosis A.

Radiographic Abnormalities

Diseases involving the upper respiratory tract, nasal cavity, infraorbital sinuses, cervicocephalic air sacs, and trachea may show no radiographic abnormalities.

Localized soft tissue densities are often abscesses (Figure 1) and may involve the nasal and oral cavities, periorbital region, or trachea. They are most commonly associated with hypovitaminosis A. Neoplasia is infrequent, but squamous cell carcinoma with bone involvement has been reported.[1] Fibrosarcomas often invade the beak and cause a significant soft tissue mass. Granulomas are the result of chronic rhinitis of bacterial[2] or fungal infection (Figure 2). Parasitic granulomas[3] are infrequent. Localized subcutaneous air pockets and granulomas are reported in association with disease of the cervicocephalic air sac system.[4]

Positive-contrast rhinography and sinography may aid in radiographic evaluation[5] (Figure 3). Studies of normal radiographic patterns in psittacines demonstrate communication between the infraorbital sinus and the nasal cavity, beak, opposite sinus, periorbital region, and tympanic region. This communication helps explain the beak deformities and massive swelling evident around the ocular and aural regions and associated with some of the upper respiratory diseases.

Radiographic changes commonly are caused by lower respiratory tract disorders. These include changes in normal reticular pulmonary pattern, bronchial thickening, abnormal air sac density, subcutaneous emphysema, aerophagia, and discrete masses.

Parabronchial infiltrates cause a blotchy appearance to the usually uniform pulmonary pattern. This change is seen frequently in birds with avian pneumonia along the caudal midlateral aspects of the lungs[6] and is best visualized in ventrodorsal radiographs (Figure 4). Aerodynamics in the

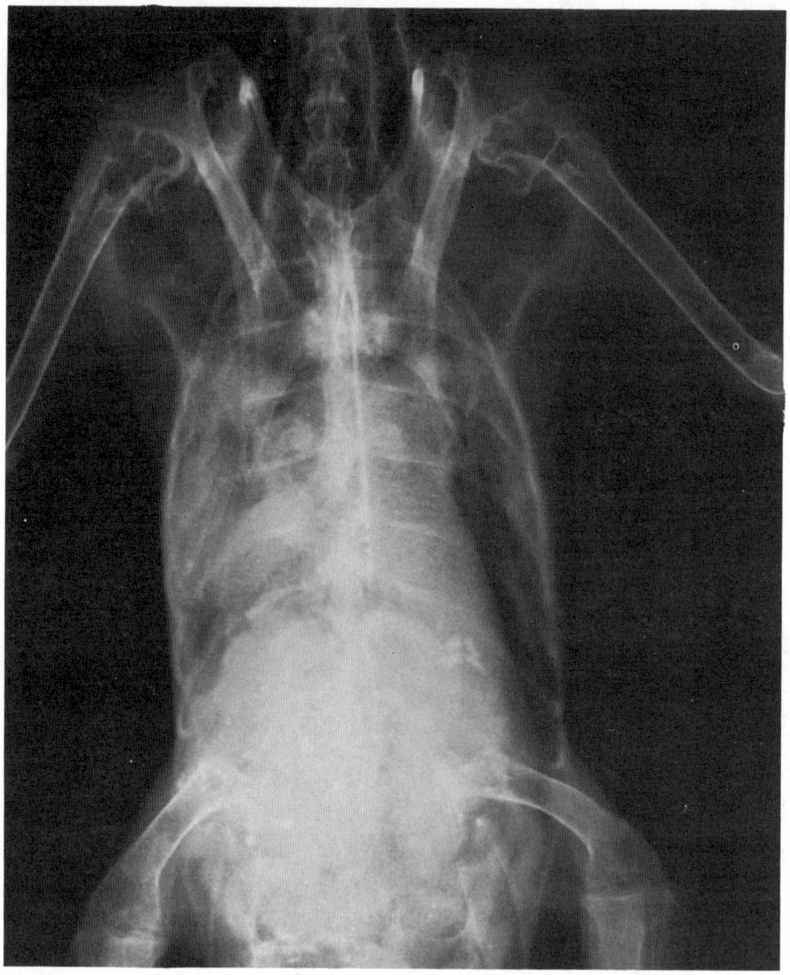

Figure 5—Consolidation present in the right lung of this mynah bird obliterated the normal reticular pattern. The lesion was caused by aspergillosis.

neopulmo contribute to the depositing of pathogens in this region. Focal areas of consolidation obliterate the parabronchial pattern so that, instead of a pronounced parabronchial wall with an air-filled center, the air is replaced by a soft tissue density. Caseous exudate or fluid, such as hemorrhage or edema, also may obliterate the parabronchi. Abscesses, fungal granulomas, or tumors also may cause discrete, well-defined, soft tissue masses that replace the normal pulmonary pattern (Figure 5). In ventrodorsal radiographs, the peripheral portions of the avian lung normally have greater density than the central portions. With the development of the neopulmo, the lateral portion of the lung increases,[7] causing increased soft tissue density. Infiltration around the bronchi results in an ability to visualize parallel walls of the air-filled bronchi. This infiltration occurs within the pulmonary parenchyma and extends into the air sacs (Figure 6).

Air sac disease may cause a barrel-shaped appearance to the avian thorax (Figure 7). Thickened and consolidated air sacs do not change in size as much as normal air sacs do during expiration, thus resulting in relatively fixed dimensions of the chest that mimic full inspiration. The abdominal air sacs become blunted, and lines across the air sacs become apparent. The normal air density becomes a subtle, gray, soft tissue density that may be homogeneous or irregular. Sharply demarcated soft tissue lines and obscured abdominal detail are present in lateral radiographs (Figure 8). Bacterial infections, hypovitaminosis A complicated by bacterial infection, and such fungal diseases as aspergillosis and mucormycosis[8] cause consolidating air sacculitis. Because viral diseases with secondary bacterial involvement play a significant role in pulmonary disease in other species, a similar situation probably exists in birds. Viruses interfere with the bactericidal action of the lung and cause direct cell damage, which may result in bacterial complications between Days 6 and 10 of infection.[9] Chlamydiosis also may cause primary air sacculitis; but it is usually a systemic disease associated with multiple-organ

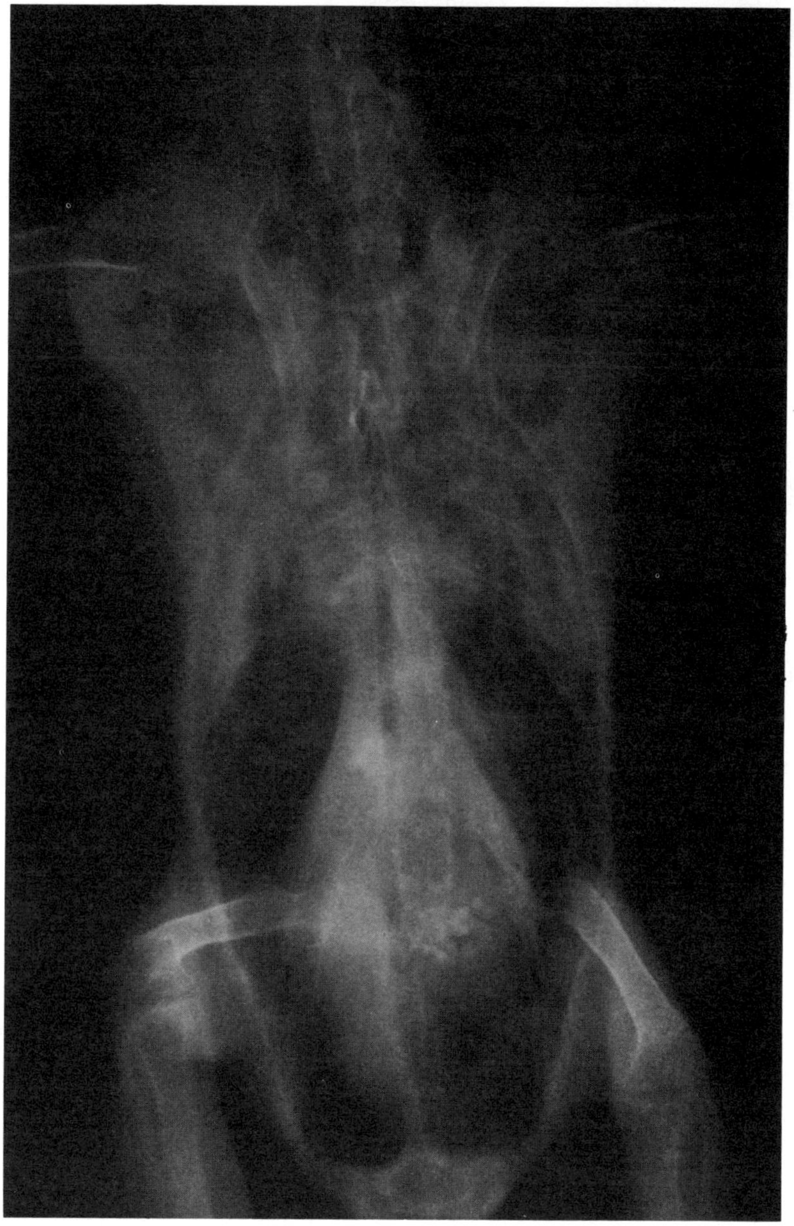

Figure 6—This view shows increased air sac density and blunting of abdominal air sacs, which were caused by air sacculitis. Prominent bronchi from wall thickening extend to clavicular air sacs.

involvement and, often, concurrent gram-negative infection.

Gas is not normally found in the gastrointestinal tract of birds. Radiographically detectable aerophagia often accompanies significant respiratory problems. In such cases, the air is uniformly distributed throughout the intestinal tract with no evidence of distention or localization (Figure 9). Subcutaneous emphysema may occur in association with traumatic air sac rupture.

Pulmonary masses are uncommon. When they do occur, they are usually abscesses or granulomas rather than neoplasms.

Summary

Radiographic changes associated with avian respiratory disorders often are subtle. The ventrodorsal view is most helpful for assessment of lung and air sac lesions. Pneumonia and air sacculitis are the most commonly encountered lower respiratory tract abnormalities. Prominence or obliteration of pulmonary reticular pattern, visualization of intrapulmonary bronchi, increased air sac density, blunted air sacs, and fixed appearance to air sacs are the radiographic changes that may be apparent. Radiographic lesions are uncommon with upper respiratory disease; but localized soft tissue masses, usually abscesses, may be apparent.

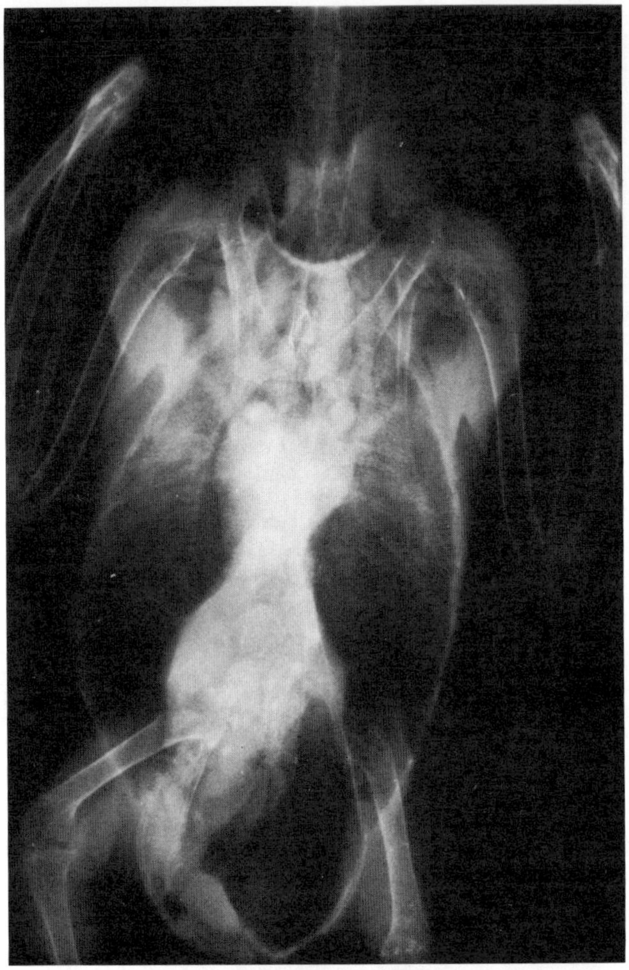

Figure 7—A barrel-shaped appearance, prominent lines across the air sacs, and increased parabronchial pattern indicate air sacculitis and pneumonia.

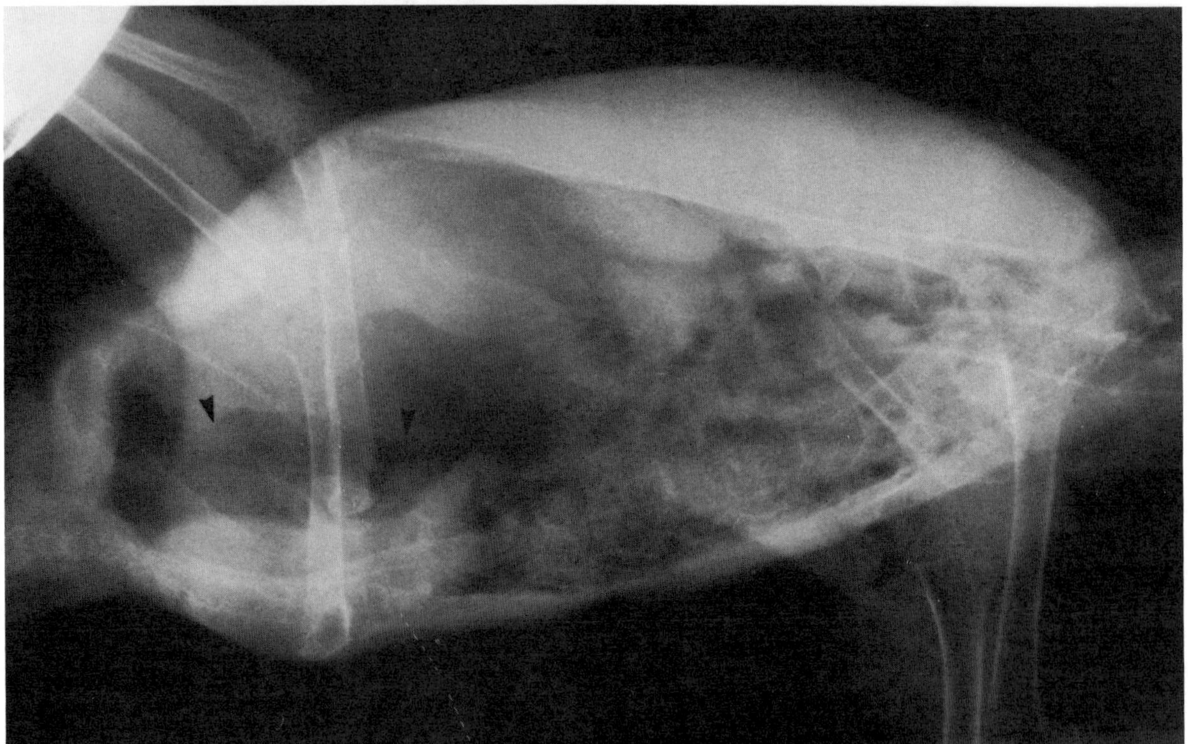

Figure 8—Ventral abdominal detail is obscured by overlying soft tissue density. Soft tissue lines in air sacs are the result of consolidating air sacculitis (*arrows*).

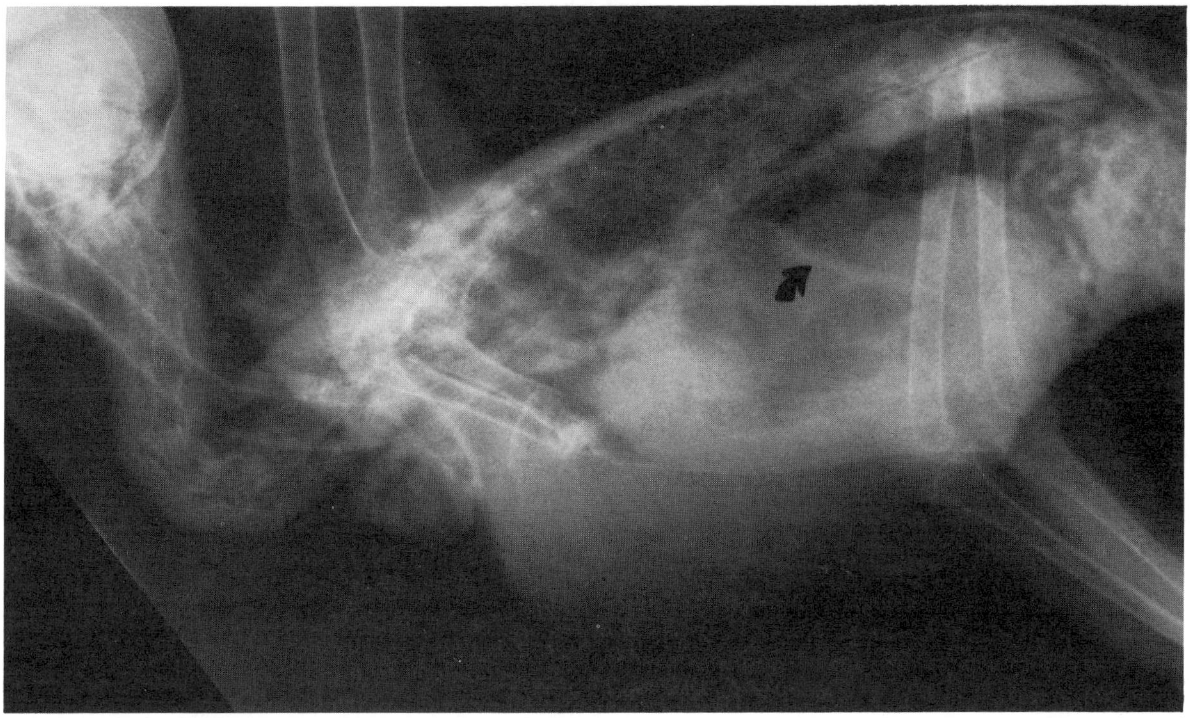

Figure 9—Gas is uniformly distributed throughout the small intestine. Air sac changes are present (*arrow*). Aerophagia is secondary to respiratory distress.

REFERENCES

1. Altman RB: Respiratory diseases of psittacine birds. *Small Anim Vet Med [Update Series]* 10:1-7, 1978.
2. Crane SW, Jacobson E, Shields RP: Cryosurgical removal of an intranasal granuloma from an African gray parrot. *VM SAC* 75(3):499-501, 1980.
3. McMillan MC: Avian radiology, in Petrak ML (ed): *Diseases of Cage and Aviary Birds*. Philadelphia, Lea & Febiger, 1982, pp 329-360.
4. Walsh MT, Mays MC: Clinical manifestations of cervicocephalic air sacs of psittacines. *Compend Contin Educ Pract Vet* 6(9):783-792, 1984.
5. McMillan MC: Unpublished radiographic studies, Angell Memorial Animal Hospital, Boston, MA, 1979.
6. Lowenstine LJ: Avian anatomy and its relation to disease processes. *Proc Annu Meet AAV*:1-9, 1984.
7. Duncker H: Structure of the avian respiratory tract. *Respir Physiol* 22:1-19, 1974.
8. Dawson CO, Wheeldon EB, McNeil PE: Air sac and renal mucormycosis in an African gray parrot (*Psittacus erimacus*). *Avian Dis* 20(3):593-600, 1976.
9. Green GM: Lung defense mechanisms. *Med Clin North Am* 57(3):547-562, 1973.

Avian Anesthesia

Robert B. Altman, DVM
A and A Veterinary Hospital
Franklin Square, New York

Avian anesthesia, because of size and anatomical and physiological variations of the avian patient, is more critical and hazardous than anesthesia in mammals. The purpose of this paper is to offer the clinician the most practical and safest choice of anesthetic agents currently available and to discuss the application of these agents.

Before considering the choice of an anesthetic agent, the clinician must decide if anesthesia is indicated for the contemplated procedure. While selection of an anesthetic agent is important, the decision whether or not to use anesthesia is of equal importance.

If, because of the physical condition of the patient or the simplicity of the procedure, anesthesia can be avoided, the procedure should be undertaken without the benefit of an anesthetic agent. With the exception of areas around the cere and legs, birds have a relatively poorly developed cutaneous sensory and vascular system and there is little apparent pain or bleeding when the skin is incised.

If the size and strength of the patient permits adequate restraint, if the procedure is of short duration, and if the anatomic site is easily accessible, the surgical procedure should be attempted without any form of anesthesia since the risk of anesthesia could be greater than the need for analgesia and restraint.

The selection of an anesthetic agent should be based on the following criteria.

1. The age and general physical condition of the bird. It is essential to examine the patient thoroughly prior to the administration of anesthesia.
2. The restraint required for the surgical procedure.
3. The anatomic site of the surgery.
4. The duration of the procedure.
5. Size and idiosyncrasies of the various avian species.

The surgical team for avian surgery should include the surgeon, an assistant to position and hold the patient during the procedure and an anesthesiologist. The anesthesiologist must administer the anesthetic agent and carefully monitor the patient throughout the procedure. The depth and rate of respiration must be visualized throughout the procedure. As a result of this requirement, draping the patient is avoided or plastic transparent surgical drapes are used. The bird's respiratory and cardiac rate should be monitored with a stethoscope, either standard or esophageal, throughout the procedure to determine the necessity for increasing or decreasing gas anesthesia. Monitoring the heart rate on an oscilloscope or electrocardiograph is of great value (Figs 1 and 2).

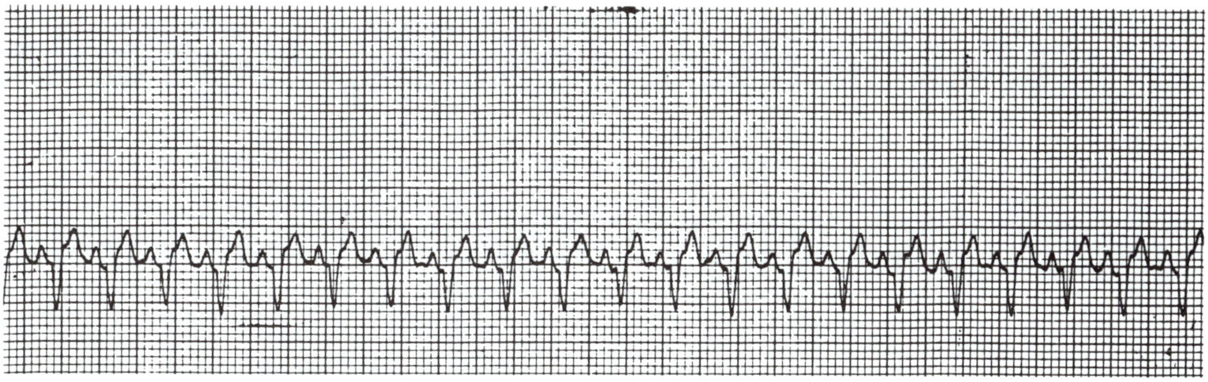

Fig 1—A Lead II standard electrocardiogram of an Amazon Parrot during induction with halothane anesthesia at a paper speed of 50 mm per second; the heart rate is 400 beats per minute. Note that the QRS complex in birds is negative in Lead II.

Unless surgery of the crop is contemplated, birds should not be fasted preoperatively. Glycogen storage in the liver of birds is poor and, as a result, glycogen depletion can occur in small species, such as canaries and budgerigars, in as little as 12 to 24 hours and in larger species, such as parrots, in 24 to 48 hours.

All surgical candidates should have a packed cell volume (PCV) and a blood glucose determination prior to surgery. Appropriate therapy can be instituted depending upon the results of these tests. Birds with a PCV above 55 to 60 percent should be given fluids before or during surgery. Anemic birds, with a PCV of less than 20, should have surgery postponed when feasible or should be transfused prior to anesthesia and surgery. If a homologous transfusion cannot be given, pigeon blood can be used effectively.

Hypoglycemic birds (glucose levels below 200 mg/100 ml) should be supplemented with 5% glucose and saline, intravenously if possible, before and during surgery.

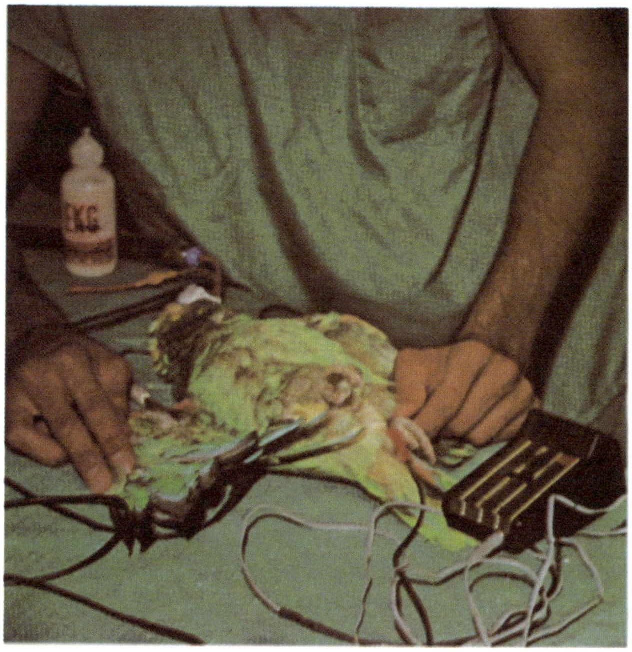

Fig 2—Limb leads for electrocardiogram Lead II and temperature probe on an anesthetized parrot. Electronic thermometer (Electro: Therm, Electromedics Inc., Denver, Colorado) monitors temperature changes throughout the anesthetic period.

Atropine should be administered at the dose of 0.04 to 0.1 mg/kg or 0.0012 to 0.003 mg/30 g to decrease respiratory secretions. The standard concentration of atropine is 0.5 mg/ml, which must be diluted.

During anesthesia, heat loss is considerable and the body temperature can drop as much as 19 degrees. It is therefore obligatory to take measures to conserve body temperatures as much as possible. Heating pads during surgery and heated recovery cages postoperatively are necessary. Fortunately, body temperature returns to normal rapidly after anesthesia is discontinued. In a recent study,[1] body temperature under halothane anesthesia dropped an average of 11.2°F and under ketamine anesthesia dropped an average of 4.2°F; body temperature returned to normal within 10 to 20 minutes after cessation of both anesthetic agents.

Heart rate also decreases sharply with general anesthesia. With halothane, the heart rate decreased an average of 223 beats per minute within the first 10 minutes and returned to normal within 5 to 10 minutes after discontinuing anesthesia.[1]

All birds large enough to be intubated should have an endotracheal tube passed even if gas anesthesia is not contemplated. Intubation is possible in birds larger than a cockatiel or lovebird (Fig 3). In small psittacine birds that cannot be intubated, some means of mechanically holding

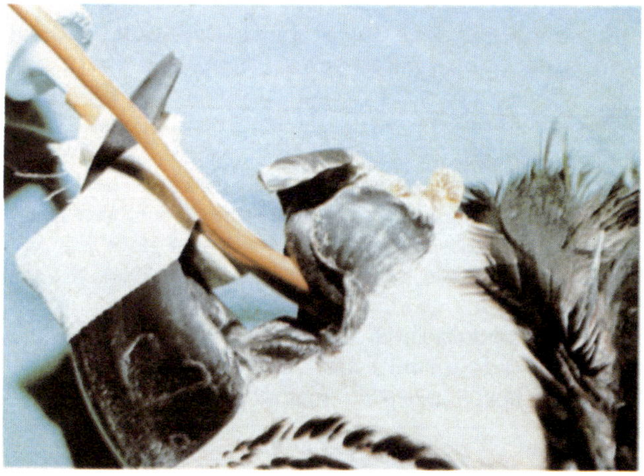

Fig 3—Endotracheal intubation in a Macaw. The endotracheal tube is taped securely to the upper bill, so that inadvertent tension on the tube can neither pull out the endotracheal catheter nor rupture the trachea as the result of tension on the cuffed end of the tube.

the large, fleshy tongue from falling back into the mouth while the bird is in dorsal recumbency will prevent the tongue from occluding the glottis. A bent paper clip can be used for this purpose.

The endotracheal tube should be moist or lubricated to facilitate entry into the glottis. If a cuffed endotracheal tube is used, care must be taken not to overinflate the cuff and injure or rupture the tracheal rings. A bird's trachea has tracheal rings which are continuous for 360 degrees and therefore the trachea has little ability to expand in diameter. Cole tubes can also be used. It is important to keep the lumen of the endotracheal tube patent, and not permit viscid respiratory secretions to accumulate and occlude the tube.

Local Anesthesia

Local anesthetics have little application in avian surgery other than for topical use. Birds display little discomfort when the skin is incised or sutured and since problems relating to shock and restraint are not overcome with local anesthetics, there is little need for this form of anesthesia. Proparacaine hydrochloride[a] is an ophthalmic topical anesthetic used in the eye during examination and for corneal staining with fluorescein. Lidocaine hydrochloride ointment[b] is used to reduce discomfort and resultant tenesmus after reduction of a prolapsed cloaca.

For large species of birds, such as water fowl, 2% procaine or lidocaine hydrochloride is used at a dose of 1 to 3 ml. In birds the size of pigeons, a dose of 0.25 to 1.0 ml has been used safely.[10,11] For small caged birds, a subcutaneous dose not exceeding 200 mg/kg of an 0.2% solution of procaine has been used.[13] The author finds little use for this form of anesthesia in small birds.

General Anesthesia

Parenteral administration of injectable anesthetics can be given safely via the intramuscular or intravenous routes.

Barbiturate Anesthetic Agents

This group of anesthetic agents is infrequently used because of the duration of anesthesia, the prolonged recovery period, the long period after recovery before the patient can eat and drink and the inability to reverse the drug after administration. The only need for this group of anesthetics is for terminal experimental surgery in which prolonged anesthesia is required.

A combination drug[c] containing chloralhydrate, sodium pentobarbital, magnesium sulfate, propylene glycol and ethanol[9,10,11] is the most reliable and safest of the long-acting barbiturate anesthetic agents. The intravenous dose is approximately 1.0 to 1.5 ml/kg but should be given to effect. The intramuscular dose is 2.5 ml/kg. Some muscle necrosis results from intramuscular injection of this drug. In obese birds, badly debilitated birds and birds that are poor anesthetic risks, the dosage should be reduced to 2 ml/kg.

Sodium pentobarbital has the same application as the combination drug and a narrower margin of safety. The dose is 1.5 mg/30 g of body weight.

Thiamylal sodium[d] has been used in the larger species such as peafowl, water fowl, falconiforms and large psittacines as a short-acting anesthetic. Its use is limited to endotracheal intubation and surgical procedures of short duration. The dose is approximately 0.2 ml/kg of a 2.5% solution given slowly, intravenously. This drug should be given to effect.

The Cyclohexylamines

This group of drugs has been used very successfully for avian anesthesia.

A combination of tiletamine and benzodiozepine,[e] during its clinical investigation, proved to be a safe and effective anesthetic agent for all size birds but this agent has not been marketed.[13]

Ketamine hydrochloride[2,8,12,13,16] is the most widely used of the cyclohexylamines. It is relatively safe and can be used in all species of birds.

Advantages of this drug over other injectable anesthetic agents are its wide margin of safety, the ability to safely administer more of the drug if the desired level of anesthesia has not been attained and its relatively smooth induction and recovery.

Disadvantages of ketamine are (1) its variable effects on different species and individuals; (2) its inability to adequately diminish muscle tone; (3) its inability to suppress ocular and oral reflexes; (4) its stimulation of fluttering, tremors and, sometimes, convulsions; and, (5) since it is a cataleptoid anesthetic, its inability to attain analgesia. The duration of anesthesia with ketamine can be prolonged. There is also an increase in salivation and cardiovascular and respiratory depression.

Tremendous variation in dosage has been reported in the literature for this dissociative drug. The author finds a range of 50 to 100 mg/kg given intramuscularly to be the most effective dose for small species weighing up to 500 g. For large species weighing over 500 g, including large psittacines, fowl, and raptors, 25 to 50 mg/kg injected intramuscularly seems to be the optimal dose.

Induction generally takes from 3 to 5 minutes and anesthesia lasts for 10 to 30 minutes. Recovery is variable and may take from 30 minutes up to 5 hours. Larger doses will result in prolonged recovery.

Ketamine is excreted in the kidneys. In dehydrated or debilitated birds and birds with renal insufficiency, fluids should accompany the administration of this drug. Ketamine has been used in conjunction with halothane at the lower dose range as a preanesthetic agent for endotracheal intubation. It has also been used in combination with xylazine[f] and diazepam.[g,17]

Methoxymol[h] is a short-acting hypnotic which has been used with good success as a restraint and anesthetic agent.[5,6,18] Its effect and margin of safety are comparable to that of ketamine and, because of fluttering, gas anesthesia is frequently used as an adjunct.

Induction is approximately 1 to 3 minutes and anesthesia lasts from 15 to 30 minutes. Doses of 10 to 40 mg/kg are

---

[a]Ophthane® 5% ophthalmic solution, E.R. Squibb and Sons, Inc., Princeton, NJ 08540.

[b]Xylocaine® ointment 5%, Astra Pharmaceutical Products, Inc., Worcester, MA 01606.

[c]Equithesin®, Jensen-Salsbery/Burroughs Wellcome, Kansas City, MO 64141.

[d]Surital®, Parke-Davis and Co., Detroit, MI 48207

[e]Tilazol®, Parke-Davis and Co., Detroit, MI 48207

[f]Rompun®, Haver-Lockhart, Shawnee, KS 66201

[g]Valium®, Roche Laboratories, Nutley, NJ 07110

[h]Metomidate®, Pitman-Moore, Inc., Washington Crossing, NJ 08560

reported to be effective with the higher ranges used for major surgical procedures.

Saffon[i,16] is a steroid anesthetic that is used in Great Britain and Europe, but is not available in the United States. It has been used in psittacine and passerine species, but its primary use has been with raptors. It is a safe anesthetic for short-term procedures in most species. Cooper and Redig[7] reported a number of deaths related to the use of this anesthetic in red-tailed hawks (*Buteo jamaicensis*).

Xylazine[14] is a sedative, analgesic and muscle relaxant. Its sedative and analgesic activity is related to depression of the central nervous system.

Xylazine can cause muscle tremors, bradycardia with partial A-V block and reduction of the respiratory rate. Salivation and movement in response to noise also occur.

When given intramuscularly at a dose of 50 to 100 mg/kg, induction time is 2 to 4 minutes. Recovery is in 30 minutes to several hours.

In psittacine birds of varying size and species, the author has encountered only one fatality out of 25 birds tested at the above dosage range. Xylazine is not as reliable an anesthetic agent as ketamine but offers much better analgesia. Pigeons do not tolerate this drug well and its use in this species should be avoided.

Inhalation Anesthesia

Of all the anesthetic agents suitable for avian use today, volatile anesthetics are the safest and most reliable. Induction is rapid and, because detoxification occurs quickly, recovery is also rapid and usually smooth. Regulation of anesthetic depth is possible, resulting in a much wider margin of safety. Administration of volatile anesthetics can be accomplished by constant flow with oxygen directed across the bird's nose or via a nose cone, or by endotracheal intubation.

Any bird in which an endotracheal tube can be passed into the glottis should be intubated. Most birds larger than a cockatiel can readily be intubated with a Cole tube or a standard cuffed tube, sized 10 French gauge or larger. All endotracheal tubes should be cut short to decrease dead space. A nonrebreathing system must be used on birds weighing less than 5 kg. The gas and oxygen flow should be high enough to prevent rebreathing of carbon dioxide. Induction is accomplished by placing the bird in a transparent chamber in which it can be observed. A fish tank or transparent nose cone is the most practical apparatus. When the desired level of anesthesia has been reached, the bird should be intubated and maintained on a nonrebreathing system. For a small bird that cannot be intubated, the head can be placed in a nose cone made from an empty syringe case or the gas flow can be directed across the bird's nose. The advantage of the latter technique is that visualization and monitoring of the patient is easier and less confining than with a nose cone and there is no accumulation of expired carbon dioxide. The primary disadvantage of this method is escape of gas into the operating room.

It is necessary to recognize and understand the planes of surgical anesthesia as defined in Table I. Corneal reflexes are recognized by the membrana nictitans flashing across the eye in response to stimulus of the cornea.

Cere reflexes are present in response to pin pricks to the cere.

Pedal reflexes (withdrawal of the foot in response to pressure stimulus to the toes) will diminish until the deep plane of anesthesia is reached and will then disappear. This reflex is not consistent in all species.

Palpebral reflexes and reflexes of the cere are the first reflexes to disappear.

The ideal plane of surgical anesthesia is characterized by slow regular and deep respirations with slight corneal and pedal reflexes. If respirations are shallow or all reflexes are absent, the bird is too deep and apnea can rapidly ensue.

Halothane[2,3,8,13,15,19] is the anesthetic of choice since it conforms to all the criteria of rapid induction and recovery and excellent control of anesthetic level. It is preferred to

ⁱCT1341, Glaxo Lab Ltd., England

TABLE I*

PROGRESSION OF SIGNS OF SURGICAL ANESTHESIA

	Stages of Anesthesia			
	Induction and Narcosis	*Light*	*Medium*	*Deep*
Signs	Eyelids closing, wings starting to droop, head lowered			
Voluntary movement	Can be aroused and is pain sensitive	Absent	Absent	Absent
Respirations	Deep, rapid and regular without stimulation	Deep and rapid	Slow, deep and regular	Slow, regular and shallow
Corneal reflexes	Present	Present	Slow or intermittent	Absent
Pedal reflexes	Present	Present	Slow or intermittent	Absent
Palpebral reflexes	Present	Present	Absent	Absent
Cere reflexes	Present	Present	Absent	Absent

*Classified and compiled by Arnall.[20]

methoxyflurane because induction and recovery time is more consistent and faster.

Induction is accomplished by the administration of a 2% to 3% concentration of halothane with a 0.5 to 2.0 liter per minute oxygen flow. Induction time is approximately 1 to 5 minutes. During induction, a brief excitation period with trembling and wing fluttering is followed by relaxation and deep regular respiration. The intubated patient should be maintained on a 0.5 to 1.0 liter per minute flow and a concentration of 0.5% to 1.5% halothane.

Recovery with a 100% oxygen flow usually takes about 3 to 8 minutes. If the patient becomes deeper than the desired level of anesthesia, the anesthetic plane can be quickly lowered by either reducing the halothane concentration or administering 100% oxygen.

Halothane causes a rapid decrease in blood pressure, heart rate and body temperature.[1] All of the above return to normal levels within a short time after the cessation of halothane administration.

Methoxyflurane[2,4,8,13,19] is successfully used for avian anesthesia although induction and recovery times are not as rapid as with halothane. One advantage of methoxyflurane is that it is possible to administer this agent without an expensive anesthetic vaporizer.

Induction requires a 3% to 4% concentration with a 2 to 3 liter per minute oxygen flow. Maintenance requires a 1.5% to 2% concentration with a 0.5 to 1 liter per minute oxygen flow.

Both halothane and methoxyflurane are nonexplosive. Nitrous oxide can be used in combination with halothane and oxygen in a 50% to 50% mixture of nitrous oxide and oxygen.

It is extremely important to monitor both induction and maintenance of gas anesthesia by observing the respiratory depth and rate and the EKG throughout anesthesia. Adjustments in anesthetic concentration should be made rapidly. If respiratory arrest occurs, the anesthetic should be stopped, the system blown out with pure oxygen and the bird resuscitated gently until respirations return.

If the bird is not intubated, artificial respiration should be administered by digital pressure on the sternum at the rate of 30 to 40 respirations per minute with 100% oxygen being directed into the bird's nostrils.

As soon as the surgical procedure has been completed, the anesthesia is discontinued; the bird should be maintained on oxygen until all reflexes have returned and the patient is able to lift its head. The time period between head movements and perching can be very short and the endotracheal tube should be removed to avoid injury to the trachea. As soon as the endotracheal tube has been removed, the bird should be placed in a heated (75°-80°F) recovery cage in sternal or lateral recumbency. It is important that the recovery cage has no obstructions, such as perches, feed cups and toys. The cage should be glass or plastic without any bars. During recovery, a wing or leg can be caught between the bars of the cage causing severe injury.

As soon as the bird is ambulatory, with reasonable stability, it should be placed on a perch and offered food and water.

REFERENCES

1. Altman RB: Effect of halothane and ketamine anesthesia on body temperature and electrocardiographic changes. Presented at the annual AAZV meeting, Denver, Colorado, October, 1979.
2. Amand WB: Avian anesthesia, in Kirk R (ed): *Current Veterinary Therapy VI*. Philadelphia, WB Saunders Co, 1977.
3. Bilo D, Best G, Schonenberger I, Nachtigall W: Zur methode der halothan-inhalationsnarkose bie vogeln (taube and wellensittich). *J Comp Physiol* 79:137–152, 1972.
4. Brinkman DC, Burch GR: Methoxyflurane anesthesia in birds. *Allied Vet* 36(2):39–40, 1964.
5. Callear J FF L: Correspondence use of the hypnotic agent methoxymol (R7315) in birds of prey. *Vet Rec* 88:242, 1971.
6. Cooper JE: Use of the hypnotic agent methoxymol in birds of prey. *Vet Rec* 87:751–752, 1970.
7. Cooper JE, Redig PT: Unexpected reactions to the use of CT1341 by red-tailed hawks. *Vet Rec* 97:352, 1975.
8. Franchetti DR, Klide AM: Restraint and anesthesia, in Fowler M (ed): *Zoo and Wild Animal Medicine*. Philadelphia, WB Saunders Co, 1978.
9. Gandal CP: Avian anesthesia and surgery. AAHA 34th Meeting Scientific Presentation, New York City, p 22, 1967.
10. Gandal CP: Avian Anesthesia Federation Proceedings *Fed Am Soc Exp Biol* 28(4):1533–1534, 1969.
11. Gandal CP: Satisfactory general anesthesia in birds. *J Am Vet Med Assoc* 128(7):332–334, 1956.
12. Kittle EL: Ketamine HCl as an anesthetic for birds. *Mod Vet Pract* 52:40–41, 1971.
13. Klide AM: Avian anesthesia. *Vet Clin North Am* 3(2):175–180, 1973.
14. Levinger IM, Kedem J, Abram M: A new anesthetic sedative for birds. *Br Vet J* 129:296–300, 1973.
15. Myers RE, Stettner LJ: Halothane anesthesia in birds. *Physiol Behav* 4:277–278, 1969.
16. Paddleford R: Anesthetic management for birds of prey, in Fowler M (ed): *Zoo and Wild Animal Medicine*. Philadelphia, WB Saunders Co, 1978.
17. Redig PT, Duke GE: Intravenously administered ketamine HCl and diazepam for anesthesia of raptors. *J Am Vet Med Assoc* 169:886, 1976.
18. Ryder-Davis P: The use of metomidate, an intramuscular narcotic for birds. *Vet Rec* 92:507–509, 1973.
19. Sanford J: Avian anesthesia, in Soma LR (ed): *Textbook of Veterinary Anesthesia*. Baltimore, William and Wilkins, 1971, pp 359–368.
20. Arnall: Anesthesia and surgery in cage and aviary birds. *Vet Rec* 73(7):139–142, 1961.

Update

Isoflurane[1] (AErrane®—Anaquest) is the safest and most efficacious of the gas anesthetic agents. The primary disadvantage is its high cost.

Induction requires a higher concentration of isoflurane, 3 to 5%, with a 2- to 3-L/min flow of oxygen. Induction generally takes approximately 1 to 4 minutes. Maintenance is accomplished with a 2 to 3% concentration with a 0.5- to 1.0-L/min oxygen flow.

Recovery is extremely rapid, because isoflurane is insoluble in blood, and birds can recover sufficiently to perch and fly in as little as 3 to 5 minutes.

1. Harrison GJ: Anesthesiology, in Harrison, Harrison (eds): *Clinical Avian Medicine and Surgery*. Philadelphia, WB Saunders Co, 1986, pp 549–558.

General Principles of Avian Surgery

Robert B. Altman, DVM
A & A Veterinary Hospital
Franklin Square, New York

It is impossible to present a comprehensive description of avian surgery in one article. The author will discuss basic avian surgical principles and describe a few of the common surgical procedures.

There are a number of anatomical and physiological factors unique to birds that affect anesthesia and surgery, and they will be briefly mentioned.

Cutaneous vascularization and innervation are not as well developed in birds as they are in other mammalian species and, therefore, skin incisions other than on the feet or around the cere result in little pain. The lack of subcutaneous connective tissue makes accessibility to muscle, bone, and underlying structures in birds simple and relatively avascular. Many cutaneous blood vessels are readily visible and can be avoided or ligated before incision, thus permitting maximal hemostasis.

Presurgical examinations should be routine and should include measurements of hematocrit (PCV), total solids, serum glucose, and serum uric acid.

Birds with serum glucose levels lower than 200 mg/100 ml should be supplemented with dextrose before and during surgery. Glycogen storage capacity in birds is considerably less than in other species, and this increases the possibility of hypoglycemia from surgical shock. It is therefore essential to take all necessary measures to reduce surgical stress and to supplement the patient with dextrose when necessary.

Birds with blood uric acid levels above 30 mg/100 ml should have surgery postponed until those levels can be reduced. If the PCV is lower than 25 to 30%, surgery should be postponed if possible, or a blood transfusion should be administered during the surgical procedure.

A total serum protein level lower than 2 mg/100 ml is a sign of impending trouble, and the prognosis for a successful surgical result must be guarded.

The cutaneous ulna vein in birds can readily be cannulated using a 25-gauge Teflon cannula. A soft, flexible cannula is preferred to a rigid one, because there is less chance of puncturing the thin-walled vessel. 2.5% dextrose in one-half strength saline or 5% dextrose in water can be administered slowly (2 to 5 drops/minute) using a microdrip delivery system.

Surgical Principles

Basic surgical principles that are applicable to all mammalian species are also applicable to birds, but several specific ones deserve emphasis.

Hemostasis is of extreme importance. Because total blood volume, particularly in the smaller avian species, is only 2 to 4 ml, the loss of a few drops of blood can represent a loss of a significant part of the bird's total blood volume. For example, four drops of blood in a small finch constitute approximately 10% of its total blood volume. Ligation of all blood vessels prior to transection is the preferred technique to maintain hemostasis, because blood loss is thus eliminated. Electrosurgery minimizes capillary bleeding.

When planning the skin incision, it is important to consider the path of the feather tracts, because skin excision can cause the incision to change direction after it is sutured. If possible, the incision should be planned so that feather tracts will not undergo any directional change after the procedure has been completed. Not only can such directional change cause unsightly feather patterns, but it can sometimes interfere with wing or leg movement. The skin incision should be started with a number 15 scalpel blade and then extended with scissors or electrosurgery. Blunt dissection should be used to separate all tissues, and blood vessels should be ligated as they are encountered.

Under gas and injectable anesthesia, body temperature in the avian patient drops precipitously,[1] and although body temperature returns to normal shortly after the cessation of anesthesia, supplemental heat should be offered during and after completion of the surgical procedure. Although it has been found that supplementary heat does not curtail the fall in temperature, it seems that the temperature drop is not as rapid when supplementary heat is given. Hot water jackets and electric heating pads are suitable warming devices. An incubator is an effective heat chamber for recovery. Supplemental heat should be maintained until body temperature returns to normal.

Preparation of the surgical site can be started either before or after anesthesia has been administered. The feathers should be plucked in a direction parallel to their growth and follicle direction. Plucking at an angle increases the possibility of tearing the skin. After the feathers have been removed from the surgical field, the skin should be washed with povidone-iodine or a similar surgical scrub soap. The surgical field and the surrounding feathers should then be washed with alcohol. Dousing the surrounding feathers with alcohol helps to prevent any encroachment of these feathers over the surgical field during the procedure. It is extremely important to be sure that all the alcohol has evaporated from the skin before electrosurgery is employed, as the alcohol can ignite and burn the patient. Although alcohol tends to cool the patient, it does not appear to increase temperature loss significantly. A sterile, water-soluble surgical lubricant[2] can be used to keep surrounding feathers from the surgical site. This gel can easily be washed off after completion of the procedure.

Positioning the patient depends on the location of the surgical site. A drape or towel should be placed over the table or heating appliance. The easiest position to restrain the bird in is dorsal recumbency. An assistant can hold the wings and legs or they can be taped to the table. In lateral recumbency the wings are held together in extension over the back of the bird. It is essential that thoracic movement not be impaired. During the procedure, surgeons should be aware of the position of their hands and wrists so that no pressure that might inhibit thoracic movement and breathing is exerted on the patient at any time.

Surgical drapes should be employed whenever possible, but the drapes must not interfere with the anesthetist's observation of the patient's respirations. Sterile transparent plastic drapes[3] can be used when standard cloth drapes interfere with visualization of the patient and to maintain asepsis. The disadvantages of these drapes are their inability to absorb blood and other fluids and their slippery surface.

Many of the instruments used in avian surgery are ophthalmic instruments that allow fragile tissues to be handled gently. Ligation, subcutaneous suturing, and closure of the skin incision are performed with 3-0 to 5-0 polyglycolic acid or equivalent chromic gut suture material. Polyglycolic acid suture material is preferred to chromic gut because it is stronger and easier to work with.

Skin suturing is usually accomplished with a simple continuous stitch to minimize surgical and anesthetic time. Postsurgical picking at sutures is rare and can be prevented with the use of an Elizabethan collar. The use of absorbable suture material in the skin precludes the necessity for removal. With the rapid regrowth of feathers, removal could be difficult.

During anesthetic recovery, the patient should be observed to ensure that hemostasis has been complete and there is no postoperative bleeding.

Tumors of the Ventral Body Region

Superficial tumors are frequently encountered, mostly on the ventral aspect of the body. Most of these are xanthomas and lipomas that are, often, undergoing ulceration and central necrosis; this necessitates surgical removal.

After the surgical site is prepared, a skin incision is made directly over the mass, if the mass is small.

Most of these masses are well encapsulated. The skin is bluntly dissected off the surface of the tumor and the mass is peeled out. Blood vessels are ligated as they are encountered. After the tissue has been removed, standard skin closure as described above is performed. Subcutaneous sutures are unnecessary.

If the tumor is large and the skin over the tumor is ulcerated or friable and thickened, as is often the case, an elliptical skin incision is made around the mass and the subcutaneous tissues are bluntly or electrosurgically dissected. All blood vessels should be ligated. Ligation is preferred to electrosurgical coagulation because postsurgical bleeding is much less likely to occur following ligation. In birds, postsurgical capillary bleeding persists for a much longer time than it does in mammals. Standard skin closure is performed after hemostasis is assured. If the tumor is in the thoracic inlet area, extreme care should be taken during dissection, because the crop is often adhered to the tumor capsule.

The tumor mass is frequently tightly adhered by a strong fibrous band to the pectoral muscle area, particularly directly over the sternum. This band must be dissected or incised in order to peel off the mass. If central necrosis has occurred, care should be taken not to rupture the walled-off tumor, because the necrotic liquified tissue will flow over the surgical site. There is often capillary bleeding from the muscle surface when the tumor is peeled off the surface of the pectoral muscles. This bleeding can be controlled only by electrocoagulation.

Laparotomy

The approach for a laparotomy offering the greatest intraabdominal exposure is a transverse incision halfway between the caudal end of the sternum and the cloacal opening. This incision can extend from one leg to the other. The skin, and then the combined abdominal muscles and peritoneum, are incised. Particular care should be taken not to lacerate the underlying viscera when cutting through the muscle layers. The gizzard and pancreatic intestinal loop are the most prominent organs visible after the abdomen has been entered (Figure 1). It is wise to maintain as much air sac integrity as possible when exploring the abdomen. It will be necessary to rupture the abdominal air sacs during exploration.[4] The extent of air sac disruption will depend on the intraabdominal area involved and the depth of abdominal exploration. Blood vessels within the abdomen should be ligated before transection. Closure of the abdomen is accomplished in two suture lines. The peritoneum and abdominal muscles are closed with a simple continuous stitch using 3-0 to 5-0 polyglycolic acid or chromic gut sutures. The skin is sutured the same way. Although simple interrupted sutures would be a better means of repair in the muscle layers, it is often more important to achieve as rapid a closure as possible to decrease surgical and anesthesia time.

Surgical Correction of Egg-bound Birds

When an egg-bound bird is presented, radiographs should always be taken to ascertain the number of eggs being passed in the oviduct. Often, more than one egg is present (Figures 2A and B), and if the surgeon is not aware of the second egg, it can easily be missed during the surgical procedure, particularly if a laparotomy is not performed. If an egg is in the oviduct and is not presented into the cloaca and the patient is not stressed, it is advisable to place the bird in an incubator at 80° to 85°F for at least 24 to 48 hours before considering surgical correction.[5] Often this procedure facilitates normal delivery of the egg. If the egg has not presented after 48 hours, the delivery must be made surgically via one of two surgical approaches. The size and position of the egg or eggs determines the technique used. If the egg is presented outside the cloaca wrapped in the oviduct (Figure 3A), the length of time the tissues of the oviduct have been exposed determines the ease of removal and the anticipated postsurgical sequelae. If the prolapsed oviduct is fresh and there is no drying of tissues, the exposed tissue should be cleansed and lubricated with an antibiotic ointment prior to incising the oviduct. A small incision should be made at the least vascular point over the pole of the egg. With an instrument such as a cyclodialysis spatula or a lubricated, sterile, cotton-tipped applicator, the incision should be dilated and the oviduct gently separated from the surface of the egg. Gentle digital pressure behind the egg will force it through the opening as the oviduct is separated from the egg surface. Often the surface of the eggshell is very rough and irregular and the oviduct is in spasm, making separation difficult. After the oviduct is separated from the shell, the egg is squeezed through the incision. The incision can be extended as necessary to permit passage of the egg. If the tissue of the oviduct is viable, it should be sutured with a simple continuous pattern of 5-0 Vicryl with an atraumatic needle. After suturing, the oviduct is gently placed back into the cloaca. An attempt should be made to replace the prolapsed oviduct back through the oviduct-cloacal opening.

If the oviduct has been prolapsed for more than 30 to 40 minutes, a significant amount of trauma and drying of the membranes will occur; some tissue will be edematous and other tissue will be dry and devitalized. The devitalized tissue must be excised. Often the tissue is so closely adhered to the surface of the egg that it cannot be separated and

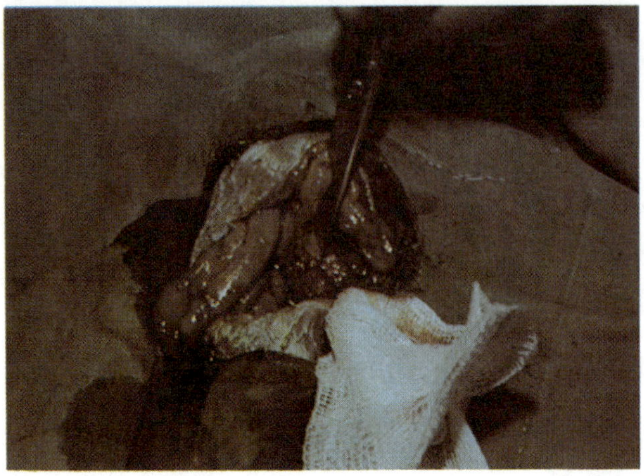

Figure 1—A standard laparotomy approach. To the left is the pancreatic loop of the small intestine. The gizzard is elevated.

must be removed with the egg. After the devitalized tissue has been dissected away, the remaining tissue should be gently teased from the shell surface and the egg should be delivered. If possible, the remaining oviduct should be sutured as described above and replaced into the cloaca. Suturing is often impossible because of the amount of tissue loss, and the oviduct must be replaced without suturing. Although one might expect peritonitis to result, if the bird is kept on systemic antibiotics, uncomplicated recovery often follows.

If a second egg is presented within a few days after surgery, the bird may be in jeopardy. If the egg presents within the cloaca but cannot be passed through the cloacal opening because of the egg's size or irregular shape and rough shell surface, instillation of a sterile lubricant followed by gentle dilation of the cloacal orifice and cloaca and digital pressure from outside the abdomen will often deliver the egg.

If the egg is in the cloaca, wrapped in prolapsed oviduct (Figure 3B), the cloaca should be dilated and lubricated as described above and the oviduct should be incised, allowing the egg to be presented.

If the egg has not been presented into the cloaca but is at the oviduct-cloacal opening (Figure 3C), dilation of the cloaca and the oviduct-cloacal opening will sometimes permit passage of the egg through the orifice into and out of the cloaca. If the orifice cannot be adequately dilated or if the egg is very large, and if the shell membranes can be visualized through the orifice, a hole should be drilled through the presented pole of the egg with an 18-gauge needle and the entire contents of the egg should be aspirated into a syringe. The eggshell should then be compacted down gently by digital pressure through the abdominal wall. In most instances, the egg will compress with particles of shell clinging to the shell membrane, and the compacted egg can be withdrawn through the ori-

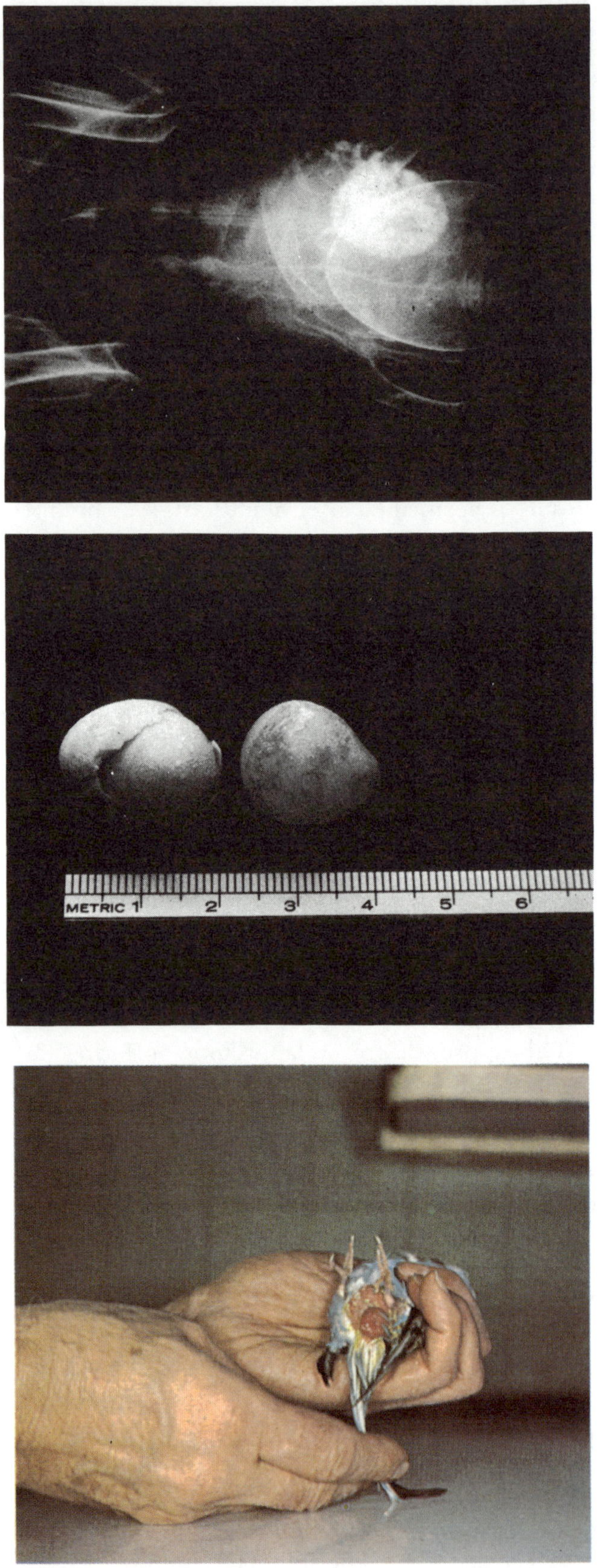

Figure 2—*(A)* Radiograph of a budgerigar in ventrodorsal position. A very large egg clearly fills the caudal abdomen. Note the second egg (broken), visible at the anterior pole of the large egg. *(B)* Two eggs removed through the cloaca in a budgerigar. The shell is very rough and irregular, and the egg shape is abnormal. *(C)* Postsurgical cloacal prolapse of a budgerigar following egg removal.

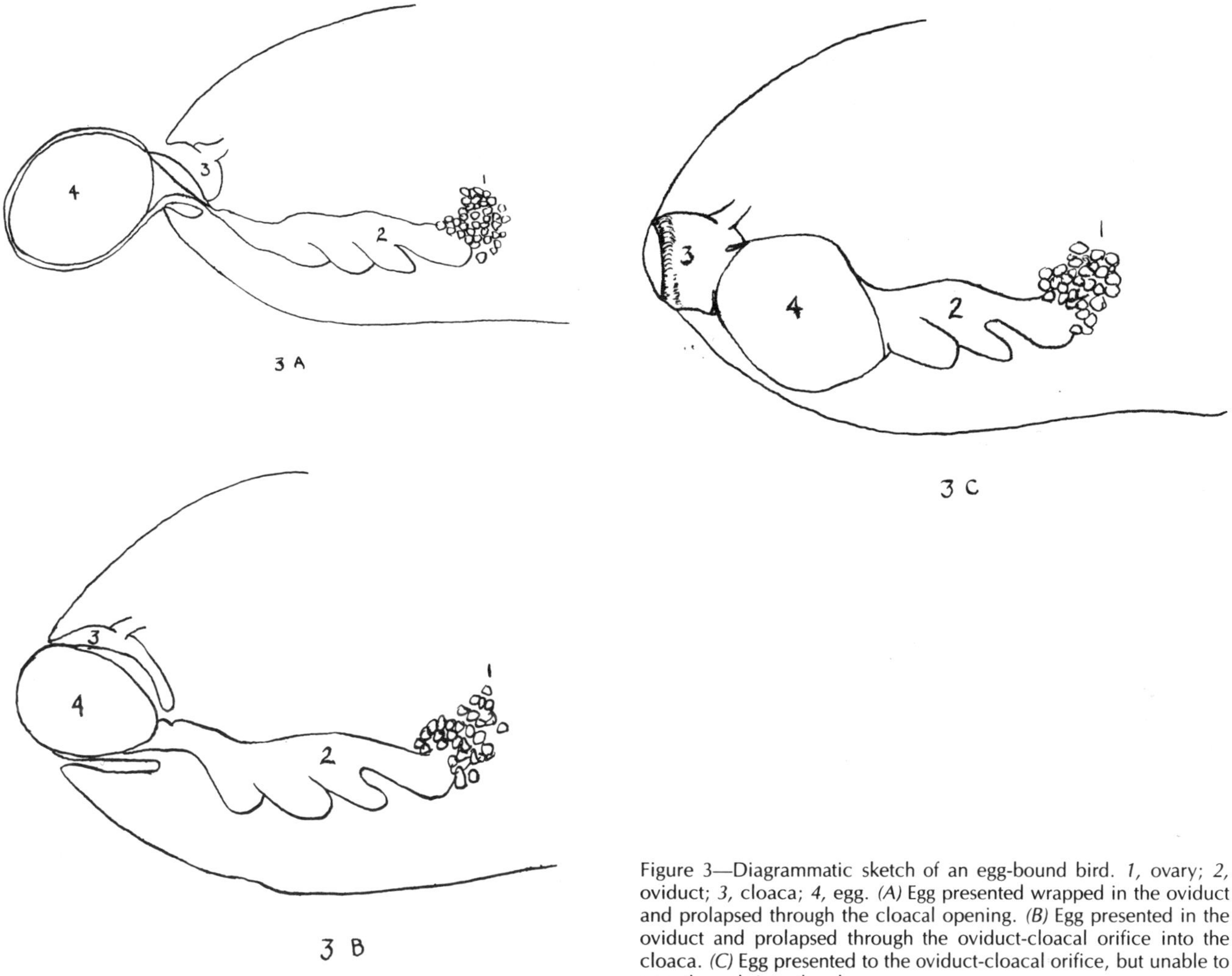

Figure 3—Diagrammatic sketch of an egg-bound bird. *1,* ovary; *2,* oviduct; *3,* cloaca; *4,* egg. *(A)* Egg presented wrapped in the oviduct and prolapsed through the cloacal opening. *(B)* Egg presented in the oviduct and prolapsed through the oviduct-cloacal orifice into the cloaca. *(C)* Egg presented to the oviduct-cloacal orifice, but unable to pass through into the cloaca.

fice with a rat-toothed iris forceps or a small Allis forceps. When extracting the broken egg, care should be taken to ease it out so that the mucosa of the oviduct is not lacerated. Often, the eggshell can be removed in toto, but sometimes piecemeal removal is necessary. It is important to remove all particles of shell from the oviduct. If there have been shell particles or any possibility of egg contents leaking into the oviduct, the oviduct should be irrigated with warm saline to avoid yolk peritonitis. All of the previously described techniques can be performed without anesthesia. Many birds are severely stressed and anesthesia can present a significant risk.

If it is determined that the egg cannot be removed by any of the above techniques, a laparotomy is undertaken. After entering the abdominal cavity, the oviduct can be found on the left side. An incision over the egg through the oviduct easily produces the egg and the incision is sutured as previously stated. If there is necrosis of the oviduct, both the oviduct and ovary are removed.[6]

One of the most consistent sequelae in egg-bound birds in which there have been trauma and devitalization of the oviduct is postsurgical prolapse of the oviduct as a result of tenesmus (Figure 2C). Tenesmus can be minimized by the use of a topical anesthetic cream to reduce sensation and by the placement of a pursestring suture in the cloacal ring. This suture should be tight enough to prevent prolapse but loose enough to permit passage of droppings. The pursestring suture should be removed in 24 hours. Systemic antibiotics should be administered for five to seven days postoperatively.

Eye Enucleation

Enucleation of the avian eye is a common procedure. It is necessitated by postorbital tumors (Figure 4), abscesses, tumors within the globe, and panophthalmitis, which often results from trauma or chronic, nonhealing keratitis and corneal ulcers.

The bird's eye is round, flattened anterioposteriorly, and larger than the opening of the orbit. As a result, the bird's eye is a tight fit for the orbit, and access behind the eye is more difficult than in most mammalian species. Enucleation must be performed under general anesthesia. A circumferential incision is made around the margin of the

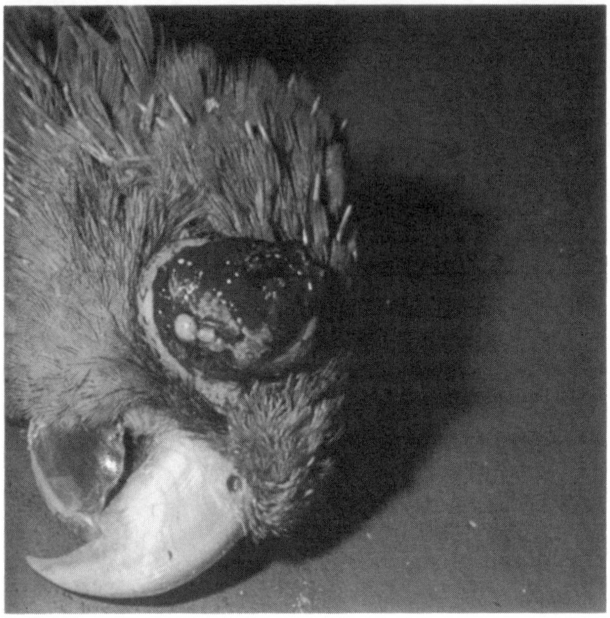

Figure 4A

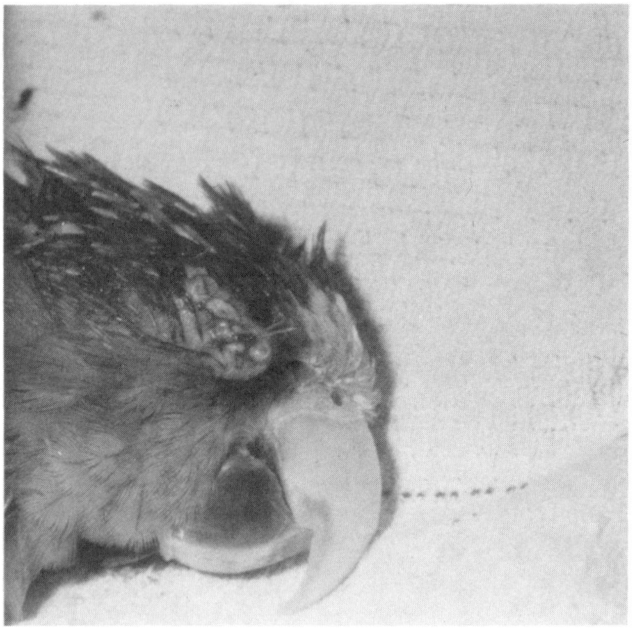

Figure 4B

Figure 4—*(A)* Half-moon parrot with a postorbital tumor proptosing the eye. *(B)* Immediately after eye enucleation.

eyelid approximately 1 to 2 mm from the margin of the lid. The only difficult area to dissect is the medial canthus, which is held by tough fibrous tissue. With blunt dissection, the palpebral conjunctiva and its adnexal tissues are separated within the orbit. By either suturing the separated eyelids together or holding them together with an Allis tissue forceps, tension can be placed on the anterior aspect of the eye, changing the shape of the globe and creating an access to the area behind the eye. The optic nerve and associated vessels are cut as close to the eyeball as possible, permitting ligation of the vessels of the remaining tissues after the eye has been removed. In smaller species, it is not always possible to pick up and ligate the vessels. Bleeding can be controlled either with electrosurgery or by packing the socket with absorbable gelatin sponge.[a] The latter method is only chosen when all other means of hemostasis fail. The incised edges of the lids are sutured together with interrupted 3-0 to 5-0 Vicryl or nylon.

Cryosurgery

Cryosurgery can be of great benefit in specific cases that are difficult to approach because of anatomical limitations or the size of the lesion.

Tumors within the nares (Figure 5) or mouths of small birds are difficult if not impossible to reach by instrumentation, and hemostasis is impossible. Small cryosurgical probes make surgery in these areas feasible. Large, broad-based tumors of the limbs or uropygial glands are amenable to

[a]Gelfoam®, The Upjohn Co., Kalamazoo, MI 49001.

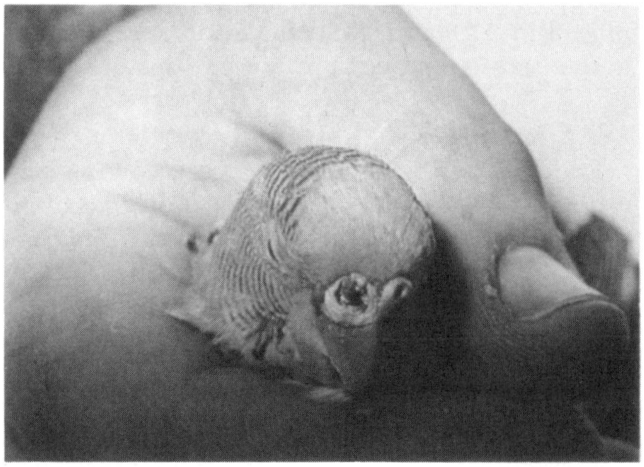

Figure 5—Tumor within the nostril of a budgerigar. This type of tumor is amenable to cryosurgery.

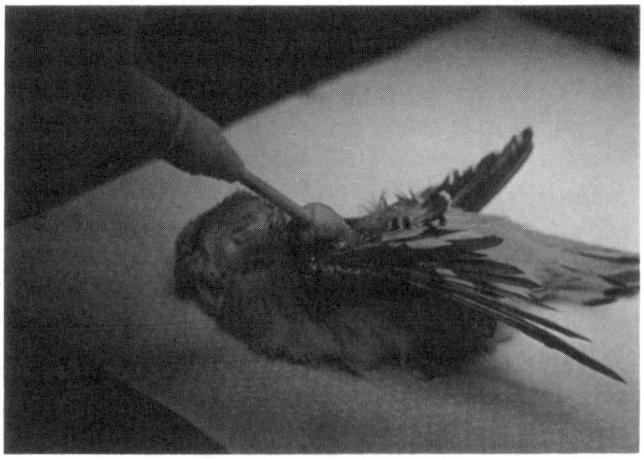

Figure 6—Cryosurgical probe freezing a broad-based tumor of the wing of a budgerigar.

cryosurgery. There is little or no skin elasticity in the region of the uropygial gland, and therefore it is rarely possible to close an incision if any of the skin of the surrounding area has to be extirpated. For very broad-based tumors of the wings (Figure 6), it is usually necessary to utilize two or three freezing procedures over a two- to three-week period.

It is important to follow the patient throughout the sloughing and granulation stages to be certain that the bird does not traumatize the area by picking at it. This is particularly true of psittacine birds. Chewing at the surgical site is common, and severe trauma resulting in significant bleeding can occur. It is therefore prudent to fit the bird with an Elizabethan collar or other device to prevent self-mutilation.

REFERENCES

1. Altman RB, Miller MS: Effects of anesthesia on the temperature and electrocardiogram of birds. *Annu Proc Am Assoc Zoo Vet Denver:* 61-62a, 1979.
2. Redig PT, Roush JC: Orthopedic and soft tissue surgery in raptorial birds, in Fowler M (ed): *Zoo and Wild Animal Medicine.* Philadelphia, WB Saunders Co, 1978, pp 246-253.
3. Wallach JD: Surgical techniques for cage birds, in *The Veterinary Clinics of North America I, Cage Birds.* Philadelphia, WB Saunders Co, 1973, pp 229-235.
4. Dolphin RE, Olsen DE: Surgery in companion birds. *VM SAC Avian Pract:* 1313-1316, 1977.
5. Amand WB: Surgical problems, in Fowler M (ed): *Zoo and Wild Animal Medicine.* Philadelphia, WB Saunders Co, 1978, pp 304-306.
6. Gandal CP: Surgical techniques and anesthesia, in Petrak M (ed): *Diseases of Cage and Aviary Birds.* Philadelphia, Lea & Febiger, 1969, pp 217-231.

Update

Corrective surgery for hyperplastic cloacal mucosal prolapse can incorporate three surgical techniques. When the hyperplastic mucosa prolapses through the cloacal opening, the mucosal surface dries and becomes traumatized and abraded, which causes a great deal of discomfort for the bird.

Surgical approach depends on the severity and amount of hyperplastic tissue. If the hyperplastic tissue is localized to a specific area of the mucosa and is somewhat pedunculated, the hyperplastic tissue can be ligated and excised. However, hyperplastic tissue will more frequently be found to involve the entire circumference of the cloaca just distal to the mucocutaneous junction at the cloacal orifice.

When ligation is not possible because of the extent of the hyperplastic tissue, then mucosal resection is necessary. The procedure can be accomplished by either electrosurgery or cryosurgery. Hemorrhage is more extensive with electrosurgery than with cryosurgery. This condition requires repeated surgical intervention because of its proliferative nature. Cryosurgery is less traumatic to the patient.

Color Atlas of Reptilian Parasites Part I. Protozoans

Susan M. Barnard, BS
Senior Keeper
Department of Herpetology
Atlanta Zoological Park
Atlanta, Georgia

It is impossible to duplicate a reptile's natural environment in captivity. Captivity therefore is stressful, predisposing reptiles to parasitic diseases.[1] Once an infected reptile is captive, those parasites having direct life cycles predominate over parasites requiring intermediate hosts. The consequence of this parasitism is competition with the host animal for food,[2] removal of tissue and fluid, blocking of lymph and blood vessels, edema, ulcerations, necrosis, and anemia.[2-4] Ultimately, death can occur.

The captive reptile's diet includes fruits, vegetables, invertebrates, birds and mammals, and a variety of amphibians and other reptiles. As a result, the feces of a captive reptile contain plant and animal artifacts that too often are mistaken for normal parasitic fauna, leading to unnecessary treatment.

Presented in this four-part series is a pictorial diagnosis of prevalent species of parasites affecting captive reptiles. Also presented are plant and animal artifacts that are commonly mistaken for parasites of reptilian hosts.

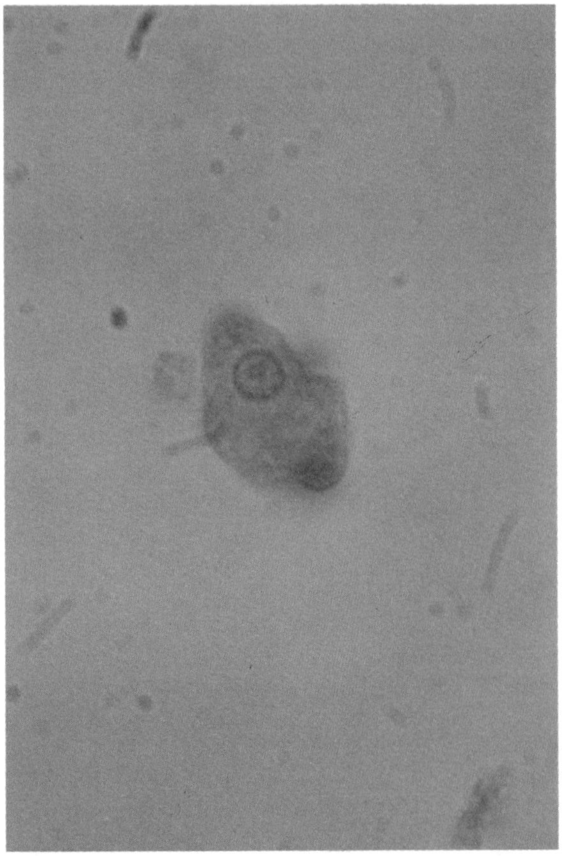

Figure 1A

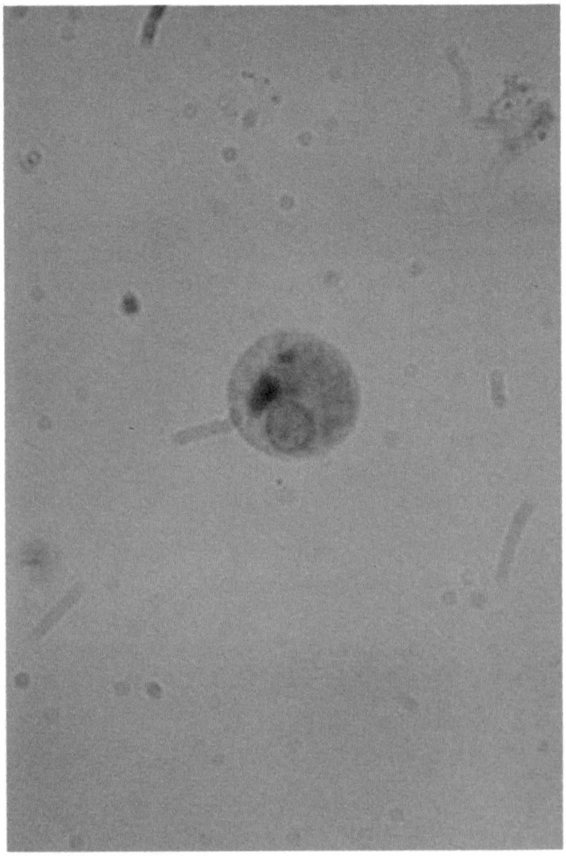

Figure 1B

Figure 1—(**A**) *Entamoeba* sp. trophozoite (×1000) and (**B**) *Entamoeba* sp. cyst (×1000). *Entamoeba invadens* is a highly pathogenic protozoan in lizards and snakes; the most severe damage occurs in the colon and liver. Clinical signs are usually limited to the terminal phase of infection and include anorexia, weight loss, blood and/or mucus in stools, and vomiting. *Entamoeba invadens* is transmitted by ingestion of infective cysts passed in feces. When chemically fixed, trophozoites average 16μ in diameter.[5,6] Cysts measure from 11 to 20μ in diameter and contain from one nucleus to four nuclei.[5,7]

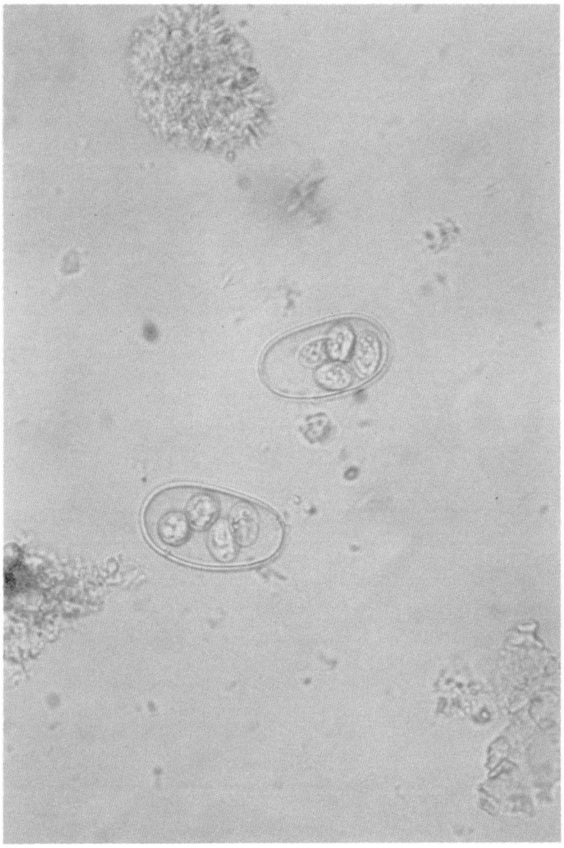

Figure 2A

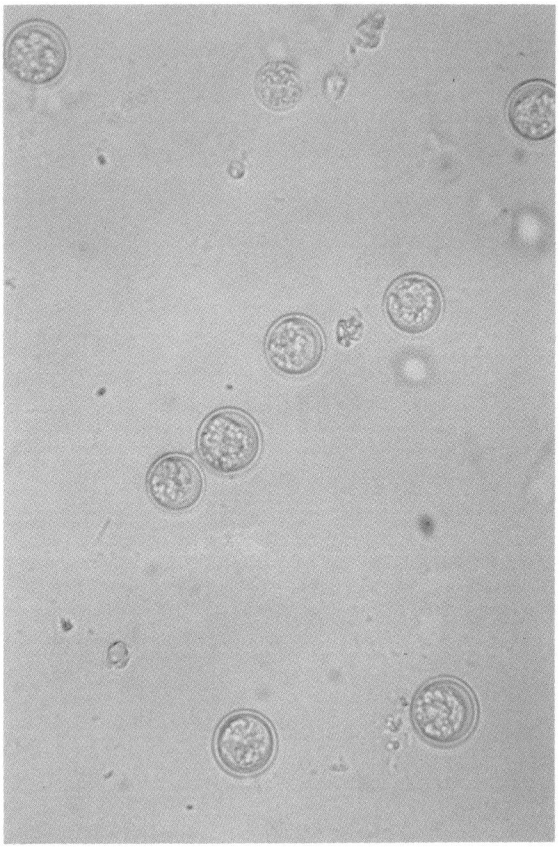

Figure 2B

Figure 2—(**A**) *Eimeria* sp. measuring 10 to 15μ by 25 to 37μ (×400) and (**B**) unsporulated oocysts of *Caryospora simplex* measuring 13.5 to 16.2μ in diameter (×400). *Eimeria* is the primary coccidian found in reptiles[4,8-10]; but several others, such as *Caryospora, Isospora,* and *Sarcocystis,* are also common.[5,11] The intestinal tract and gallbladder are primarily affected, causing such clinical signs as restlessness, anorexia, and regurgitation. Transmission occurs by ingestion of sporulated oocysts from contaminated feces or soil. Oocysts vary in size according to species.

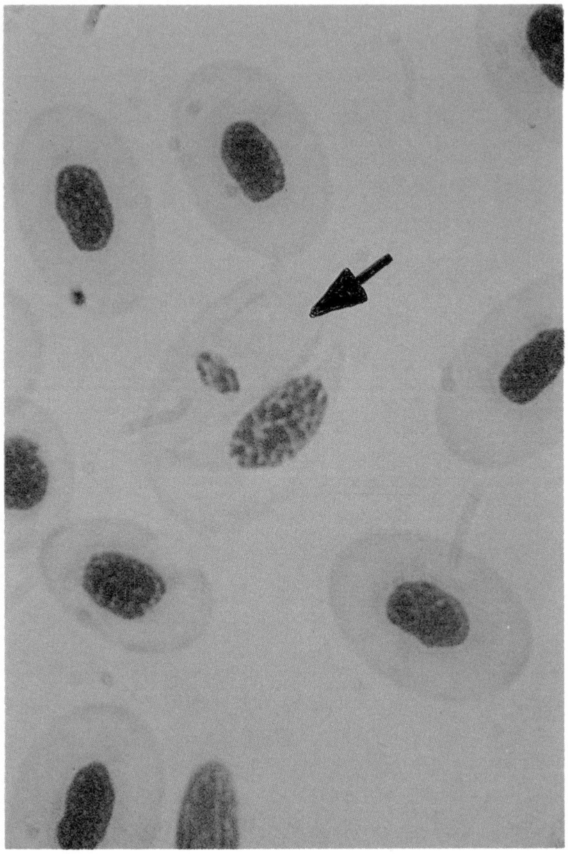

Figure 3

Figure 3—*Haemogregarina* sp. (*arrow*) (×1000). The major genera of blood sporozoans affecting reptiles include *Haemogregarina, Haemoproteus, Hepatozoon, Karyolysus, Plasmodium, Schellackia,* and *Simondia.*[7,12,13] Transmission occurs through the bites of leeches, ticks, and other blood-sucking invertebrates and by ingestion of mites.[4,7,14-16] A heavy infection of blood sporozoans has been known to cause anemia and inanition in snakes.[17,18]

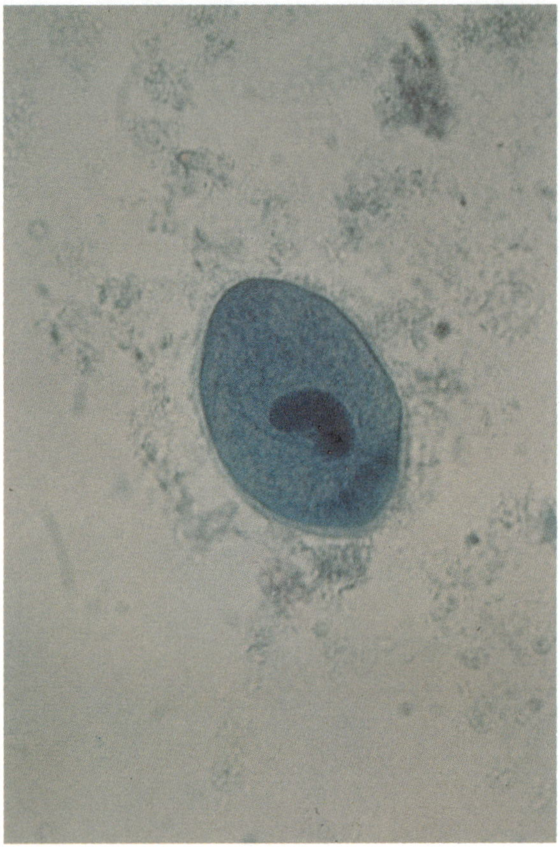

Figure 4A

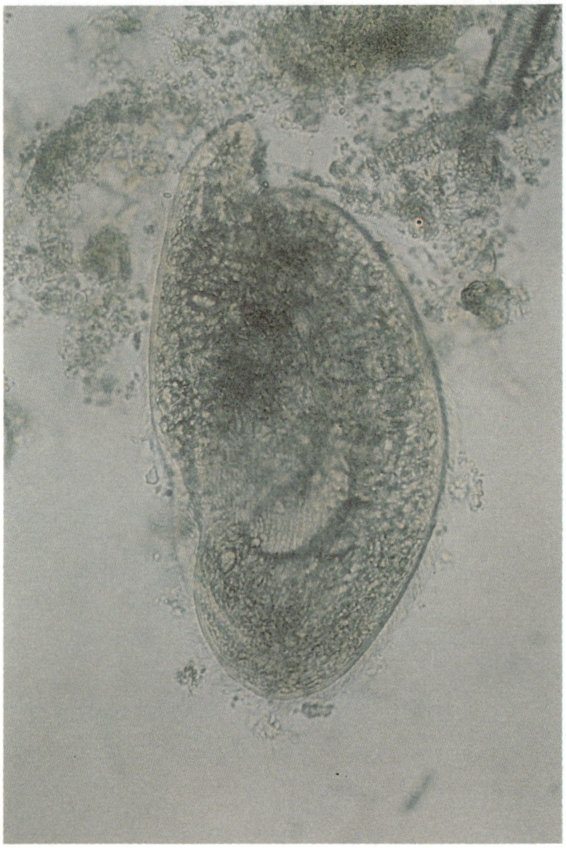

Figure 4B

Figure 4—(**A**) *Balantidium* sp. trophozoite (×400), (**B**) *Nyctotherus* sp. trophozoite (×200), and (**C**) *Nyctotherus* sp. cyst (×400). Although ciliates commonly affect tortoises, they have also been known to affect lizards and snakes. *Balantidium* and *Nyctotherus* are the two primary genera of ciliates affecting reptiles,[4] and they inhabit the host's intestines. *Balantidium* trophozoites vary in length from 70 to 300μ,[5] and *Nyctotherus* trophozoites vary in length from 60 to 190μ.[5] *Nyctotherus* is not known to be pathogenic[5,6]; however, *Balantidium* may be pathogenic in large numbers or in association with other parasites or pathogenic bacteria.[5,10] Transmission is by ingestion of the parasites passed in affected feces.

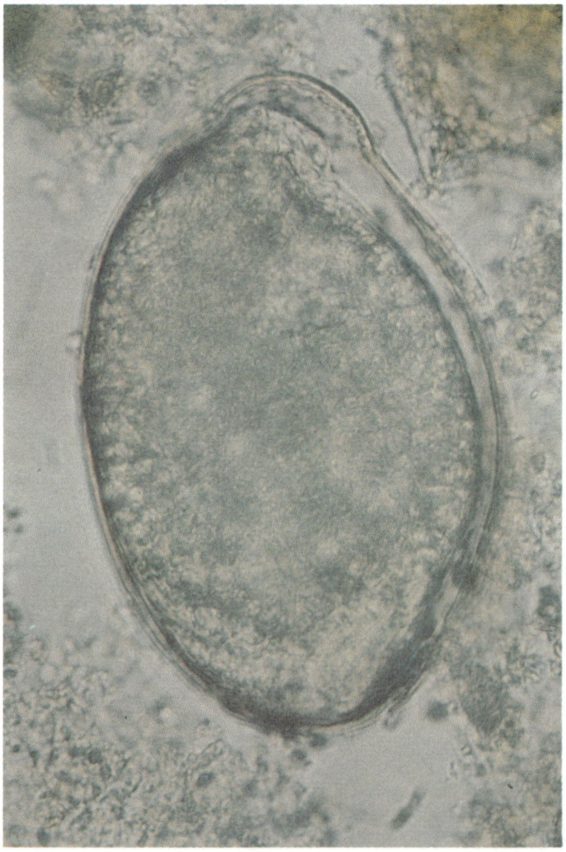

Figure 4C

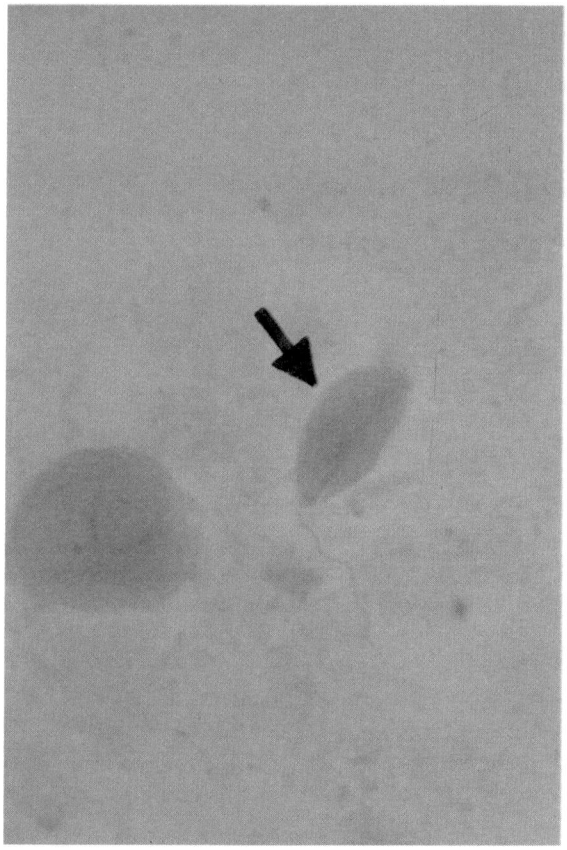

Figure 5—Trichomonad (*arrow*) (×1000). Pathogenicity caused by flagellates may vary according to a reptile's species, age, and general health. Young animals and those with other disorders are more likely to suffer deleterious effects. *Trypanosoma* and *Leishmania* commonly occur in reptiles and inhabit the circulatory system and intestines.[5,6] Flagellates affecting primarily the host's intestines include trichomonads, *Hexamastix, Hexamita, Monocercomonas,* and *Proteromonas.*[4-7] *Hexamita* also affects the urinary bladder of chelonians.[5,9] Trypanosomes are transmitted to reptiles by leeches and arthropod vectors. *Leishmania* can be contracted by either a bite or ingestion of an invertebrate intermediate host,[5,6] and the intestinal flagellates are contracted by ingestion of the organism passed in affected feces. Diagnosis is best made by direct smear because the movement of flagellates is easily observed.

Acknowledgments

This study was supported, in part, by the Society for the Study of Amphibians and Reptiles, the American Association of Zoo Keepers, and the Atlanta Zoological Society. My deepest appreciation and thanks to Dr. Daniel R. Brooks, Dr. Steve J. Upton, and Dr. Nixon Wilson for their diagnostic expertise; to Mr. Rick Etzel, Ms. Tamara Romaine, and Mr. Fred Alvey for their assistance with the literature search; and to Ms. Susanne Wahlquist, Dr. Susan Wade, and the many individuals and institutions submitting fecal material, parasites, and prepared slides.

REFERENCES

1. Telford SR Jr: Parasite diseases of reptiles. *JAVMA* (11)159:1644-1652, 1971.
2. Soulsby EJL: *Helminths, Arthropods, and Protozoa of Domestic Animals (Monnig).* Philadelphia, Lea & Febiger, 1968.
3. Frank W: Endoparasites, in Cooper JE, Jackson OF (eds): *Diseases of the Reptilia,* vol 1. New York, Academic Press, 1981.
4. Reichenback-Klinke H, Elkan E: *The Principal Diseases of Lower Vetebrates.* New York, Academic Press, 1965.
5. Flynn RJ: *Parasites of Laboratory Animals.* Ames, IA, Iowa State University Press, 1973.
6. Frye FL: *Biomedical and Surgical Aspects of Captive Reptile Husbandry.* Edwardsville, KS, Veterinary Medicine Publishing Co, 1981.
7. Marcus LC: *Veterinary Biology and Medicine of Captive Amphibians and Reptiles.* Philadelphia, Lea & Febiger, 1981.
8. Bovee EC, Telford SR Jr: *Eimeria sceloporis* and *Eimeria molochis* ssp. n. from lizards. *J Parasitol* 51:85-94, 1965.
9. Keymer IF: Protozoa, in Cooper JE, Jackson OF (eds): *Diseases of the Reptilia,* vol 1. New York, Academic Press, 1981.
10. Kiel JL: A review of parasites in snakes. *Southwestern Vet* (3)28:209-220, 1975.
11. Pellerdy LP: *Coccidia and Coccidiosis.* Budapest, Akademiae Kiado, 1965.
12. MacKerras MJ: Hematozoa of Australian reptiles. *Aust J Zool* 9:61-122, 1961.
13. McGhee RB: Diseases caused by *Protista,* in Weinman D, Ristic M (eds): *Infectious Blood Diseases of Man and Animals.* New York, Academic Press, 1968.
14. Booden T, et al: Transfer of *Hepatozoon* sp. from boa constrictor to a lizard, *Anolis carolinensis* by mosquito vectors. *J Parasitol* 56:832-833, 1970.
15. Chao J, Ball GH: Transfer of *Hepatozoon rarefaciens* (Sanbon and Seligman, 1907) from the indigo snake to a gopher snake by a mosquito vector. *J Parasitol* 55:681-682, 1969.
16. Hazen TA, et al: The parasite fauna of the American alligator (*Alligator mississippiensis*) in South Carolina. *J Wildl Dis* 14:435-439, 1978.
17. Fantham HB, Porter A: The endoparasites of some North American snakes and their effects on the Ophidia. *Proc Zool Soc Lond* 123:867-898, 1953.
18. Fiennes RN T-W: Report of the society's pathologist for the year 1957. *Proc Zool Soc Lond* 132:129-146, 1959.

Color Atlas of Reptilian Parasites Part II. Flatworms and Roundworms

Susan M. Barnard, BS
Senior Keeper
Department of Herpetology
Atlanta Zoological Park
Atlanta, Georgia

Flukes (class Trematoda) and tapeworms (class Cestoidea) are dorsoventrally flattened parasites that belong to the phylum Platyhelminthes. All flukes are parasitic, either as external parasites or as endoparasites. Two types of trematodes affecting reptiles are those requiring a single host (the monogenic flukes) and the more numerous digenic flukes. Digenic trematodes must parasitize two or more hosts before completing their life cycle.

The eggs of tapeworms vary considerably in form and size. Some eggs pass from the reptilian host intact within the proglottids; others escape from the tapeworm's uterine pore into the host's intestinal tract, where they can be observed in feces microscopically.

Parasitic nematodes (class Nematoda) of reptiles range in length from a few millimeters to over 30 centimeters. Their eggs may be observed microscopically in reptilian feces, uric acid, or sputum, depending on the species.

Some commonly occurring flatworm and roundworm eggs observed in reptiles after captivity are presented in this article. The other nematode genera will be reviewed in Part III of this series.

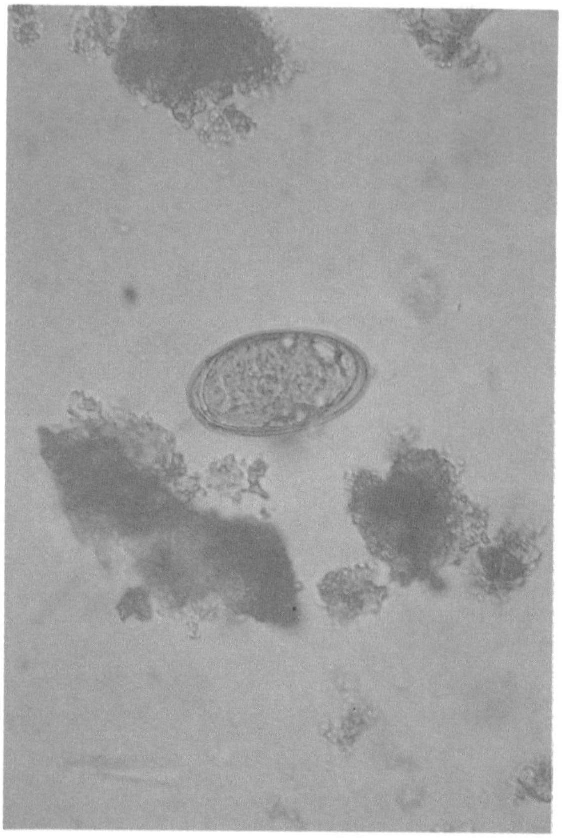

Figure 1—*Ochetosoma* sp. (×400). Flukes of the genus *Ochetosoma* are digenic trematodes that primarily inhabit a reptile's intestinal tract. Other commonly parasitized areas are the lungs, liver and gallbladder, circulatory system, and genital tract; trematodes also may be found free within the coelomic cavity.[5-10] Larval forms locate in the host's muscle, bile duct, skin, and various other tissues.[7,8] Transmission occurs when the reptile ingests such intermediate hosts as amphibians and crayfish. Severe infections can cause listlessness, anorexia, weight loss, dyspnea, uremia, pressure necrosis, and ultimately death. Digenic fluke eggs are gold to dark brown in color and measure 20 to 40μ long.[10]

Figure 2—(**A**, **B**, **C**, and **D**) Eggs from various cestodes observed in the feces of reptiles (×400). Cestodes affecting reptiles are hermaphroditic[9] and non-host specific.[8] Humans can become infected with some species by introducing contaminated material from their hands into their eyes.[8] Transmission to the reptile occurs by ingestion of intermediate hosts, such as ticks, copepods, fish, frogs, tadpoles, or other reptiles. Cockroaches can mechanically transfer cestode infections and are also a potential intermediate host.[8] Adult worms compete for nutrients and can cause chronic enteritis; large species may be pathogenic because of their size. Larval forms cause sparganosis in reptiles, and tissue damage can occur as larvae migrate throughout the body. Sparganosis should be suspected when subcutaneous or intramuscular lumps are detected on palpation.

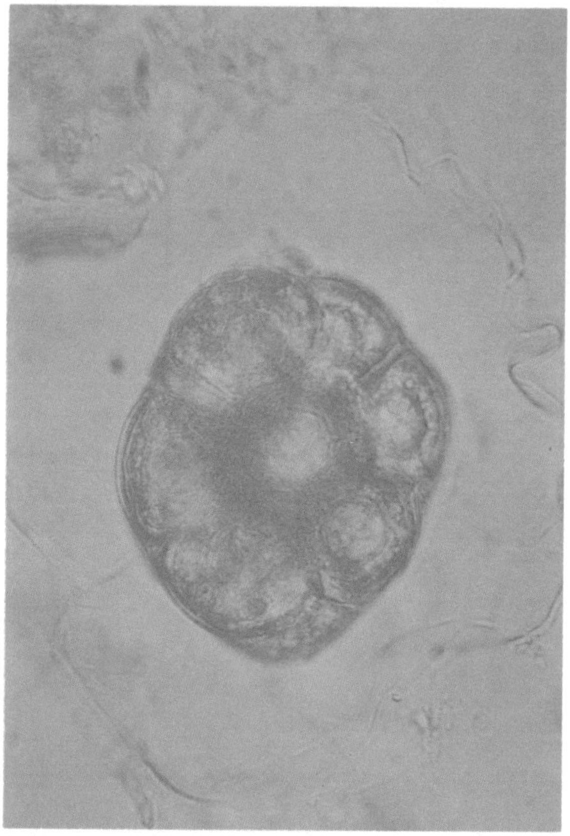

Figure 2A

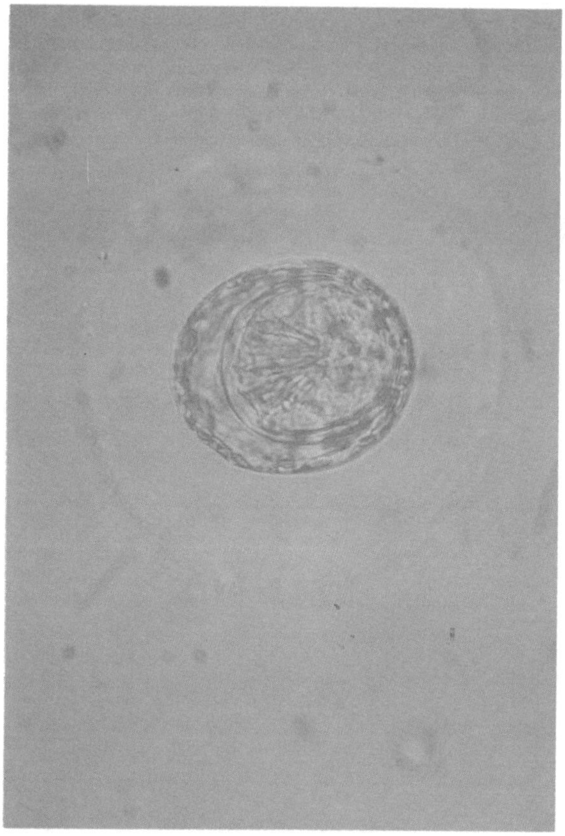

Figure 2B

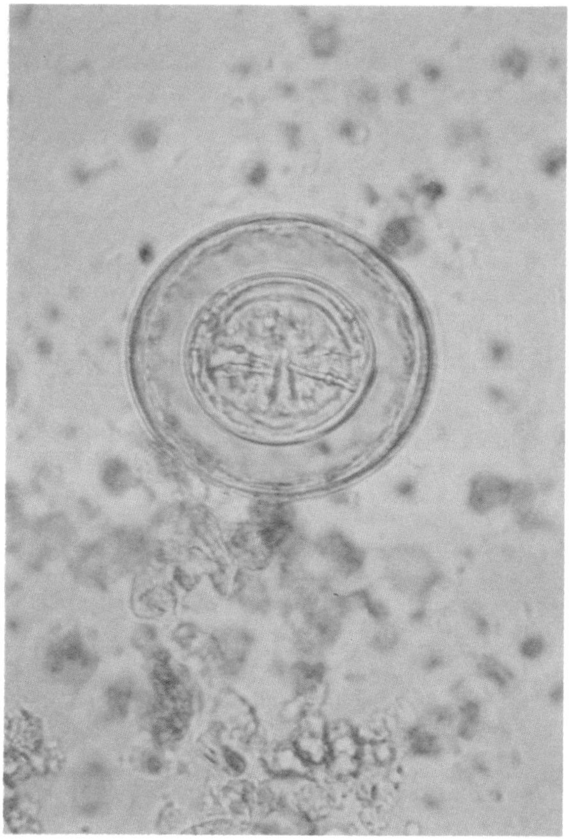

Figure 2C

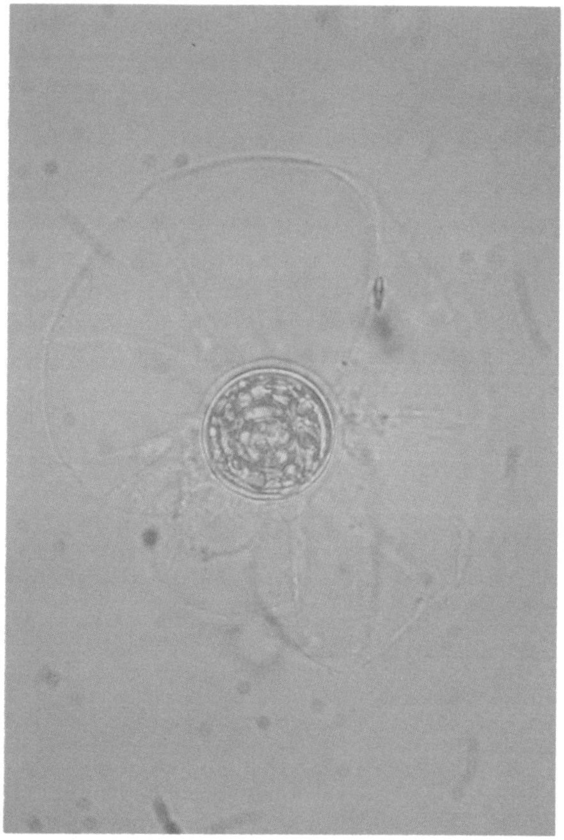

Figure 2D

Figure 3—(A) *Strongyloides* sp. egg (×400) and **(B)** *Strongyloides* sp. larva (×400). Based on egg size and description, the parasites in the genera *Strongyloides* and *Rhabdias* are impossible to differentiate solely on microscopic examination. If *Rhabdias* is suspected, diagnosis is possible if eggs can be demonstrated in wet mounts from tracheal washings. *Strongyloides* inhabits the small intestine or esophagus, while *Rhabdias* inhabits the host's lungs. Transmission occurs (1) by ingestion of embryonated eggs or infective third-stage larvae or (2) possibly by penetration of infective larvae through the skin. In both genera, the parasite can survive in a free-living form for several generations. Clinical signs of *Strongyloides* may be diarrhea, while *Rhabdias* may cause respiratory distress. Both parasites cause anorexia resulting in weight loss or death.

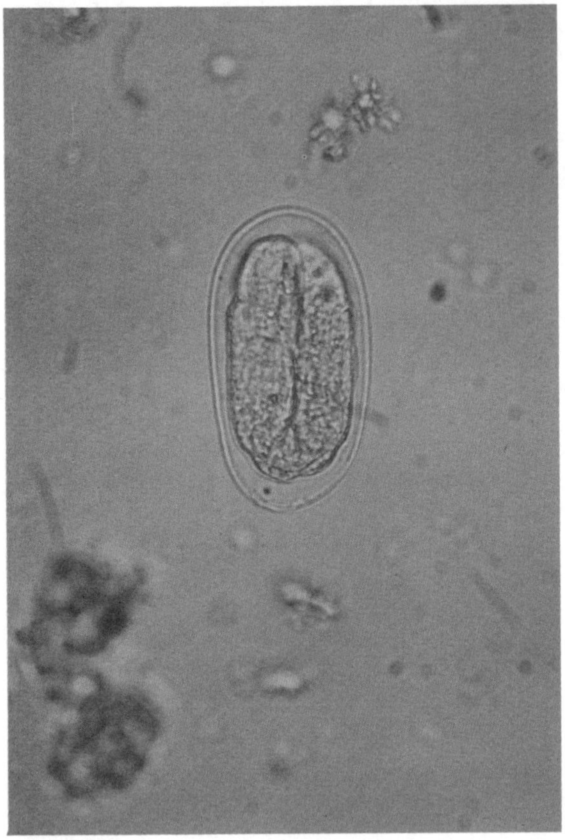

Figure 3A

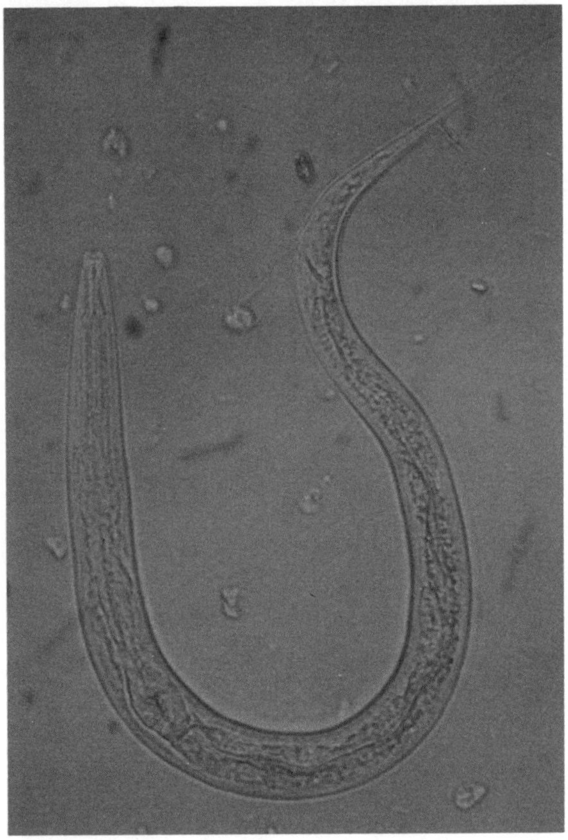

Figure 3B

Acknowledgments

This study was supported, in part, by the Society for the Study of Amphibians and Reptiles, the American Association of Zoo Keepers, and the Atlanta Zoological Society. My deepest appreciation and thanks to Dr. Daniel R. Brooks, Dr. Steve J. Upton, and Dr. Nixon Wilson for their diagnostic expertise; to Mr. Rick Etzel, Ms. Tamara Romaine, and Mr. Fred Alvey for their assistance with the literature search; and to Ms. Susanne Wahlquist, Dr. Susan Wade, and the many individuals and institutions submitting fecal material, parasites, and prepared slides.

REFERENCES

1. Cheng TC: *The Biology of Animal Parasites.* Philadelphia, WB Saunders Co, 1964.
2. Yorke W, Maplestone PA: *The Nematode Parasites of Vertebrates.* Philadelphia, Blakiston, 1926.
3. Ortlepp RJ: Observations on the nematode genera *Kalicephalus, Diaphanocephalus,* and *Occipitodontus* g.n., and on the larval development of *Kalicephalus philodryadus* sp. n. *J Heminthol* 1:165-189, 1923.
4. Harwood PD: The helminths parasitic in the amphibia and reptilia of Houston, Texas and vicinity. *Proc US Natl Mus* 81:1-71, 1932.
5. Frank W: Endoparasites, in Cooper JE, Jackson OF (eds): *Diseases of the Reptilia,* vol I. New York, Academic Press, 1981.
6. Reichenback-Klinke H, Elkan E: *The Principal Diseases of Lower Vertebrates.* New York, Academic Press, 1965.
7. Flynn RJ: *Parasites of Laboratory Animals.* Ames, IA, Iowa State University Press, 1973.
8. Frye FL: *Biomedical and Surgical Aspects of Captive Reptile Husbandry.* Edwardsville, KS, Veterinary Medicine Publishing Co, 1981.
9. Marcus LC: *Veterinary Biology and Medicine of Captive Amphibians and Reptiles.* Philadelphia, Lea & Febiger, 1980.
10. Kiel JL: A review of parasites in snakes. *Southwestern Vet* 28(3):209-220, 1975.

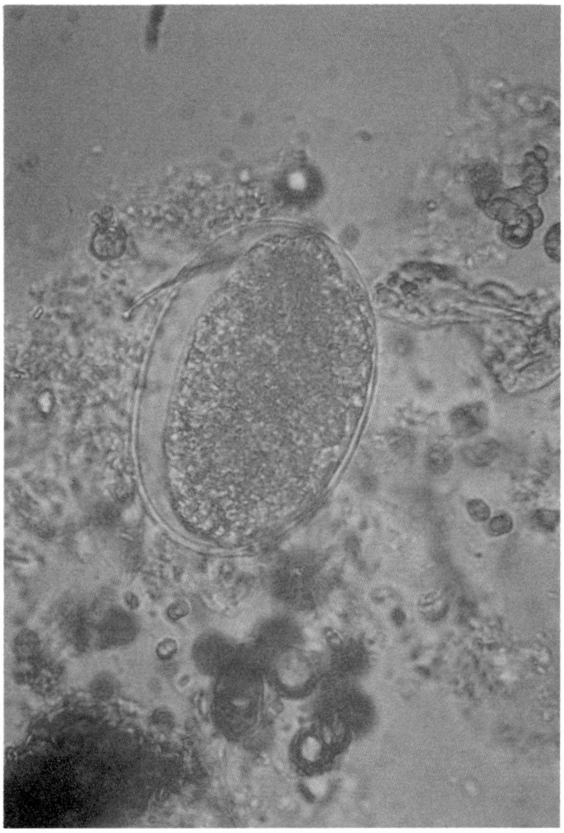

Figure 4A

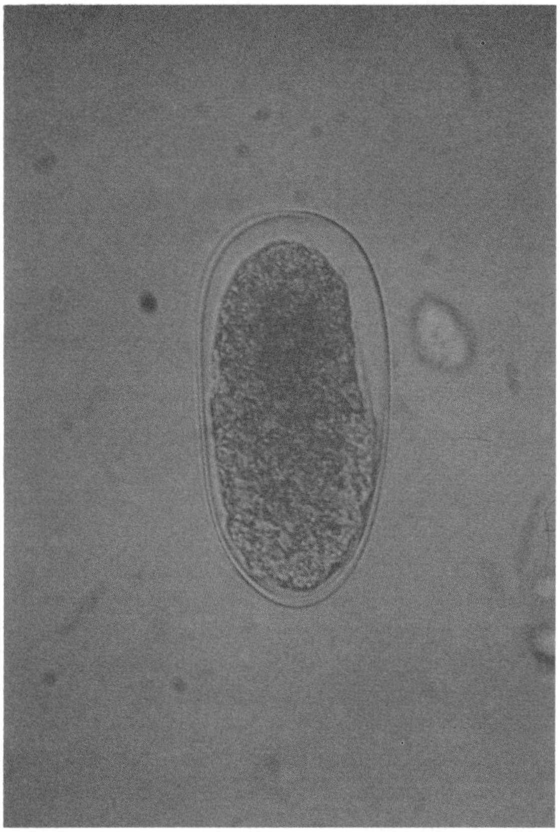

Figure 4B

Figure 4—(**A**) *Oswaldocruzia* sp. (×400) and (**B**) *Kalicephalus* sp. (×400). *Oswaldocruzia* and *Kalicephalus* are hookworms that occur in reptiles worldwide and that inhabit the host's digestive tract. The two genera are similar in appearance. Transmission of *Oswaldocruzia* is probably direct, but little is known about its life cycle.[1,2] Transmission of *Kalicephalus* is (1) by ingestion of ova or infective third-stage larvae or (2) possibly by penetration of infective larvae through the skin. Severe infections of *Oswaldocruzia* may cause intestinal obstruction and peritonitis. *Kalicephalus* may cause anemia, hemorrhagic ulcers, and intestinal obstruction. A *Kalicephalus* organism measures 55 to 100μ long and 27 to 50μ wide[3]; *Oswaldocruzia* measures 75 to 80μ long by 42 to 50μ wide.[4]

Color Atlas of Reptilian Parasites. Part III. Miscellaneous Endoparasites and Ectoparasites

Susan M. Barnard, BS
Senior Keeper
Department of Herpetology
Atlanta Zoological Park
Atlanta, Georgia

Part III of this four-part series features diagnostic photomicrographs of nematode eggs (class Nematoda) commonly observed in reptilian feces as well as photomicrographs of a pentastomid egg (class Pentastomida) and the snake mite, *Ophionyssus natricis*.

Some pentastomid infections may infect reptiles for only about a year if the reptile is maintained under optimum hygienic conditions; however, those species of pentastomids that are capable of autoinfection may survive within the captive reptilian host for many years.

Ectoparasites often transmit other parasites and may be vectors for such diseases as Q fever, tularemia, and Russian spring and summer encephalitis. Common places where ectoparasites may be found are under a reptile's scales in the areas of the chin, eyes, cloaca, body folds, and buccal cavity.

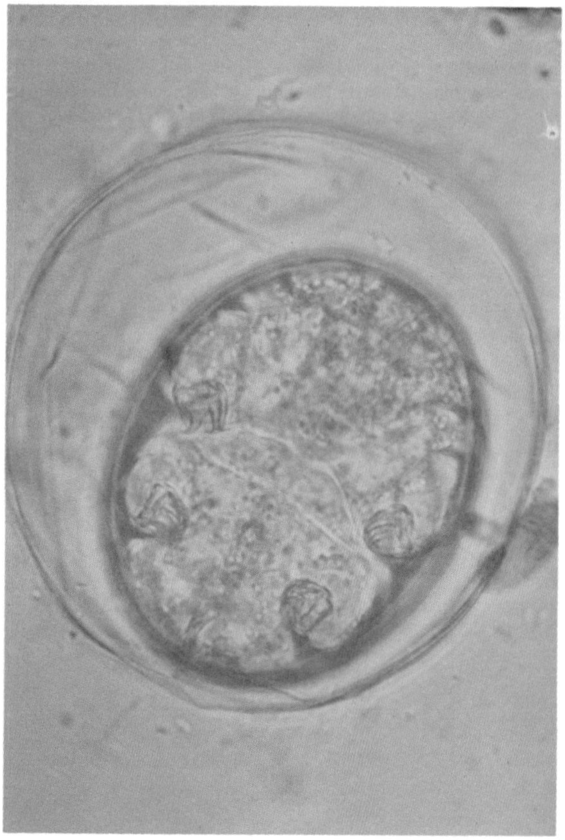

Figure 1—Pentastomid egg (×400). Pentastomids, also called *tongue-worms,* possess the qualities of both annelids and arachnids. The most common are *Porocephalus, Armillifer, Kiricephalus,* and *Raillietiella.* The lung is the primary host location for *Porocephalus* and *Armillifer.*[1,2] Adult *Raillietiella* and *Kiricephalus* also inhabit the lung,[1] while larvae and nymphs are found in subcutaneous tissue and the stomach wall.[3,4] All stages of *Raillietiella* have been reported in the lungs of a fer-de-lance snake (*Bothrops atrox*).[5] Transmission occurs from ingestion of an intermediate mammalian host. Therefore, feeding captured wild rodents to captive reptiles should be avoided. Because humans are an accidental host,[3] care should be exercised when handling infected animals. Clinical signs include lethargy, anorexia, dyspnea, and blood-tinged sputum. Some reptiles do not suffer deleterious effects from a pentastomid infection. Others, however, may suffer from hemorrhagic, acute inflammatory, or chronic granulomatous reaction in the colon, liver, or lungs from migrating larvae, nymphs, and adults.[3,6] Eggs measure approximately 130 to 140 μ.[7]

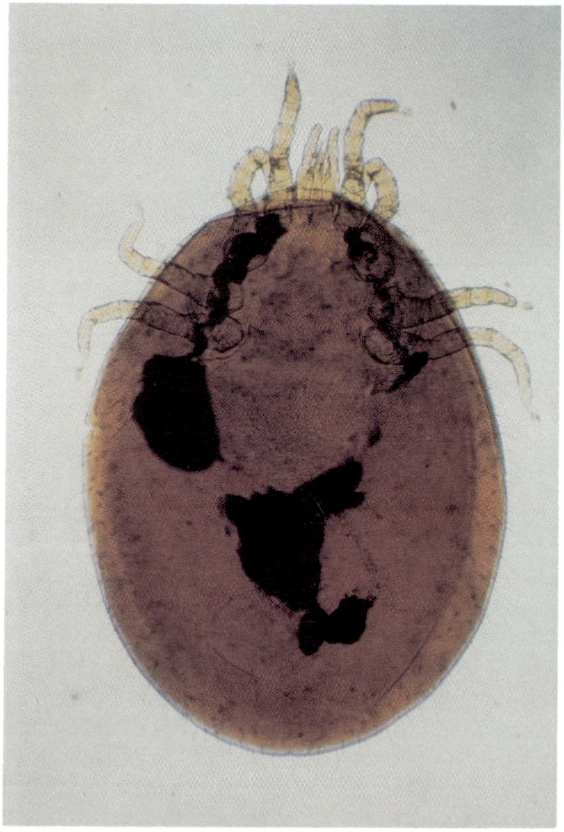

Figure 2

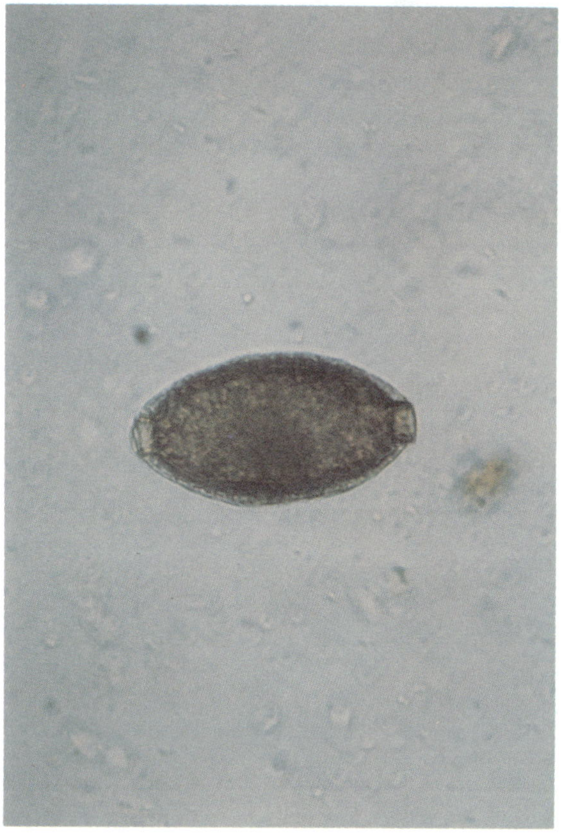

Figure 3

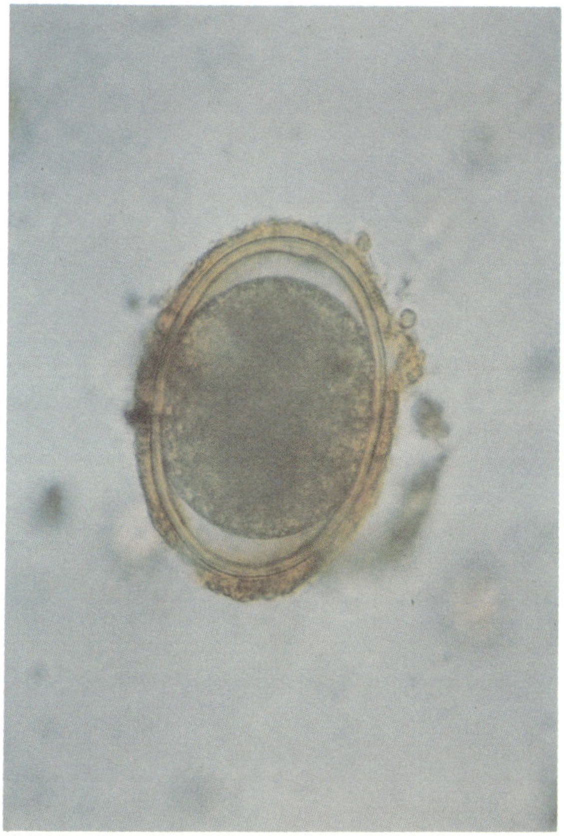

Figure 4

Figure 2—The snake mite, *Ophionyssus natricis* (×40). Of the 250 species of mites that affect reptiles, *O. natricis* is the most common to occur in captive reptiles. It is a mechanical vector for *Aeromonas hydrophila,*[8] the major causative organism of pneumonia. This ectoparasite is transmitted easily from one animal to another and causes irritation to the affected reptile. Infested animals may be observed soaking themselves excessively in their water-bowls or continually rubbing and twisting. Severe infestations can cause anemia and death.

Figure 3—*Capillaria* sp. (×400). *Capillaria* is the only known genus of trichurids to infect lizards and snakes.[3,5] These organisms primarily inhabit the host's intestines but have been observed in other organs.

Figure 4—*Ophidascaris* sp. (×400). *Ophidascaris* and *Hexametra* are the two most common genera of ascarids found in snakes.[3,4] They inhabit the host's stomach, esophagus, and/or small intestine. Severe infections of adult worms can occlude the stomach, causing the animal to regurgitate.[5] Diarrhea[3] and purulent pneumonia[9] are other frequent problems. The most probable source of infection in nature is by ingestion of such intermediate hosts as frogs and rodents.[10,11] Both genera measure 83 μ in diameter.[12]

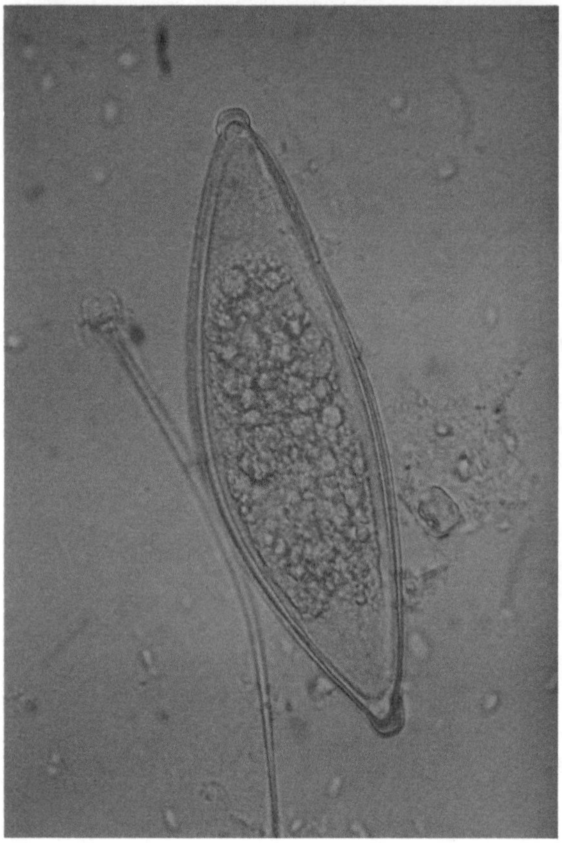

Figure 5A

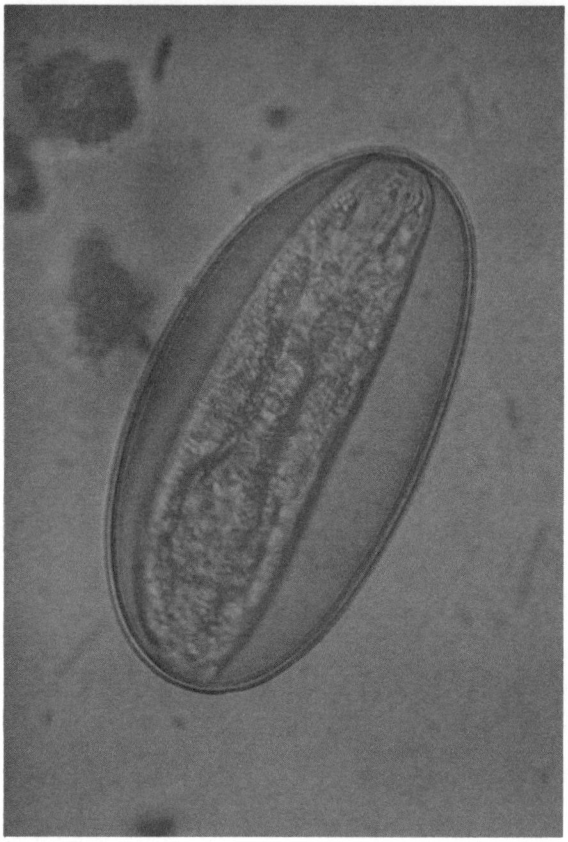

Figure 5B

Figure 5—(**A, B,** and **C**) Oxyurids commonly observed in the feces of reptiles (×400). *Falcaustra* and *Parapharyngodon* have been reported to be the most common oxyurids of reptiles in the United States.[13-16] Also common are (**A**) *Pharyngodon* in lizards and (**B**) *Tachygonetria* in chelonians of the family Testudinidae and lizards in the genus *Uromastix*.[1,5] Generally, oxyurids are nonpathogenic. They have a direct life cycle and inhabit the host's colon. (**C**) Oxyurid eggs are one of the most common helminths observed in lizards.

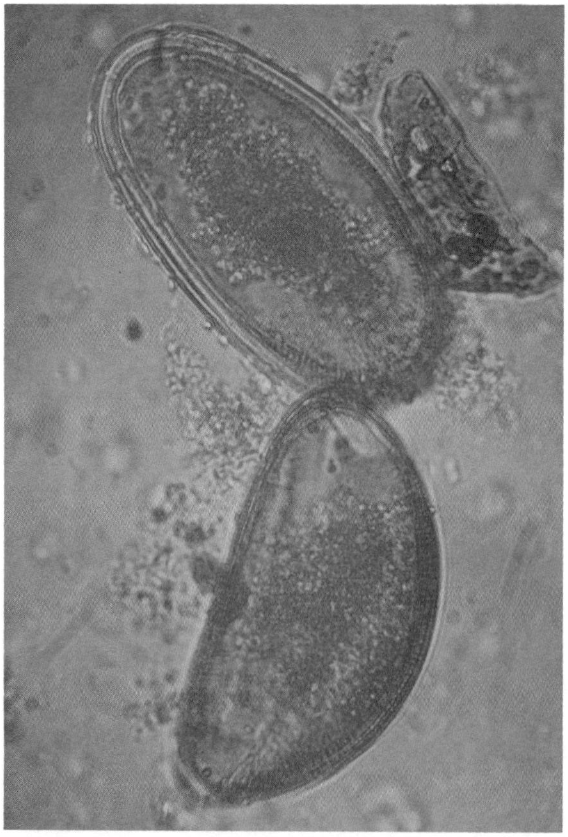

Figure 5C

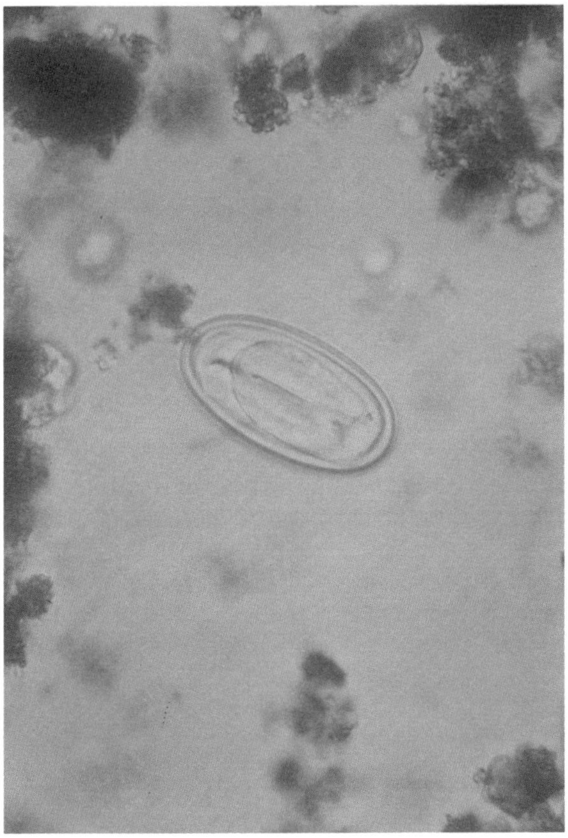

Figure 6—Spirurid ovum measuring 32.5 μ by 52.5 μ (×400). The life cycles of spirurids include two or more hosts.[1] Reptiles may either act as the intermediate hosts for birds and mammals or serve as the final hosts.[1,4,5] Aquatic reptiles become infected by ingesting the larval stages when feeding on copepods. Insects and other arthropods serve as a source of infection for terrestrial reptiles. Ants are a common source of infection, and captive reptiles may become infected if ants gain access to caging. Some commonly occurring spirurids are *Abbreviata*, which infect lizards, and *Gnathostoma*, which parasitize crocodilians and other reptiles.[1] *Physaloptera*, *Skrjabinoptera*, and *Thubunaea* commonly infect snakes and other reptiles.[1,3] *Proleptus* is known to infect chelonians.[1] Spirurids are parasites of the mouth and gastrointestinal tract.

Acknowledgments

This study was supported, in part, by the Society for the Study of Amphibians and Reptiles, the American Association of Zoo Keepers, and the Atlanta Zoological Society. My deepest appreciation and thanks to Dr. Daniel R. Brooks, Dr. Steve J. Upton, and Dr. Nixon Wilson for their diagnostic expertise; to Mr. Rick Etzel, Ms. Tamara Romaine, and Mr. Fred Alvey for their assistance with the literature search; and to Ms. Susanne Wahlquist, Dr. Susan Wade, and the many individuals and institutions submitting fecal material, parasites, and prepared slides.

REFERENCES

1. Reichenback-Klinke H, Elkan E: *The Principal Diseases of Lower Vertebrates*. New York, Academic Press, 1965.
2. Frye FL: *Biomedical and Surgical Aspects of Captive Reptile Husbandry*. Edwardsville, KS, Veterinary Medicine Publishing Co, 1981.
3. Kiel JL: A review of parasites in snakes. *Southwestern Vet* 28(3):209-220, 1975.
4. Marcus LC: *Veterinary Biology and Medicine of Captive Amphibians and Reptiles*. Philadelphia, Lea & Febiger, 1981.
5. Frank W: Endoparasites, in Cooper JE, Jackson OF (eds): *Diseases of the Reptilia*, vol I. New York, Academic Press, 1981.
6. Deakins DE: Diagnosis and treatment of parasites of amphibians and reptiles. *Am Assoc Zoo Vet Ann Proc*:37-46, 1972-1973.
7. Slocombe JO, Budd J: *Armillifer brumpti* (Pentastomida) in a boa in Canada. *J Wildl Dis* 9:352-355, 1973.
8. Camin JH: Mite transmission of a hemorrhagic septicemia in snakes. *J Parasitol* 34:345-354, 1948.
9. Wallach JD: Medical care of reptiles. *JAVMA* 155:1017-1034, 1969.
10. Sprent JF: Studies on ascaridoid nematodes in pythons: The life history and development of *Ophidascaris moreliae* in Australian pythons. *Parasitology* 60:97-122, 1970.
11. Sprent JF: Studies on ascaridoid nematodes in pythons: The life history and development of *Polydelphis anoura* in Australian pythons. *Parasitology* 60:375-397, 1970.
12. Harwood PD: The helminths parasitic in the Amphibia and Reptilia of Houston, Texas and vicinity. *Proc US Natl Mus* 81:1-71, 1932.
13. Rausch R: Observations on some helminths parasitic in Ohio turtles. *Am Midl Nat* 38:434-442, 1947.
14. Walton AC: The parasites of amphibia. *J Wildl Dis* 40:(microcard), 1964.
15. Williams RW: Helminths of the snapping turtle, *Chelydra serpentina*, from Oklahoma, including the first report and description of the male of *Capillaria serpentina* (Harwood, 1932). *Trans Am Microsc Soc* 72:175-178, 1953.
16. Yamaguti S: The nematodes of vertebrates, in Yamaguti S (ed): *Systema helminthum*, vol 3. New York, Interscience Publications, 1961.

Color Atlas of Reptilian Parasites Part IV. Pseudoparasites

Susan M. Barnard, BS
Senior Keeper
Department of Herpetology
Atlanta Zoological Park
Atlanta, Georgia

The diet of a captive reptile comprises various plant material and animals, including fruits, vegetables, invertebrates, birds, mammals, amphibians, and other reptiles. Consequently, the feces of reptiles contain remnants and/or spurious parasitic eggs from the food they eat; these artifacts can be mistaken for normal reptilian parasites, leading to unnecessary treatment.

The final part of this four-part series presents some common parasitic eggs of animals fed to reptiles in captivity. Also featured are the plant and animal artifacts frequently observed in reptilian feces. For additional information, the reader may wish to review the article by Habermann and Williams[1] and the book by Flynn.[2]

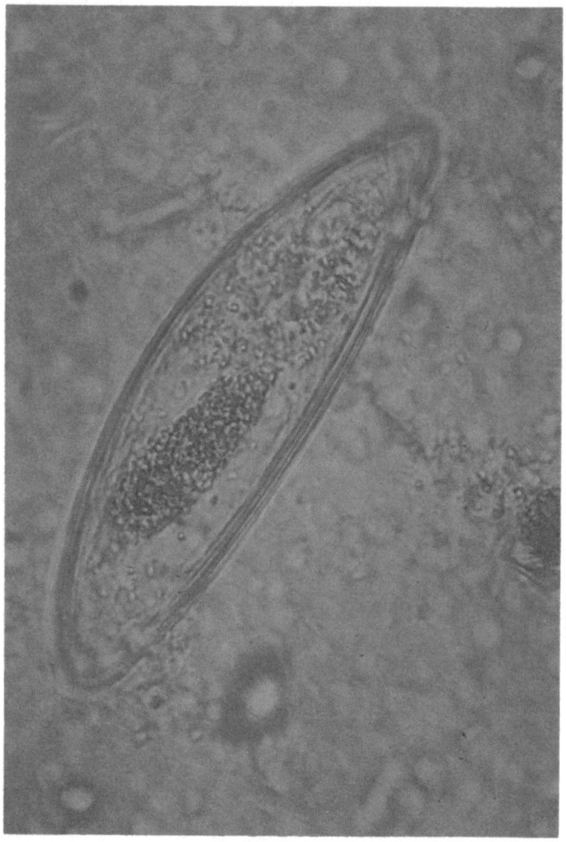

Figure 1A

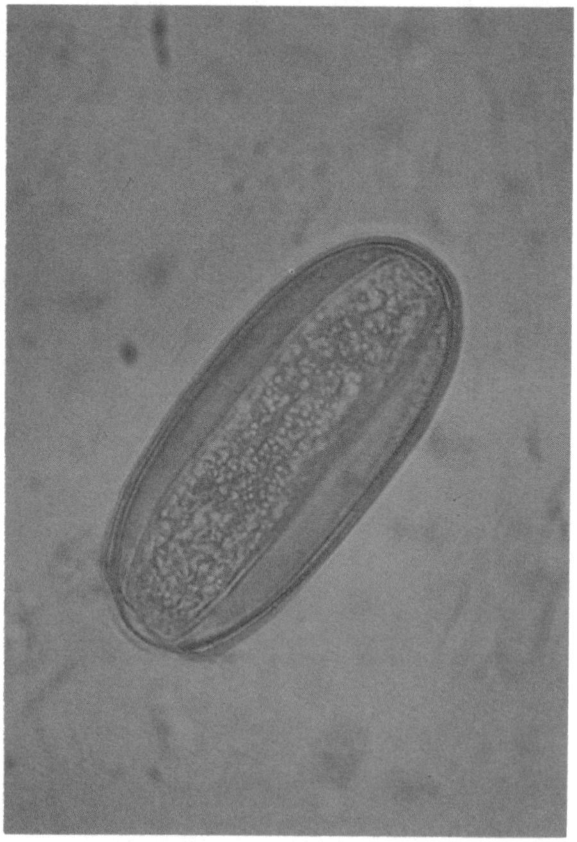

Figure 1B

Figure 1—(A) *Syphacia obvelata* (×400) and **(B)** *Aspiculuris tetraptera* (×400). *Syphacia obvelata* and *Aspiculuris tetraptera* are pinworms of mice. Their eggs are the most commonly found in the feces of captive carnivorous reptiles. If observed, sequential fecal examinations should be performed. A series of negative findings may indicate that an infection was spurious, since these parasites would be expected to appear intermittently.[3] Ova of *S. obvelata* measure 118 to 153 μ by 33 to 55 μ and those of *A. tetraptera* measure 89 to 93 μ by 36 to 42 μ.

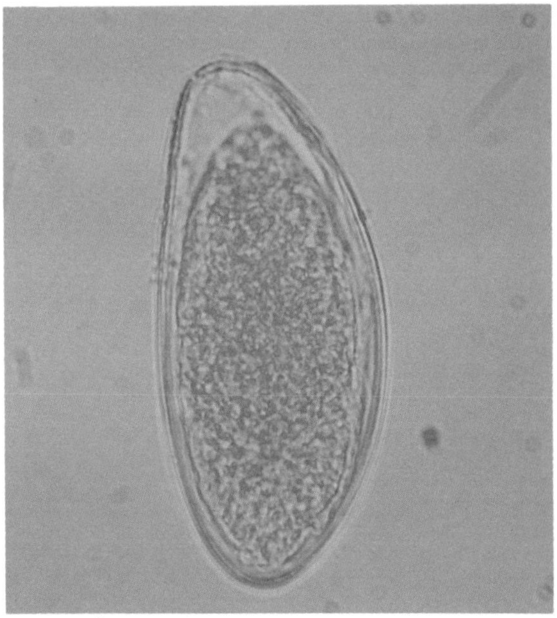

Figure 2A

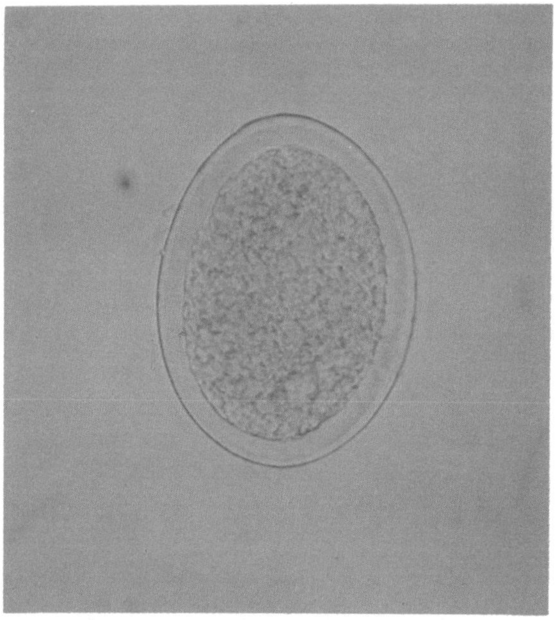

Figure 2B

Figure 2—(A) *Passalurus ambiguus* (×400) and **(B)** *Ascaridia galli* (×400). Giant snakes, such as boas and pythons, are frequently fed rabbits and chickens and may exhibit parasites of these prey animals in their stools. Microscopic examination of the stools of prey animals before they are fed to a reptile may be beneficial in detecting spurious parasites. The eggs of *P. ambiguus*, a common pinworm of rabbits and hares, measure 95 to 103 μ by 43 μ. The eggs of *A. galli*, the common roundworm of domestic and wild birds, measure 70 to 80 μ by 45 to 50 μ.

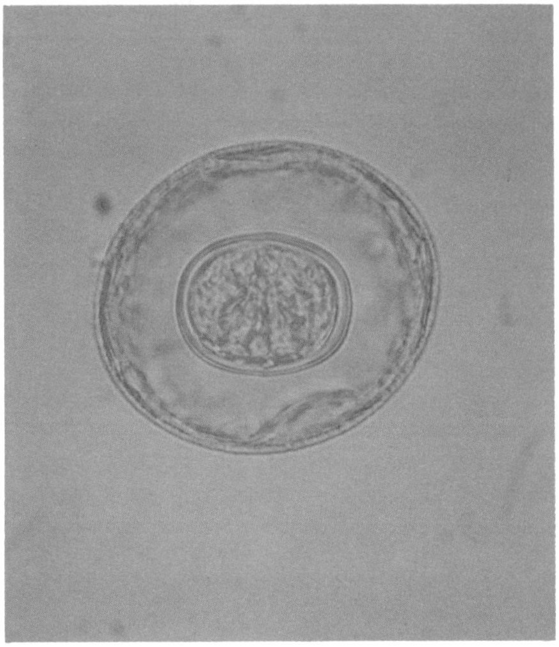

Figure 3A

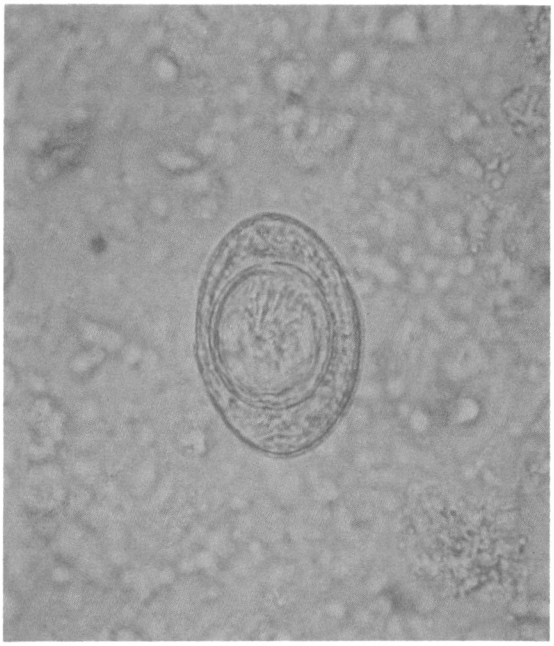

Figure 3B

Figure 3—(A) *Hymenolepsis diminuta* (×400) and **(B)** *Hymenolepsis nana* (×400). Although the tapeworm, *H. diminuta*, has an indirect life cycle, institutions breeding their own rodents may observe *H. diminuta* in the feces of captive reptiles when rodent colonies are exposed inadvertently to invertebrate intermediate hosts.[3] The dwarf tapeworm, *H. nana*, is the only known cestode with both direct and indirect life cycles.[4,5] *Hymenolepsis nana* ova are especially prevalent in the feces of carnivorous captive reptiles. Eggs of *H. nana* measure 44 to 62 μ by 30 to 55 μ, possess polar filaments, and contain an embryo measuring 24 to 30 μ by 16 to 25 μ. Ova of *H. diminuta* measure 62 to 88 μ by 52 to 81 μ, lack polar filaments, and contain an embryo measuring 24 to 30 μ by 16 to 25 μ.

Figure 4—(**A**) Partially digested mite (×100) and (**B**) invertebrate egg (×400). Mites commonly infest laboratory rodents. Invertebrate parts or eggs frequently appear in stools of reptiles. Although the mites parasitizing prey animals pose no threat to reptiles, the possibility of lethal consequences from the snake mite, *Ophionyssus natricis*, demands a thorough external examination of the reptile in question.[3]

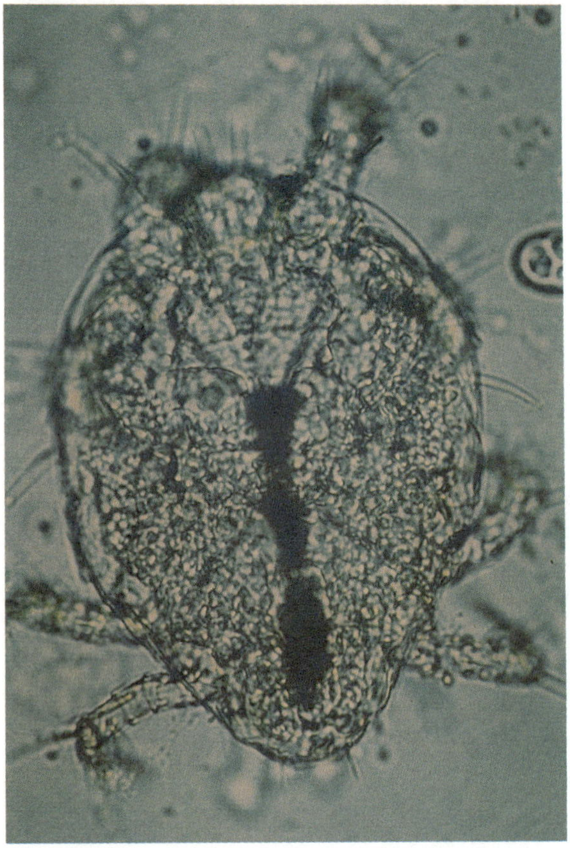

Figure 4A

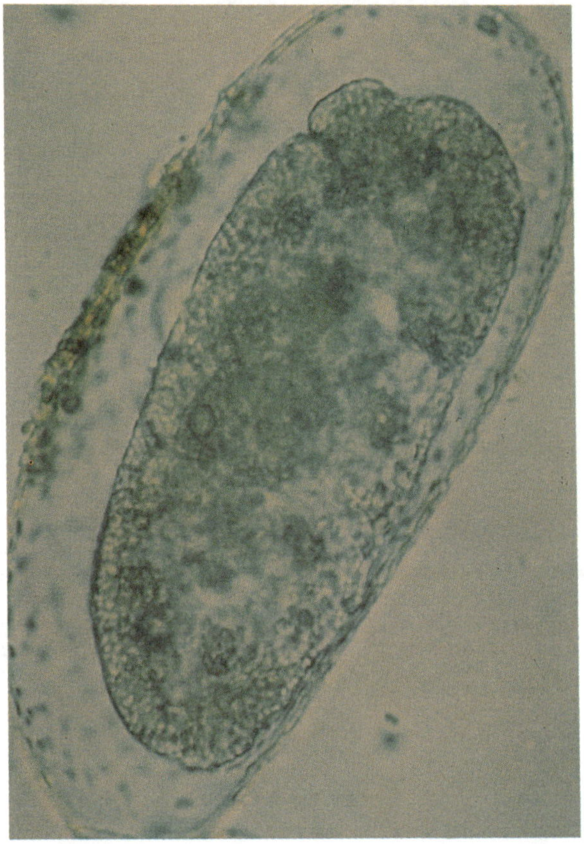

Figure 4B

→

Figure 5—(**A**) Banana seeds (×100), (**B**) plant hair (×400), (**C**) animal hairs (×100), and (**D**) pine pollen (×400). Common artifacts observed in the feces of herbivorous reptiles include banana seeds and plant hairs. Animal hairs are routinely observed in the stools of carnivores, and pine pollen may be observed in the feces of all reptiles. Banana seeds can be mistaken for segmented tapeworms, while both plant and animal hairs have been confused with nematode larvae. The observer should note the obvious lack of internal structures in these artifacts, and their disparate sizes and shapes should minimize the possibility of mistaken identity.[3]

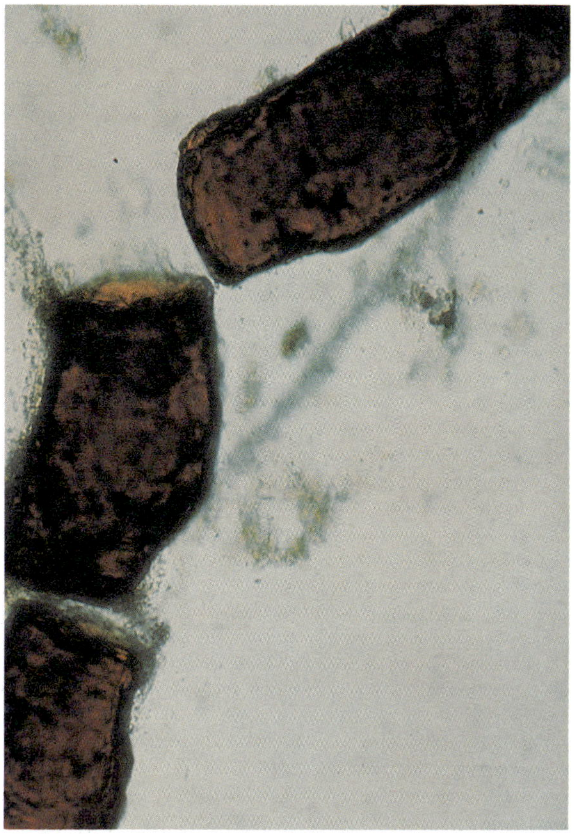

Figure 5A

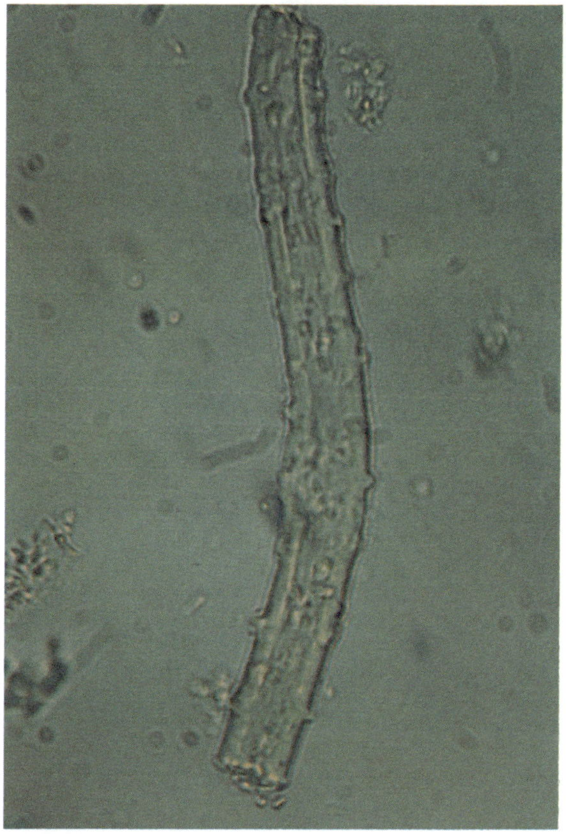

Figure 5B

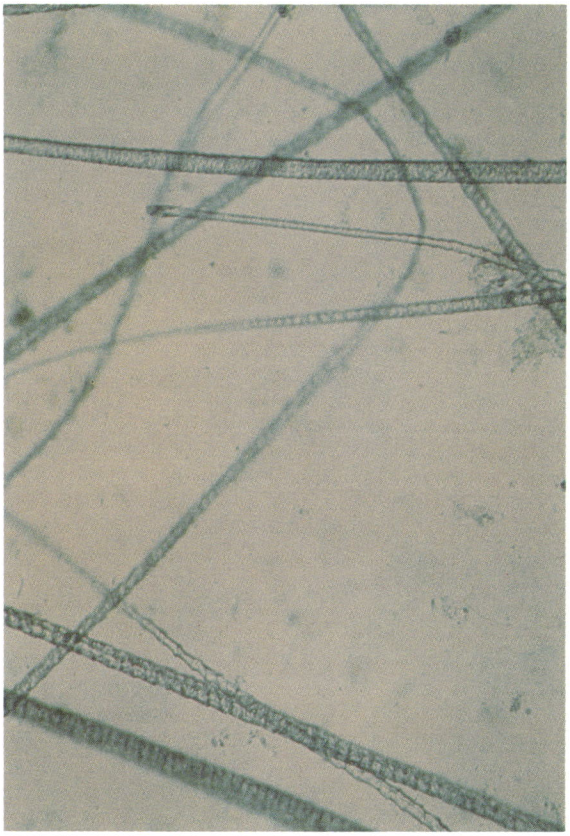

Figure 5C

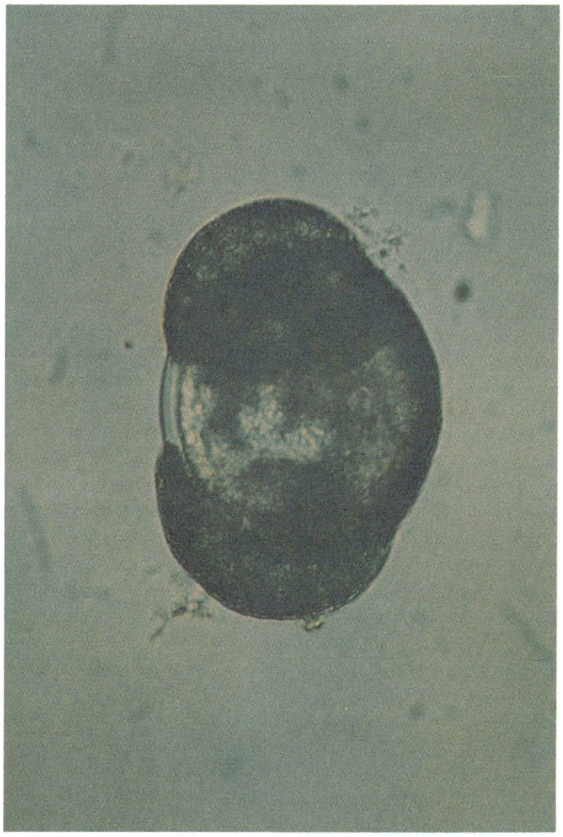

Figure 5D

Acknowledgments

This study was supported, in part, by the Society for the Study of Amphibians and Reptiles, the American Association of Zoo Keepers, and the Atlanta Zoological Society. My deepest appreciation and thanks to Dr. Daniel R. Brooks, Dr. Steve J. Upton, and Dr. Nixon Wilson for their diagnostic expertise; to Mr. Rick Etzel, Ms. Tamara Romaine, and Mr. Fred Alvey for their assistance with the literature search; and to Ms. Susanne Wahlquist, Dr. Susan Wade, and the many individuals and institutions submitting fecal material, parasites, and prepared slides.

REFERENCES

1. Habermann RT, Williams FP Jr: The identification and control of helminths in laboratory animals. *J Natl Cancer Institute* 20:979-1009, 1958.
2. Flynn RJ: *Parasites of Laboratory Animals*. Ames, IA, Iowa State University Press, 1973.
3. Barnard SM: A review of some fecal pseudoparasites of reptiles. *J Zoo Ann Med* 14:79-88, 1983.
4. Cheng TC: *The Biology of Animal Parasites*. Ames, IA, Iowa State University Press, 1973.
5. Wardle RA, McLeod JA: *The Zoology of Tapeworms*. Minneapolis, MN, University of Minnesota Press, 1952.

Diseases of Reptiles Part I. Noninfectious Diseases

Elliott R. Jacobson, DVM, PhD
Assistant Professor
Department of Laboratory Animal and Wildlife Medicine
College of Veterinary Medicine
University of Florida
Gainesville, Florida

Reptiles are phylogenetically the first vertebrate group adapted to a terrestrial life-style. The evolution of the amniotic egg, which could be deposited in a nonaquatic environment, represented a major biologic development that separated this group from antecedent amphibians. Oviparity, ovoviviparity, and viviparity are reproductive strategies of present-day reptiles. Thermoregulation of egg clutch temperature in Burmese pythons and maternal behavior of crocodilians exemplify refined techniques of reproductive behavior. Crocodilians, aquatic turtles, and many snakes have secondarily evolved adaptations to an aquatic environment. Marine turtles, several crocodilians, sea snakes, and the Galapagos iguana are the only present-day reptiles adapted to a saltwater existence. For more descriptive biology, the reader is referred to a herpetology text.[1]

Reptiles are second only to fishes with regard to numbers of imported animals. Numerous native species are also collected and distributed through the pet trade. Ultimately, reptiles that survive beyond the importer and distributor are maintained in either private collections, zoologic collections, or academic institutions. Reptiles remain an important group of research animals for basic biologists.

The stress of shipment and mismanagement continue to account for considerable mortality in recently imported reptiles. These animals often succumb to secondary infections following maintenance under suboptimal environmental conditions. Often the pet owner who purchases a reptile has little guidance as to the proper care and husbandry of the newly acquired pet. Certain species such as true chameleons are almost impossible to maintain beyond one year in captivity because of fastidious environmental and nutritional requirements. Few veterinarians have received formal education in the medical needs of sick reptiles, and certainly the abnormal conditions cannot be appreciated without knowledge of the normal condition. Reptiles often remain a diagnostic challenge, even for the clinician who has years of experience; many new diseases are yet to be described. As a starting point for the veterinarian interested in initiating a new career in reptile medicine, the commonly encountered noninfectious diseases will be reviewed in Part I of this paper, and infectious diseases will be discussed in Part II.

Environmental Requirements and Problems

Reptiles are ectothermic vertebrates that regulate body temperature by behavioral and physiologic processes.[2,3] Most species operate at a preferred optimum temperature range that, in the wild, preferably shows seasonal variation. The class Reptilia shows a range in this temperature preferendum. The cool-adapted tuatara from New Zealand has an optimum temperature range of 12.8° to 21.0°C. Many temperate aquatic turtles feed and are active in water at body temperatures of 13° to 17°C, although periods of basking behavior may raise body temperature to levels of 26° to 30°C. Although many snakes and lizards are adapted to rather high environmental temperatures, some species are specialists and adapted to cool montane temperatures. Knowing the preferred optimum temperature is imperative for long-term captive maintenance of a particular species. Additionally, many species may require a period of vernalization to elicit reproductive behavior and successful reproduction in captivity.

Captive reptiles will become lethargic and anorectic if environmental temperatures are suboptimal. Even if the reptile feeds at suboptimal temperatures, an optimal temperature range is necessary for digestion, assimilation, and defecation. Suboptimal environmental conditions may lead to a depressed humoral immune response[4] with possible invasion of saprophytic organisms.

Exposure to temperatures above the preferred optimum can result in localized burns, systemic effects, and death. The critical thermal maximum is a few degrees above the upper limit of the normal activity range and may be visualized as a value that is the arithmetic mean of the collective thermal points at which locomotor activity becomes disorganized and animals lose their ability to escape from conditions that will promptly lead to death.[5] Prolonged exposure to the critical thermal maximum will result in physiologic heat death. Heat sources in captivity should originate from above and outside the cage of the animal, and ideally the cage should be large enough to permit a thermal gradient. Snakes will invariably be burned by contact with incandescent bulbs placed inside the cage.

Humidity is another important environmental consideration. A relative humidity of 50 to 60% is ideal for many reptile species. A humidifier should be used if the humidity is too low. Clinical evidence of maintenance at suboptimal relative humidity includes dysecdysis, and, with snakes, retained spectacles (Figure 1).[6]

If a snake has not molted properly it should be soaked in a container having just enough water to cover the body. Retained spectacles can be gently removed with forceps or rubbed free with moistened cotton.

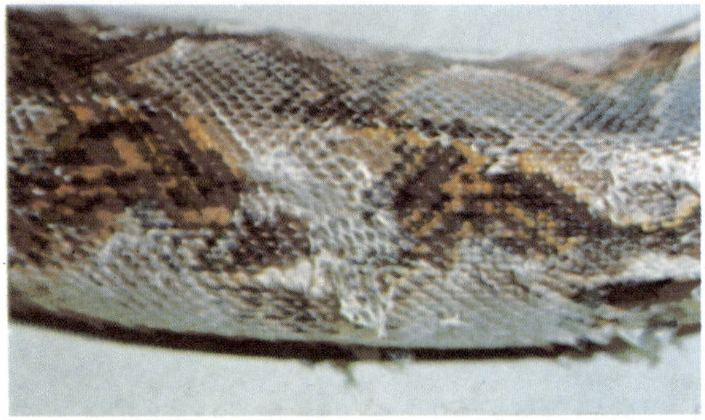

Figure 1A

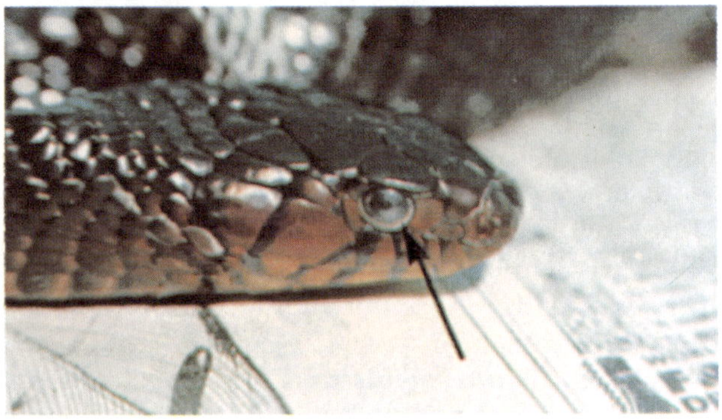

Figure 1B

Figure 1A and B—Dysecdysis in a reticulated python and retained spectacle in an indigo snake. (From Jacobson E: Histology, endocrinology, and husbandry of ecdysis in snakes: A review. *VM SAC* 72:275-280, 1977. Reprinted with permission.)

For some species an excessively high humidity can be harmful.[7] Absorbent substrates may become damp and promote the growth of opportunistic pathogens. Blister disease is commonly seen in snakes, particularly in water snakes, garter snakes, and king snakes that are maintained under moist conditions (Figure 2). Blister disease is clinically

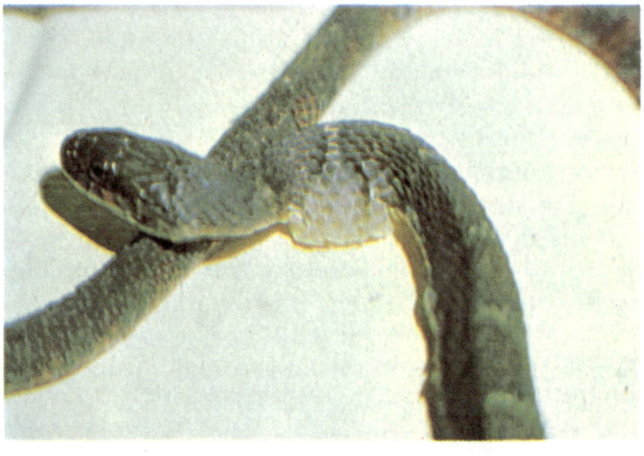

Figure 2—A common water snake with an extreme case of blister disease.

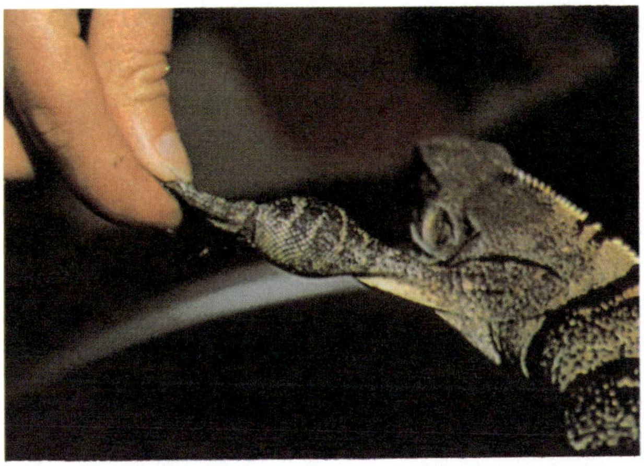

Figure 3—A ctenosaur (spiny iguana) with nutritional osteodystrophy. The diaphyseal region of the radius and ulna is extremely thickened.

seen as large, fluid-filled vesicles developing in the epidermal layer of body scales. The exact pathophysiology of this disease has not been described. Treatment includes drainage and flushing the lesions with an organic iodine solution.

Nutritional Requirements and Problems

Although most reptiles are either carnivores, insectivores, or omnivores, several species are strict herbivores. Strict herbivores are difficult to maintain in captivity and empirically appear to have complex nutritional requirements that are seldom fulfilled with captive diets. Insectivores have their own set of problems with captive maintenance. Often these animals are fed solely on mealworms and crickets which, because of inverse Ca:P ratios, are not nutritionally complete. Mealworms also are high in nondigestable chitinous material. Whole animal (mammal) feeders such as varanid lizards (monitors) and snakes seldom manifest nutritional diseases.

One of the most commonly encountered nutritional deficiencies of captive reptiles is metabolic bone disease. Dietary imbalances of calcium and phosphorus may ultimately result in nutritional secondary hyperparathyroidism and osteodystrophy.[8] A deficiency of vitamin D_3 may add to the pathogenesis of this disease. Ideally a diet should have a calcium:phosphorus ratio of 1:1 to 2:1. Skeletal muscle, visceral organs, and many vegetables contain extremely low quantities of calcium and rather high levels of phosphorus. An excess of phosphorus and a deficiency of calcium in the diet usually result in hyperphosphatemia and concomitant stimulation of parathormone which induces reabsorption of calcium from hydroxyapatite crystals in bone matrix. The cortical bone will be thin and become surrounded by a collar of proliferating cartilage.[8] This condition is commonly seen in captive green iguanas. Lizards presented with this condition may exhibit loss of movement of the rear limbs, which may show diaphyseal thickenings of the femur, radius, and ulna (Figure 3). Pathologic fractures may occur. Therapy should include an improved diet to correct the inverse Ca:P ratio. Common iguanas should be fed moistened dog chow and high-quality vegetables. Many adult iguanas will also feed on whole animals such as mice and small rats.

Crocodilians and turtles fed solely on skeletal muscle meat will also manifest metabolic bone disease. Crocodilians will develop curvatures of the spine and abnormalities in growth of jaw bones and teeth which may grow outward at oblique angles. Turtles may show abnormalities in shell growth, development of a *soft* shell, and parrot jaw (Figure 4).

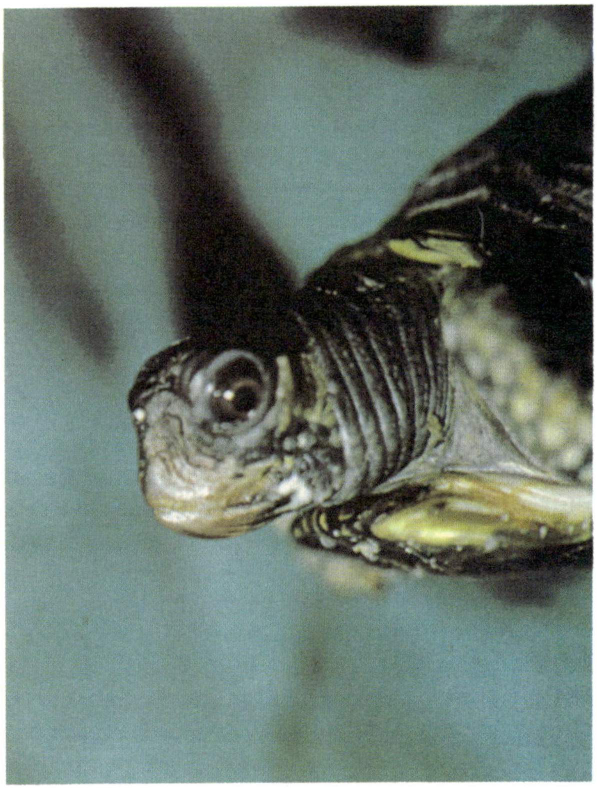

Figure 4—A young box turtle with nutritional osteodystrophy (parrot jaw). This turtle was fed only ground beef for one year prior to this photograph.

A variety of hypovitaminoses has been described for reptiles. Hypovitaminosis A is frequently seen in captive young aquatic turtles fed on skeletal muscle meat and poor-quality vegetables. The respiratory and ocular adnexal structures are often affected.[9] Since vitamin A is necessary for normal growth and integrity of epithelial structures, a deficiency results in pathologic changes in these tissues. The harderian gland and duct system may undergo squamous metaplasia with a concomitant

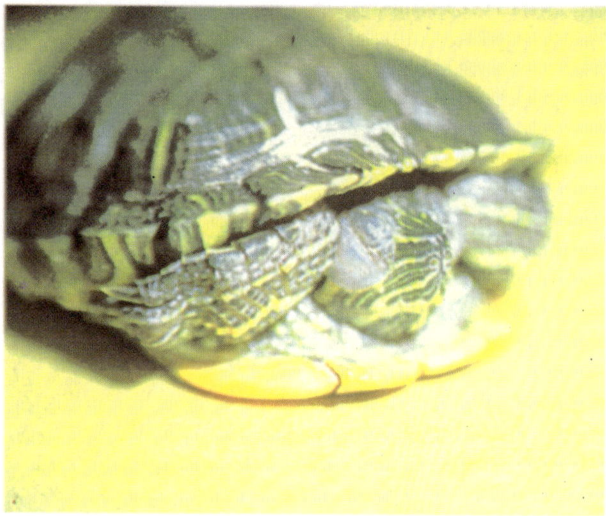

Figure 5—A young red-eared slider suffering from hypovitaminosis A. The palpebrae are edematous and closed.

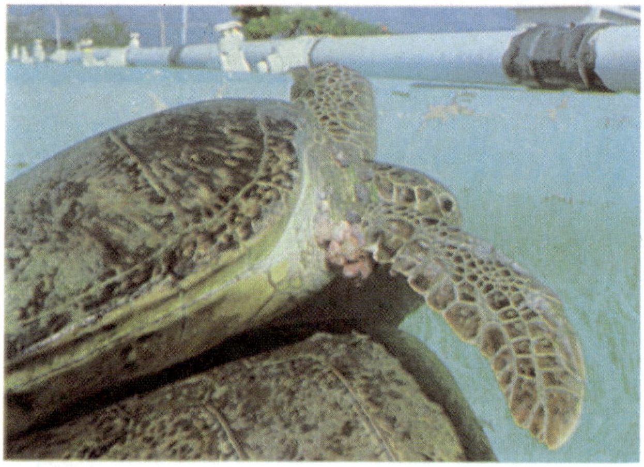

Figure 6—Adult green turtle with numerous papillomas in the axis of the forelimbs.

decrease in normal secretory activity followed by conjunctivitis and palpebral edema. The turtle suffering from hypovitaminosis A is usually anorexic, with palpebrae swollen and closed (Figure 5). The respiratory tract may show loss of ciliated epithelial cells. Treatment must include an improved diet and administration of injectable vitamin A.

Hypovitaminosis E has been described in captive crocodilians whose diet consisted primarily of fishes high in unsaturated fatty acids and also in snakes fed obese laboratory rats.[7,10] The unsaturated fatty acids, without adequate amounts of available vitamin E, are peroxidized to a pigment called ceroid. Wherever this pigment accumulates there is an inflammatory response. When fat is involved the condition is termed *steatitis.* Dietary or parenteral administration of vitamin E has been recommended,[7] and the diet should be changed so as to avoid unsaturated fatty acid containing fishes such as mackerel, mullet, and smelt.

Hypervitaminoses have also been reported in reptiles. Hypervitaminosis D has been identified in common iguanas and is associated with overzealous supplementation of the diet with commercial vitamin D.[11] Pathologic lesions include medial calcification of elastic blood vessels. Advanced cases are diagnosed radiographically. Metastatic mineralization may occur at a wide variety of soft tissue sites.

Neoplastic Disease

Although in a review of the literature and in their own findings in 1948 Schlumberger and Lucke listed only 25 reptile neoplasms,[12] a current report cites approximately 159 descriptions.[13] All of the major groups of neoplasms found in mammals have been reported in reptiles except primary neoplasms involving the central nervous system. Most neoplasms appear more commonly in old, long-term captive animals. Papillomas involving the periorbital tissues and integument in the axis of the hindlimbs and forelimbs are common in wild and mariculture-reared green sea turtles (Figure 6). Electron microscopic evaluation of papillomas has failed to demonstrate virus particles. Leeches (*Ozobranchus* spp.) usually parasitize the surface of these lesions, and histologic sections often reveal spirorchid trematode eggs within dermal capillaries.

Virus particles have been found associated with several reptile neoplasms. A C-type RNA virus was identified by electron microscopy to be budding from spleen tissue cultures in the 48th and 52nd passage, from a Russel's viper diagnosed as having a precardial myxofibroma.[14] Electron microscopic examination of an embryonal rhabdomyosarcoma in a corn snake represented the first report describing virus particles within primary tumor tissue of a reptile.[15] Recently, viruslike particles were seen in neoplastic lymphoid cells of a California king snake that had a lymphosarcoma associated with viruslike intranuclear inclusions.[16]

Suspected neoplasms should be biopsied for histopathologic evaluation. There are a variety of other pathologic inflammatory and noninflammatory changes that may grossly resemble neoplastic disease. These pseudoneoplasms must always be considered in differential diagnosis. Bacteria, fungi, and metazoan parasites typically result in a granulomatous inflammatory response in reptiles, and the clinician must be able to differentiate these lesions from true neoplasms.

Toxicological Problems

Although the aminoglycoside antibiotic gentamicin sulfate has potential nephrotoxic effects in a wide variety of animals, certain bacterial infec-

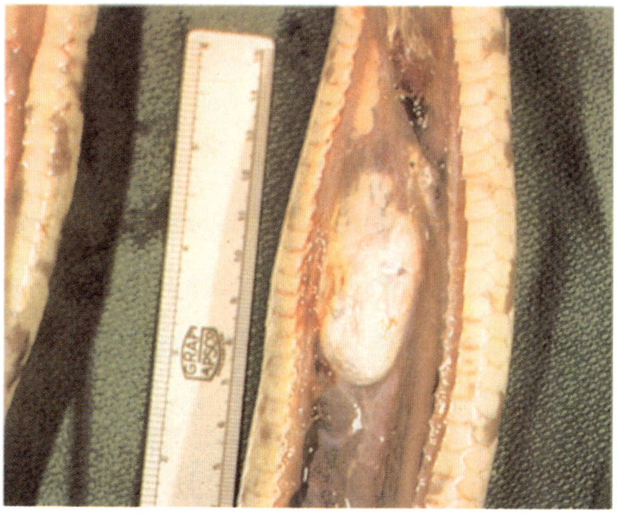

Figure 7—Uric acid precipitate in the pericardial sac of a ball python. (From Jacobson E: Gentamicin-related visceral gout in two boid snakes. *VM SAC* 71:361-363, 1976. Reprinted with permission.)

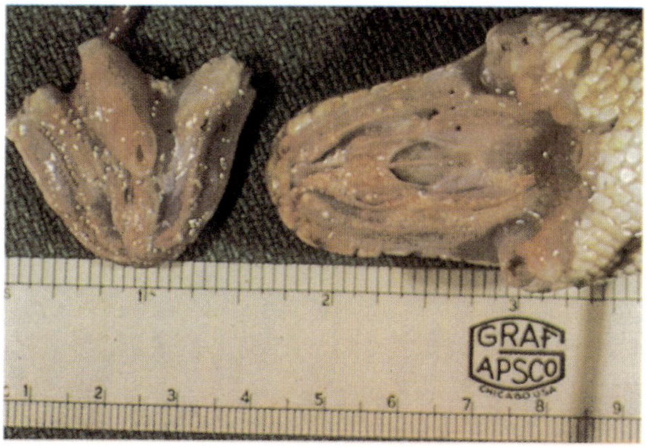

Figure 8—Uric acid precipitate seen as small white foci (tophi) along the palatine veins of a ball python. (From Jacobson E: Gentamicin-related visceral gout in two boid snakes. *VM SAC* 71:361-363, 1976. Reprinted with permission.)

tions, specifically *Pseudomonas* spp., warrant its use. Since reptiles often succumb to secondary gram-negative bacterial infections, gentamicin sulfate is often the drug of choice. Gentamicin nephrotoxicity has been reported clinically and experimentally in several species of snakes.[17,18] Since snakes have developed a system of eliminating uric acid as the principal nitrogenous waste product, renal damage may result in a condition termed *visceral gout,* in which uric acid precipitates at a variety of extrarenal sites including the vascular system, pericardial sac, liver, and lung (Figure 7). Tophi may be seen deposited along vessels in the roof of the mouth of affected snakes (Figure 8).

Blood half-lives of gentamicin following intramuscular injection have been described for several reptile species. For gentamicin in bullsnakes maintained at 24°C, 2.5 mg/kg body weight every 72 hours is the recommended treatment regimen, while for turtles in the genus *Chrysemys* kept at 26°C, 10 mg/kg body weight every 48 hours has been suggested.[19] Acclimation temperature has effects on blood half-life and extent of renal damage.[18]

Because of the potential nephrotoxic effect of gentamicin, reptiles should be fasted or food intake should be reduced during the period of treatment. This should effectively reduce the circulating uric acid levels. It has been suggested that water administration via stomach tube may aid in increasing glomerular filtration and in reducing circulating uric acid salts.

REFERENCES

1. Porter K: *Herpetology.* Philadelphia, WB Saunders Co, 1972.
2. Cowles RB, Bogert CM: A preliminary study of the thermal requirements of desert reptiles. *Bull Am Mus Natur Hist* 83:291-296, 1944.
3. Brattstrom BH: Body temperatures of reptiles. *Am Midl Natur* 73:376-422, 1965.
4. Evans EE: Comparative immunology. Antibody response in *Dipsosaurus dorsalis* at different temperatures. *Proc Soc Exp Biol Med* 112:531-533, 1963.
5. Lowe CH, Vance V: Acclimation of the critical thermal maximum of the reptile *Urosaurus ornatus. Science* 122:73-74, 1955.
6. Jacobson ER: Histology, endocrinology, and husbandry of ecdysis in snakes (a review). *VM SAC* 72:275-280, 1977.
7. Wallach JD: Environmental and nutritional diseases of captive reptiles. *JAVMA* 159:1632-1643, 1971.
8. Anderson MP, Capen CC: Nutritional osteodystrophy in captive green iguanas *(Iguana iguana). Virchows Archiv [Cell Pathol]* 21:229-247, 1976.
9. Elkan E, Zwart P: The ocular disease of young terrapins caused by vitamin A deficiency. *Pathol Vet* 4:201-222, 1967.
10. Wallach JD, Hoessle C: Steatitis in captive crocodilians. *JAVMA* 153:845-847, 1968.
11. Wallach JD, Hoessle C: Hypervitaminosis D in green iguanas. *JAVMA* 149:912-914, 1966.
12. Schlumberger HG, Lucke B: Tumors of fishes, amphibians, and reptiles. *Cancer Res* 8:657-753, 1948.
13. Jacobson ER: Neoplastic diseases of reptiles, in Cooper JE, Jackson OF (eds): *Diseases of the Reptilia.* London, Academic Press, in press.
14. Zeigel RF, Clark HF: Electron microscopic observations on a "C"-type virus in cell cultures derived from a tumor-bearing viper. *J Natl Cancer Inst* 43:1097-1102, 1969.
15. Lunger PD, Hardy WD, Clark HF: C-type particles in a reptilian tumor. *J Natl Cancer Inst* 52:1231-1235, 1974.
16. Jacobson ER, Seely JC, Novilla MN: Lymphosarcoma associated with virus-like intranuclear inclusions in a California king snake (Colubridae:Lampropettis). *J Natl Cancer Inst* 65:577-583, 1980.
17. Jacobson ER: Gentamicin related visceral gout in two boid snakes. *VM SAC* 71:361-363, 1976.
18. Hodge MK: The effect of acclimation temperature on gentamic nephrotoxicity in the Florida banded water snake. *Am Assoc Zoo Vet Annu Proc,* 1978, Knoxville, TN. Topeka, Hill's Pet Products, Inc, 1979, pp 226-237.
19. Bush M: Antibiotic therapy in reptiles, in Kirk RN (ed): *Current Veterinary Therapy VII.* Philadelphia, WB Saunders Co, 1980.

Diseases of Reptiles Part II. Infectious Diseases

Elliott R. Jacobson, DVM, PhD
Assistant Professor
Department of Laboratory Animal and Wildlife Medicine
College of Veterinary Medicine
University of Florida
Gainesville, Florida

Reptiles are susceptible to infectious agents similar to those that result in disease in higher vertebrates. Since the immune system of reptiles is temperature dependent, suboptimal environmental conditions may predispose reptiles to infection with opportunistic pathogens that under *normal* conditions exist as saprophytic microorganisms. The gram-negative bacteria, particularly *Pseudomonas* and *Aeromonas*, are commonly identified as pathogens in immunocompromised reptiles. Reptiles are also susceptible to a variety of mycotic agents that rarely result in disease in higher vertebrates. Again, suboptimal environmental conditions may predispose reptiles to mycotic infections. Within the last few years several viral agents have been incriminated as primary pathogens in reptile disease. The following is a review of infectious agents, including viruses, bacteria, and fungi, responsible for disease in reptiles.

Viral Diseases

As recently as 10 years ago, very little information was available concerning viral diseases of reptiles. Since that time several interesting viral agents have been identified, some of which were associated with disease. One of the best studied is that of *gray patch disease* in green turtles reared in a mariculture farm in the Cayman Islands.[1] The disease is caused by a herpesvirus that may infect up to 100% of young green sea turtles between 56 and 90 days after hatching. Skin lesions begin as small, circular, papular lesions that eventually coalesce into patches (Figure 1). Basophilic intranuclear inclusions are readily demonstrated in histologic section stained with hematoxylin and eosin (Figure 2). The severity of outbreaks is influenced by crowding, high water temperature, and increased fecal contamination of water. There is evidence that the virus is transmitted via the egg.

The only identified viral disease of crocodilians is caiman pox.[2] Infected caimans have gray white, circular, raised skin lesions scattered over the body surface and particularly prominent on the palpebrae (Figure 3) and rostrum. Histopathologic evaluation of lesion sites reveals hypertrophied epithelial cells containing eosinophilic intracytoplasmic inclusions when stained with hematox-

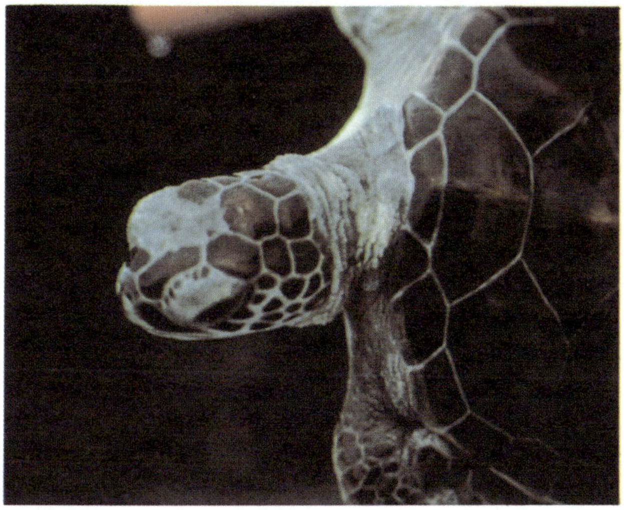

Figure 1—Juvenile green turtle with gray patch disease. Note the prominent lesions on the head and cervical region.

ylin and eosin. This disease has only been seen in young caimans, and most individuals show a spontaneous regression of lesions within several months of onset. The virus appears to be transmitted between individuals through contaminated water.

The first-described viral epizootic of snakes involved a colony of fer-de-lance housed at a serpentarium in Switzerland. This was the only species affected, although other species were housed in the same room. Snakes initially exhibited a loss of muscle tone and eventually died of severe respiratory disease manifested by openmouthed breathing with a discharge from the glottis. Although *Pseudomonas* was initially suspected as the causative agent, lung suspensions of affected snakes injected into embryonic reptile eggs resulted in the isolation and identification of a paramyxovirus.[3] Cytopathic effects in reptile cell lines have been reported for this virus.[4] Recently a paramyxolike virus has been isolated from a rock rattlesnake that had a clinical history of progressive central nervous system disease.[5] This snake was a member of a breeding group of which eight additional members died manifesting similar clinical signs. Histopathologic findings included an interstitial pneumonia, multifocal areas of gliosis in the hindbrain, and demyelination of brain stem axons. Groups of virus particles were demonstrated by electron microscopy in extracellular spaces of brain stem tissue.

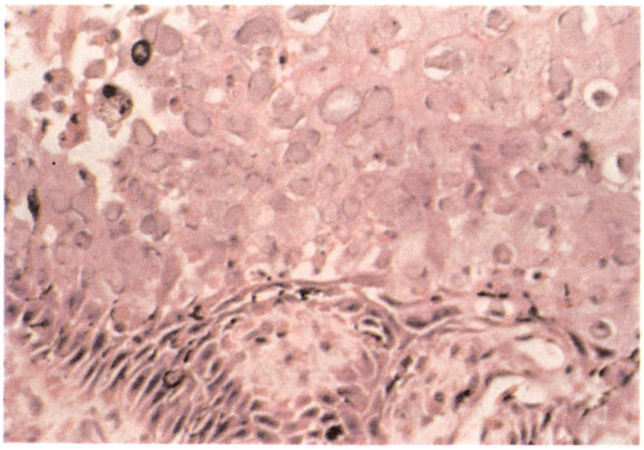

Figure 2—Photomicrograph of a gray patch lesion. Epithelial cells are enlarged and contain basophilic intranuclear inclusions.

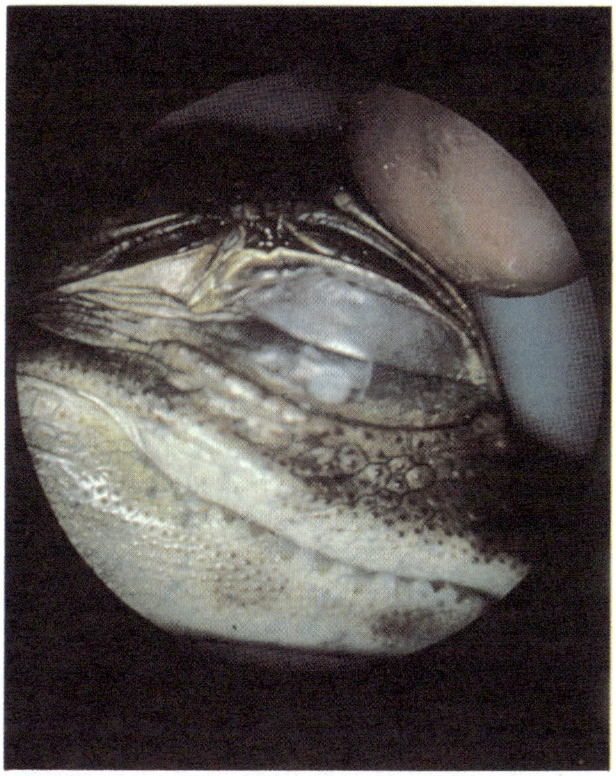

Figure 3—Juvenile caiman with a single, circular pox lesion on the palpebra.

Herpeslike particles have been found in crude snake venom obtained from kraits and cobras.[6] Histopathologic examination of venom glands from Siamese cobras with a history of chronic venom gland infections revealed degeneration and necrosis of epithelial tubules, which were often replaced by fibrous connective tissue.[7] Electron microscopy demonstrated naked and enveloped herpesviruslike particles in necrotic and ruptured epithelial cells.

Bacterial Diseases

Numerous bacterial diseases have been reported for reptiles. Although most cases involve gram-negative microorganisms that are opportunistic secondary invaders, disease can occur with gram-positives. The most important reptile zoonotic disease is salmonellosis of turtles in the genus *Chrysemys* that have been sold by the millions by the pet industry. Although *Salmonella* rarely results in overt disease in these animals, the public health aspect of salmonellosis has resulted in a ban of interstate shipment of turtles in the U.S.

One of the best-documented bacterial diseases of turtles is septicemic cutaneous ulcerative disease (SCUD) of aquatic chelonians.[8] Clinically the disease is seen as a necrotizing ulcerative dermatitis with both shell and skin lesions (Figure 4). There may be a septicemia with involvement of the liver, heart, blood, kidney, and spleen. Although the organism *Citrobacter freundii* has been incriminated as the etiologic agent, *Serratia* may be necessary to initiate the infection.[9] This disease is most often seen in chelonians that are kept in unfiltered aquatic systems that have excess accumulations of fecal material. Chloramphenicol is considered the antibiotic of choice.

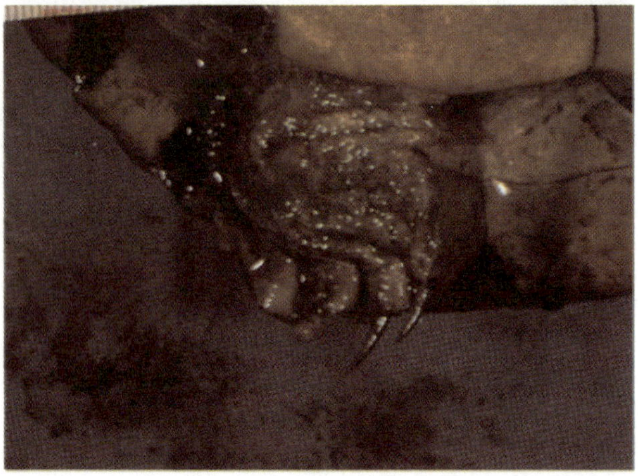

Figure 4—*Chrysemys* spp. with ulcerative skin lesions typical of SCUD.

Middle and inner ear infections are commonly seen in captive and wild box turtles (Figure 5). Lesions may be unilateral or bilateral and consist of caseous, laminated debris surrounded by a fibrous tissue capsule. A variety of gram-negative microorganisms have been isolated from these lesions; the route of infection may be via the eustachian tube. Treatment consists of draining the lesion and flushing the area with an organic iodine solution. In advanced cases in which there is bony involvement, systemic antibiotic therapy is recommended.

Local or systemic *Aeromonas* and/or *Pseudomonas* infections are common in alligators, lizards, and snakes. *Pseudomonas* spp. are commonly isolated from the oral cavity and intestinal tract of healthy squamates, and thus they are considered part of the normal fauna. Disease results from an interplay of factors that tend to simultaneously increase the virulence of the microorganism and immunosuppress the host. Environmental conditions, nutritional status of the host, and traumatic injury to tissues are all important factors that may influence the initiation of lesions and the course of disease.

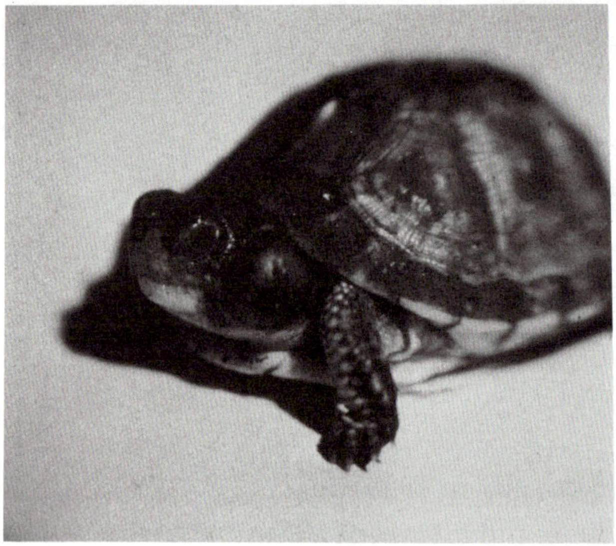

Figure 5—Juvenile box turtle with middle ear infection.

Aeromonas hydrophila was responsible for the death of American alligators in a eutrophic inland lake in Florida.[10] *Aeromonas* infections are not uncommon in alligators that are exposed constantly to environmental temperatures at the upper limit of the preferred optimum range. Bite wounds between cage-mate lizards often become infected with *Pseudomonas aeruginosa*. *Pseudomonas* spp. have been found to be associated with necrotizing enteritis and ulcerative stomatitis of snakes in zoologic collections. *Pseudomonas* spp. were isolated from 23 of 127 snakes that died of a septicemic disease in an East African snake farm.[11] Invasive burn wound sepsis with *Pseudomonas aeruginosa* has been seen in several snakes following burning of the integument (Figure 6).

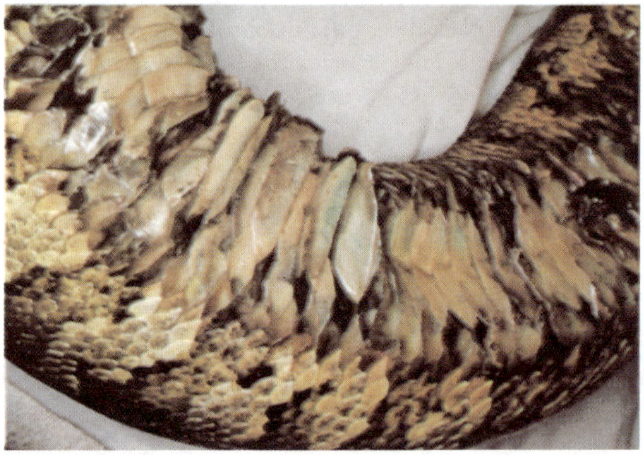

Figure 6—*Pseudomonas aeruginosa* invasive burn wound sepsis in a Burmese python.

The most significant bacterial disease of snakes in captivity is a condition called ulcerative stomatitis or *mouth rot*. Although a variety of agents have been cultured from oral lesions, *Aeromonas* and

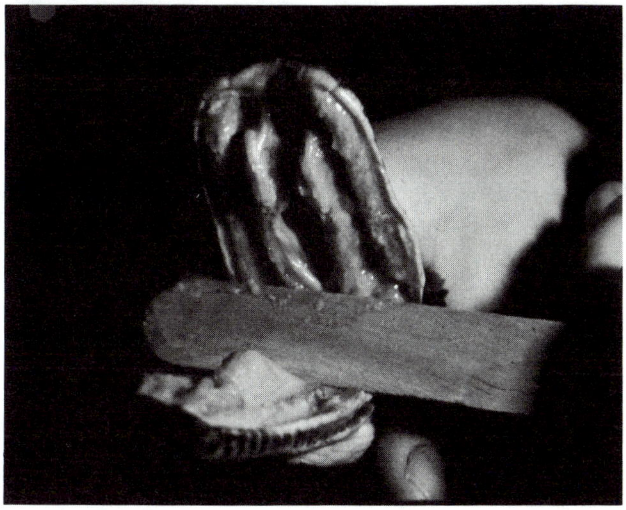

Figure 7—Blood python with chronic infectious stomatitis.

Pseudomonas are commonly isolated. Predisposing factors, including malnutrition, suboptimal environmental temperatures, and trauma, are all involved in the pathogenesis of this disease. The oral lesions consist of accumulated caseous material in the mucous membranes surrounding the teeth (Figure 7). The mucous membranes become edematous and ulcerations may eventually result in osteomyelitis of the jaw bones. Pneumonia may follow aspiration of necrotic oral debris. Oral lesions and lung washings (Figure 8) of animals with respiratory disease should be routinely cultured and followed by antibiotic sensitivity determinations.

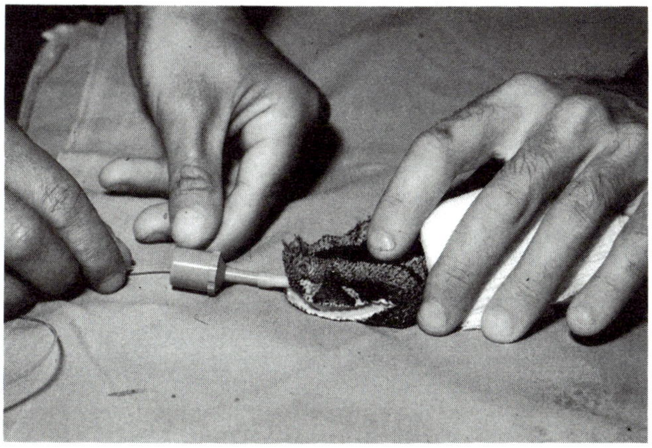

Figure 8—Lung washing taken from a rhinoceros viper. The snake was anesthetized with a halothane/O_2 mixture and a cannula is passed through the endotracheal tube into the lung.

Treatment of infectious stomatitis involves not only treating the sick animal but also eliminating the underlying predisposing factors. Often affected animals are off feed, and force feeding combined with the administration of subcutaneous/intracoelomic fluids and the appropriate antibiotics is necessary. Based upon sensitivities of isolated *Pseudomonas* and *Aeromonas*, chloramphenicol, carbenicillin, and gentamicin are the antibiotics of choice. Gentamicin sulfate (2.5 mg/kg every 72 hours for a minimum of three treatments) is usually combined with the administration of carbenicillin (400 mg/kg once per day for nine days). Administration of vitamin C has been suggested.[12] Reptiles suffering from respiratory disease can be nebulized with gentamicin and acetylcysteine. Response to treatment is a very slow process and requires several weeks for good evaluation.

Mycotic Diseases

Numerous mycotic agents have been identified as a cause of disease in all major groups of reptiles. Most reports involve disease of the integumentary and respiratory systems. The dermatophytes responsible for mammalian skin disease are seldom identified as agents of disease in reptiles. The systemic mycotic disease of mammals including histoplasmosis, cryptococcosis, blastomycosis, and coccidioidomycosis have not been reported for reptiles.

Ulcerative shell lesions of turtles are often associated with Phycomycetes. An outbreak of mucormycosis was responsible for considerable mortality in a group of Florida soft-shelled turtles.[13] Lesions typically start as small, white ulcerations in the

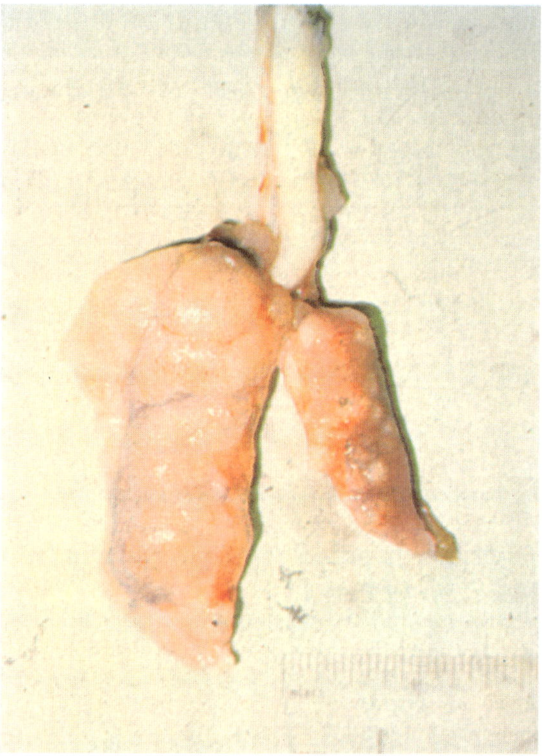

Figure 9—Lungs of a turtle with mycotic pulmonary disease. The right lung is consolidated and nodular, whereas the left lung is emphysematous. (From Jacobson ER, Gaskin JM, Shields RP, White FH: Mycotic pneumonia in mariculture-reared green sea turtles. *JAVMA* 175:929-933, 1979. Reprinted with permission.)

carapace and eventually coalesce into patches. Scrapings of these lesions stained with lactophenol cotton blue reveal nonseptate branching hyphae. Immersing the turtles in a malachite green solution (0.15 mg/liter of water) has been an effective treatment.

A variety of mycotic agents including *Aspergillus, Beauvaria, Cladosporium,* and *Paecilomyces* have been isolated from turtles with respiratory disease. Aquatic turtles with respiratory disease show signs of openmouthed breathing and swimming at an angle to the surface of the water. Necropsy generally reveals that one lung is emphysematous while the other is consolidated (Figure 9). GMS-stained sections of lung tissue reveal hyphae within the center of the granulomatous lesions. Predisposing factors for mycotic pneumonias in turtles include suboptimal environmental temperatures, debris buildup in the environment, and prior bacterial or viral disease. Antemortem diagnostic techniques should include the identification of hyphae in lung washings.

Beauvaria bassiana, a pathogen of insects, was isolated from pulmonary lesions in several alligators that were maintained under suboptimal environmental temperatures.[14] The fact that this pathogen does not grow at 37°C but does grow at low temperatures explains why it has not been reported as a pathogen in homeotherms.

Mycotic necrotizing skin disease has been described in captive snakes (Figure 10).[15] *Geotrichum, Fusarium, Trichoderma,* and *Penicillium* have been incriminated as etiologic agents. Often the lesions commence at the hinge region between adjacent scales and may penetrate into the dermis where a granulomatous inflammatory response is elicited. Suspected cases of mycotic skin diseases are easily confirmed by submitting biopsied scales for culture and histopathologic evaluation. Biopsied scales should be thoroughly ground prior to inoculation on mycotic media.

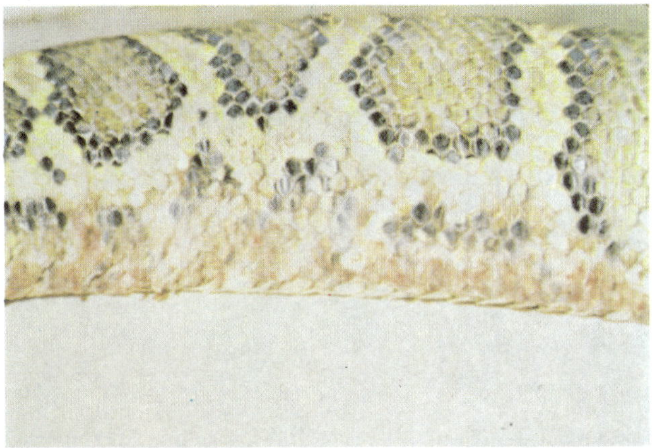

Figure 10—Necrotizing mycotic *(Fusarium)* skin disease in a Burmese python. (From Jacobson ER: Necrotizing mycotic dermatitis in snakes: Clinical and pathologic features. *JAVMA* 177:838-841, 1980. Reprinted with permission.)

Predisposing factors for mycotic skin disease in snakes include unsanitary environmental conditions, maintenance at a suboptimal temperature, and excess humidity. Spontaneous regression of lesions may occur following improvement of environmental conditions. Topical application of organic iodine ointments and 1% tolnaftate cream has been effective in treating several cases. Surgical removal of dermal granulomas may be necessary. There are no reports of treating systemic mycosis with amphotericin B.

REFERENCES

1. Rebell G, Ryulin A, Haines HG: A herpesvirus-type agent associated with skin lesions of green sea turtles in aquaculture. *Am J Vet Res* 30:1221-1224, 1975.
2. Jacobson ER, Popp JA, Shields RP, Gaskin JM: Pox-like skin lesions in captive caimans. *JAVMA* 175:937-940, 1979.
3. Leloup P, Foelsch DW, Nyler RR: Fer-de-lance virus: A probable paramyxovirus isolated from a reptile. *J Gen Virol* 44:405-418, 1979.
4. Lunger PD, Clark HF: Morphogenesis of fer-de-lance virus (FDLV) cultured at optimal cell growth temperature. *J Comp Pathol* 89:265-279, 1979.
5. Jacobson ER, Gaskin JM, Simpson CF, Terrell TG: Paramyxo-like virus infection in a rock rattlesnake. *JAVMA,* in press.
6. Monroe JH, Shibley GP, Schidlovsky G, et al: Action of snake venom on Rauscher virus. *J Natl Cancer Inst* 40:135-145, 1968.
7. Simpson CF, Jacobson ER, Gaskin JM: Herpesvirus-like infection of the venom gland of Siamese cobras. *JAVMA* 175:941-943, 1979.
8. Kaplan HM: Septicemic cutaneous ulcerative disease of turtles. *Lab Anim Care* 7:273-277, 1957.
9. Jackson CG, Fulton M: A turtle colony epizootic apparently of microbial origin. *J Wildl Dis* 6:446-468, 1970.
10. Shotts EB, Gaines JL, Martin L, Prestwood AK: *Aeromonas* induced deaths among fish and reptiles in an eutrophic inland lake. *JAVMA* 161:603-607, 1972.
11. Cooper JE, Leakey JHE: A septicemic disease of East African snakes associated with enterobacteriaceae. *Trans R Soc Trop Med Hyg* 70:80-84, 1976.
12. Wallach JD: Environmental and nutritional disease of captive reptiles. *JAVMA* 159:1632-1643, 1971.
13. Jacobson ER, Calderwood M, Clubb S: Mucormycosis in Florida soft-shell turtles. *JAVMA,* in press.
14. Fromtling RA, Jansen JM, Robinson BE, Bulmer GS: Fatal mycotic pulmonary disease of captive American alligators. *Vet Pathol* 16:428-431, 1979.
15. Jacobson ER: Necrotizing mycotic dermatitis of snakes: Clinical and pathologic features. *JAVMA,* in press.

Selected Integumentary Diseases of Tropical Freshwater Fish

Andrea P. Pesut, VMD
Mechanicsburg, Pennsylvania

Michael Goldschmidt, MSc, BVMS, MRCVS
Department of Pathobiology
University of Pennsylvania
School of Veterinary Medicine
Philadelphia, Pennsylvania

Common Diseases Affecting the Skin

Viral Disease

Lymphocystis is the only viral disease that has been identified in freshwater tropical fish.[1] It is caused by an iridovirus and is a common disease of many fish. It is characterized clinically by the presence of multiple pearllike nodules in the fins, tail, and other skin surfaces (Figure 1). Histopathological examination has shown that each nodule is an enormously hypertrophied epithelial cell. Nodules can become desquamated and secondarily infected by bacteria and fungi. High mortality can then be expected.

Fish experiencing no secondary complications eat well, show no evidence of skin irritation, and have low mortality. The nodules may persist for several months but eventually will slough off. Infected fish remain carriers, however, and will be a source of infection if introduced into a susceptible tank. Transmission may occur by ingestion or by entry of the virus into the gills or skin wounds.[2] Lesions usually develop within two to four weeks after exposure.

Diagnosis of lymphocystis can be made rapidly by direct microscopic examination of an unstained smear of tissue from the affected area. The presence of very large cells with greatly thickened hyaline cell walls is diagnostic (Figure 2). Typically, a greatly enlarged irregular nucleus is noted in each cell. The cytoplasm is granular and may contain inclusion bodies.[3]

There is no treatment for lymphocystis. Attempts have been made to surgically resect localized lesions, but the lesions recurred within two months.[1] The severity of the disease can be controlled by preventing parasitism and traumatic injury to the skin, avoiding overstocking of fish in the aquarium, and decreasing water temperature.[3]

Skin Parasites

Wild fish usually have a great diversity of parasites at low burdens when they are captured. The life cycle of some of these parasites will be arrested as a result of the lack of a needed intermediate host. Others will die and fall off the host fish because of the environmental change. Still others will build up to large numbers as a result of the stress of handling

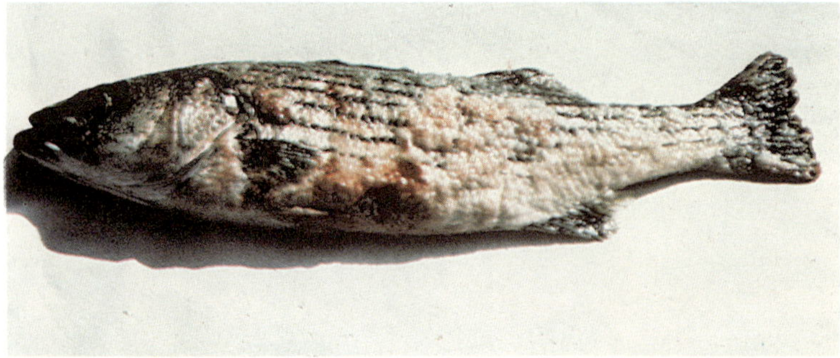

Figure 1—Lymphocystis in a striped bass is characterized by the presence of multiple pearllike nodules in the fins, tail, and other skin surfaces. (Courtesy of AH Walsh, Pfizer, Inc., Groton, Connecticut)

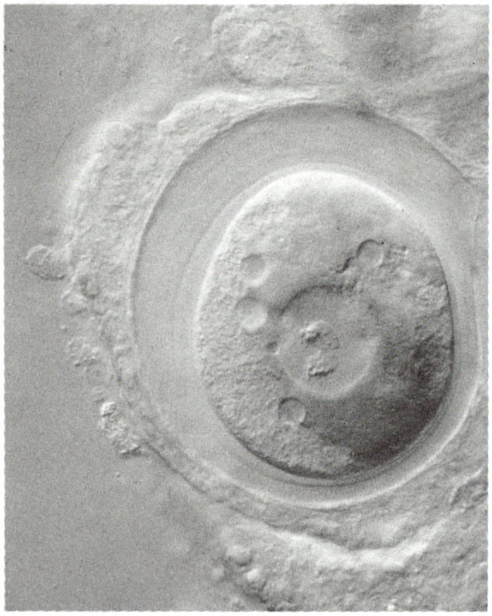

Figure 2—Microscopic view of an unstained smear of tissue from a lymphocystis-infected fish. Note the thick hyaline cell wall, enlarged nucleus, and granular cytoplasm with intracytoplasmic inclusion bodies. (× 125) (From Leibovitz L: Lymphocystis disease. *JAVMA* 176(3):202, 1980. Reprinted with permission.)

and the mixing of many carrier and susceptible fish in the static water of holding and breeding areas during export.[4] Therefore, newly acquired tropical fish often carry parasites which, within a closed aquarium system, can have devastating results.

Ichthyophthirius multifiliis and Chilodonella

Ichthyophthiriasis (ich, or white spot) is one of the best known, most common, and easily diagnosed of all parasitic skin diseases. It is caused by a ciliated protozoan, *Ichthyophthirius multifiliis*. Young stages of the parasite (trophozoites) are found in the epidermis of skin, fins, and gills. They feed on epithelial cells until they reach maturity, at which time the skin ruptures, releasing the adult parasites into the water. In an aquarium, the parasites sink to the gravel substrate and divide multiple times to produce a cystlike structure containing 500 to 2000 ciliated infective stages called *tomites*. When the cyst ruptures, the tomites are released and then reinfect the fish.

Clinical signs in acute infections may include only sudden mortality without gross evidence of disease. In more chronic infections, the skin becomes inflamed, and localized granulomas form which enclose the parasites.[5] The encysted organisms are seen clinically as white spots on the surface of the fish (Figure 3). In heavy infestations, white spots may also be seen in the corneal, buccal, and esophageal epithelia.[6] The parasite appears to be severely irritating to fish, which adopt a characteristic substrate-rubbing behavior termed *flashing*.[4] Affected fish may also evidence respiratory distress if the gills are involved. Ichthyophthiriasis is one of the most commonly fatal diseases of aquarium fish. Infected individuals may develop a dirty gray color prior to death. This is at least partly due to the osmoregulatory failure that occurs with epithelial erosion. Other parasitic or fungal infections may occur secondarily.

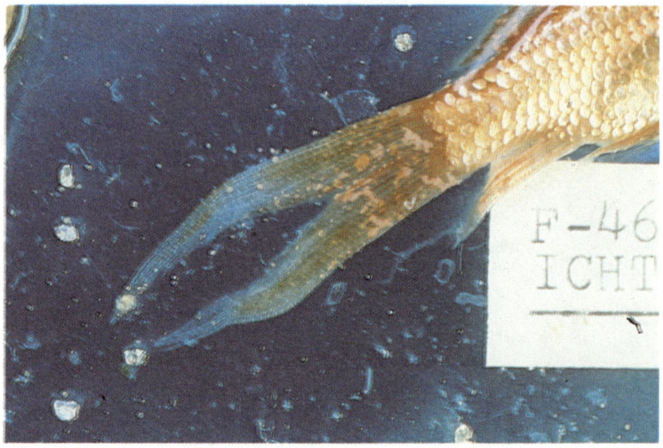

Figure 3—Infection of a goldfish with *Ichthyophthirius multifiliis*. Encysted trophozoites are seen as white spots in the tail. Rupturing cysts and tomites are present in the aquarium water. (From Leibovitz L: Ichthyophthiriasis. *JAVMA* 176(1):30, 1980. Reprinted with permission.)

Definitive diagnosis of ichthyophthiriasis can be made by direct microscopic examination of an unstained smear taken from affected areas (Figure 4). The parasite is spherical and large in diameter (50 μm to 1 mm). It is ciliated and demonstrates a constantly rotating motion. Most characteristic is its easily seen horseshoe-shaped macronucleus. It is possible to diagnose the disease by histopathology also, but this is far less sensitive and certainly more time-consuming.[5]

The length of the life cycle of *Ichthyophthirius* is directly related to the water temperature. At 4.4°C (40°F) the parasite completes its life cycle in six to eight weeks. At 21°C (70°F), the life cycle is shortened to 7 to 10 days.[7] Raising the temperature to 30°C (86°F), or greater if the fish can tolerate it, is an important part of therapy for the disease. Not only can this be directly lethal to the parasites, but it also effectively speeds the life cycle. Forms encysted on the fish mature rapidly and develop

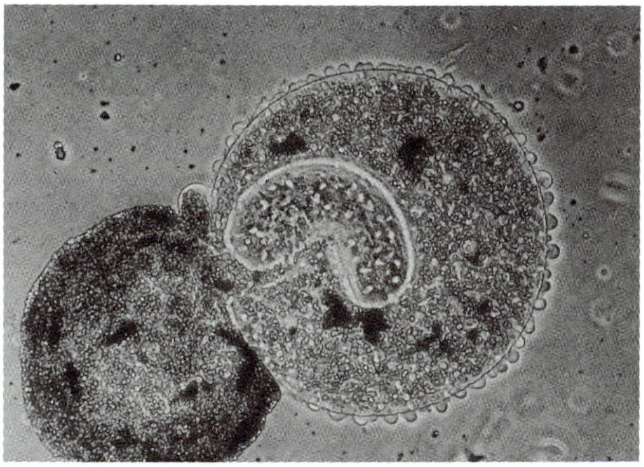

Figure 4—Microscopic view of an unstained wet mount of *Ichthyophthirius multifiliis*. Large, spherical, ciliated profile with a large horseshoe-shaped macronucleus is characteristic. (×63) (From Leibovitz L: Ichthyophthiriasis. *JAVMA* 176(1):30, 1980. Reprinted with permission.)

into the free water forms. There are no safe drugs available that can kill the encysted parasites. Free water forms however, are very susceptible to a wide variety of chemicals (discussed below). Chemical treatment of the aquarium water at elevated temperatures for 7 to 10 days should be effective in eliminating the disease.

Recovered fish may remain carriers. Disease can recur whenever the immune system is compromised or the fish are stressed. This problem has given rise to recent interest in developing a vaccine. Because *Ichthyophthirius* attacks only surface epithelial cells, it produces a poor immune response in fish. However, another ciliate, *Tetrahymena pyriformis*, when injected parenterally into fish, induces a high degree of immunity which is nonspecific. It is thought that the nonspecificity may be due to antibody against antigenic cilia components that all ciliates share. This one vaccine may prove to be protective against not only *Ichthyophthirius* but also against other ciliated protozoans such as *Chilodonella*.[8]

Chilodonella is another parasite of fish integument (Figure 5). It is colorless, oval, and about 70 μm long and is covered by rows of cilia that allow it to glide over the epithelial cells of the fins, body, and gills. It feeds by extruding its pharynx, penetrating host cells, and sucking out their contents. *Chilodonella* multiply maximally at 5 to 10°C.[6]

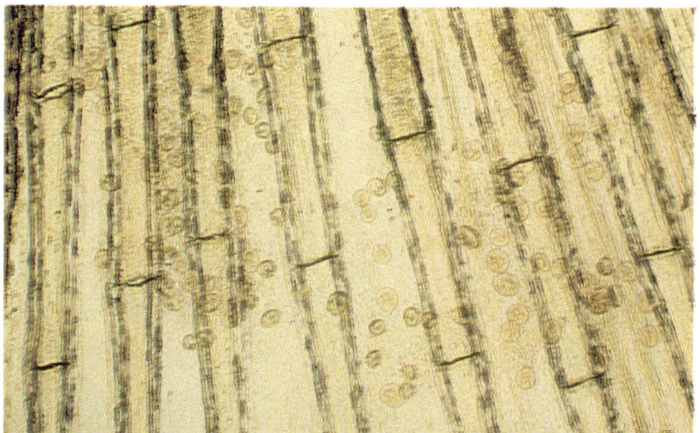

Figure 5—*Chilodonella* infection in the tail of an angelfish. Note the colorless, oval parasites present between the bony tail spines. (Courtesy of L Leibovitz, Marine Biological Laboratory, Woods Hole, Massachusetts)

Oodinium

Oodinium is a dinoflagellate which causes velvet disease in freshwater tropical fish. It also feeds directly on skin and gills. The adult parasite is pear shaped and measures approximately 150 μm in length by 70 μm in width. The cell cytoplasm of this parasite contains red, yellow, brown, or green chlorophyll. The condition caused by infestation with this parasite usually manifests itself as a gold brown skin discoloration seen as dustlike particles when examined under a hand magnifying lens.[9] This manifestation is responsible for the condition's other names: *rust disease* or *gold dust disease*. Mature trophonts leave the fish host and divide to form swarms of dinospores which then reinfect the fish. Explosive epizootics in aquaria can cause high mortality through gill and skin damage.

Ichthyobodo (Costia) necatrix

Ichthyobodo or *Costia necatrix* is a small flagellate, 10 to 15 μm long, which causes the disease costiasis in fish. The attached stage penetrates epithelial cells of fish by means of a holdfast (Figure 6). The parasite feeds on the epithelial cells and reproduces on the fish, thereby causing epidermal cell necrosis, irritation, and hypersecretion of mucus. *Ichthyobodo* may cause mortality with no clinical signs, although the skin and gill epithelium are destroyed. In other cases, there may be gray patches evident on the skin, which represent areas of excess cuticle production (Figure 7). Heavily infected fish will rub against the substrate presumably to relieve irritation but will lose scales and increase their chances of developing bacterial and fungal infections secondarily.[6]

Monogenetic Flukes

Monogenetic flukes are very common parasites of fish skin. They feed on mucus, skin, and sometimes

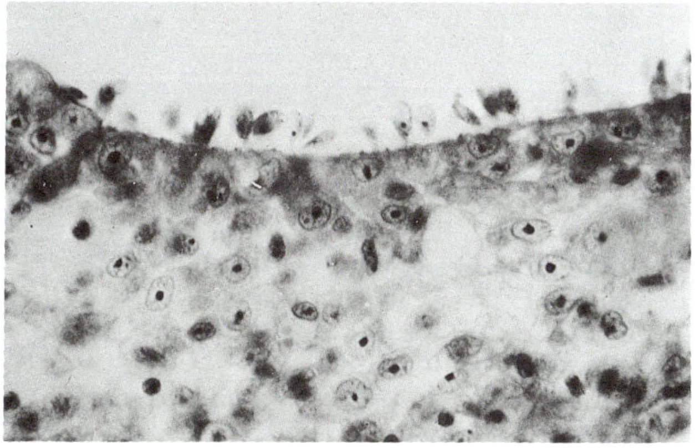

Figure 6—*Ichthyobodo necatrix* organisms attach by means of their holdfasts to the epithelial cells of a fish. (Courtesy of AH Walsh, Pfizer, Inc., Groton, Connecticut)

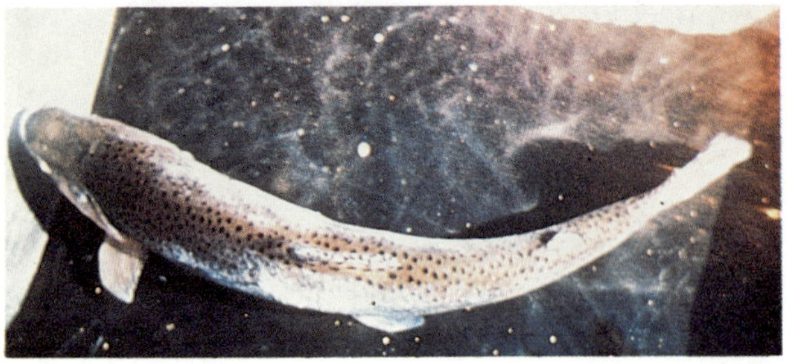

Figure 7—Gray slime evident on the sides of this rainbow trout is the characteristic gross appearance of costiasis. (Courtesy of AH Walsh, Pfizer, Inc., Groton, Connecticut)

blood. Most damaging to fish is their holdfast which bears two large centrally placed hooks and an assortment of surrounding hooklets (Figure 8). Of the two main families that parasitize tropical freshwater fish, only one involves the skin. These are the Gyrodactylidae, small flukes 0.3 to 1 mm long, found on the skin, gills, and fins. Each species is host specific. They are viviparous and can reproduce extremely rapidly. An epizootic occurrence of these parasites is usually associated with poor husbandry. Other protozoan parasites often will be present simultaneously. Heavy infections are characterized by increased cuticle production, frayed fins, skin ulcers, and damaged gills. The gyrodactylids seldom cause mortality.[7]

Digenetic Trematodes

Digenetic trematodes are another group of parasites that afflict fish skin. The life cycle of these parasites includes several larval stages, some of which encyst in fish skin as well as in various visceral organs. The host responds to the parasite by forming a pigmented connective tissue capsule (Figures 9 and 10). The color of

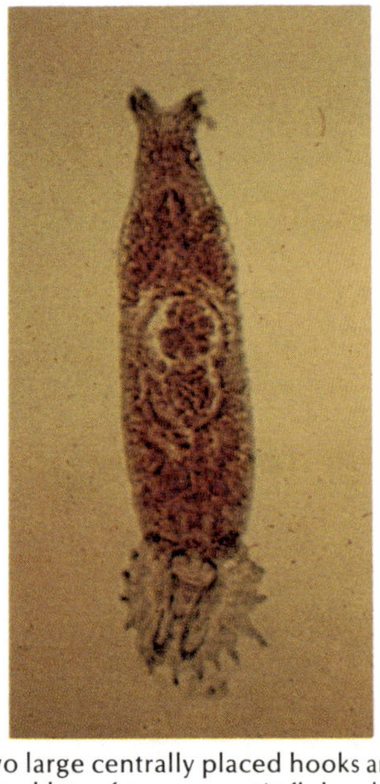

Figure 8—The two large centrally placed hooks and an assortment of surrounding hooklets of monogenetic flukes damage the skin of their fish hosts. (Courtesy of AH Walsh, Pfizer, Inc., Groton, Connecticut)

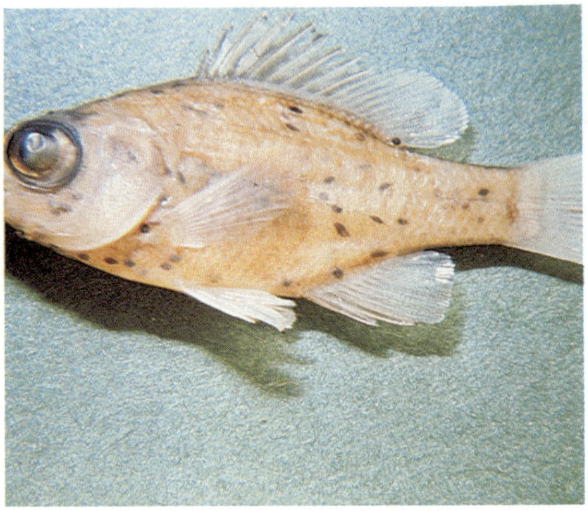

Figure 9—Larval stages of the digenetic trematodes can encyst in fish skin and cause black spot disease. (Courtesy of AH Walsh, Pfizer, Inc., Groton, Connecticut)

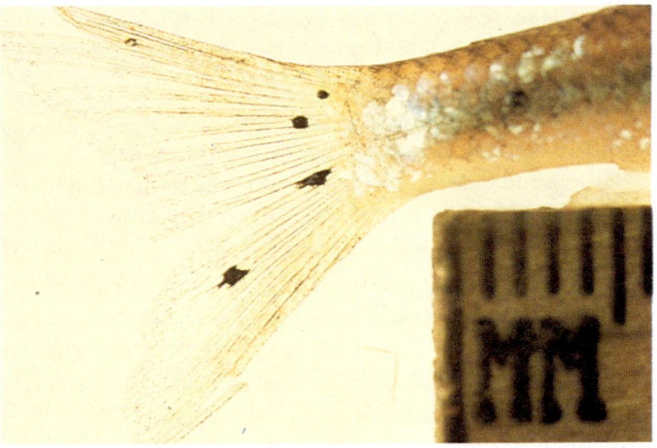

Figure 10—The color of the connective tissue capsule formed around digenetic trematode parasites depends on the parasite-host tissue interactions. (Courtesy of L Leibovitz, Marine Biological Laboratory, Woods Hole, Massachusetts)

the cyst depends on the parasite and host tissues. Specific trematode species tend to elicit specific color responses; these differing color responses have led to the several names for this disease—*black, white,* or *yellow spot disease.* An intermediate mollusk host is nearly always required for the digenetic trematodes to complete their life cycles. Newly purchased aquarium fishes may carry a heavy infestation into a tank, but the disease is self-limiting as long as there are no mollusks present. *Corydoras* species (smooth-armored catfish) are commonly heavily infected at the time of purchase and may show significant mortality at first. Those that survive may continue to harbor adults and encysted larval forms, but the parasite life cycle will remain aborted as long as no mollusks are present in the tank. Aquarium infections may also be acquired if fish are fed infected mollusk material such as fresh ground mussels or snails.[10]

Occasionally, encysted larval forms can be seen grossly on the skin surface, but definitive diagnosis of this parasite is best done at necropsy when a quantitative and qualitative assessment of worm burden can be made. A dissecting microscope is necessary to see the adults. They can be found most commonly in the lumen of the gastrointestinal tract, gall bladder, and swim bladder. Encysted forms may be present anywhere in the fish (Figure 11). Dissecting needles are used to free the cysts for identification of the parasite. Histologic sections of the brain and voluntary muscle may also reveal the cysts.[10]

Infections with digenetic trematodes can be avoided by buying healthy fish and not keeping mollusks and fish together in the same aquarium. Treatment of a disease outbreak involves removal of aquarium mollusks. Drugs are not recommended since infestation can be controlled by proper management.[10]

Copepods

Copepods of the genus *Lernaea* are easily recognized crustacean parasites of fish skin (Figure 12). These organisms are worldwide in distribution and, although they are not host specific, they are particularly common in goldfish *(Carassius auratus)* and tropical cichlids (family Cichlidae).[9] The head of these so-called anchor worms is branched and is used to embed the parasite into the integument of the fish. On physical examination, only a little of the wormlike body and a pair of external egg sacs can be seen protruding from a hole in the skin of the fish. Such lesions usually induce ulceration and eventually the formation of a fibrous nodule. In some cases, the parasite has been known to penetrate the body musculature and embed itself into internal viscera.[6] Young fish can be killed by just a few of these parasites. Older fish suffer emaciation and develop unsightly skin lesions which may become secondarily infected with bacterial or fungal agents.[7]

Another external crustacean that infects fish is *Argulus,* the fish louse. This is a large parasite (6 to 22 mm

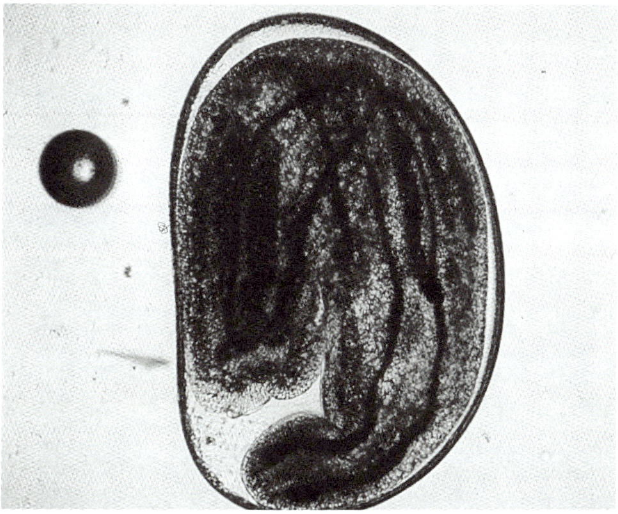

Figure 11—This encysted larval form of a digenetic trematode was removed from the intestinal serosa of a fish at necropsy. (From Leibovitz L: Digenetic trematode infection. *JAVMA* 177(1):42, 1980. Reprinted with permission.)

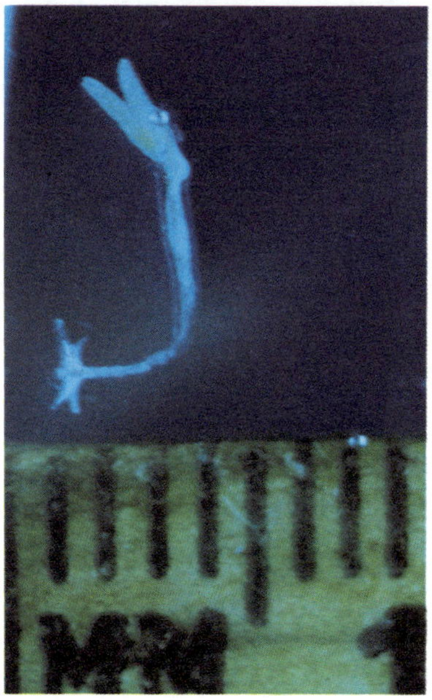

Figure 12—Copepod parasites of the genus *Lernaea* are identified by their multibranched head and two long trailing egg sacs. (Courtesy of L Leibovitz, Marine Biological Laboratory, Woods Hole, Massachusetts)

long) which can be seen grossly as it moves freely over the surface of fish (Figures 13 and 14). *Argulus* is dorsoventrally flattened and has two very conspicuous sucking disks which may be easily mistaken for large eyes. Using these suction cups and a pair of curved hooks to attach to fish, it inserts its proboscis into the epidermis and underlying tissues and feeds by injecting cytolytic toxin through its oral sting.[11] Necrotic, ulcerative lesions that are open to secondary infections are created which can cause mass mortality in young fish. Clinical signs of infection include weakness, erratic swimming, flashing, and, if the lateral line has been damaged, inability to maintain equilibrium. Argulids leave the fish host to molt and reproduce. Eggs are laid on any solid substrate.[11]

Leeches

Leeches are another visually obvious parasite common on ornamental carp (Figure 15). They can be accidentally

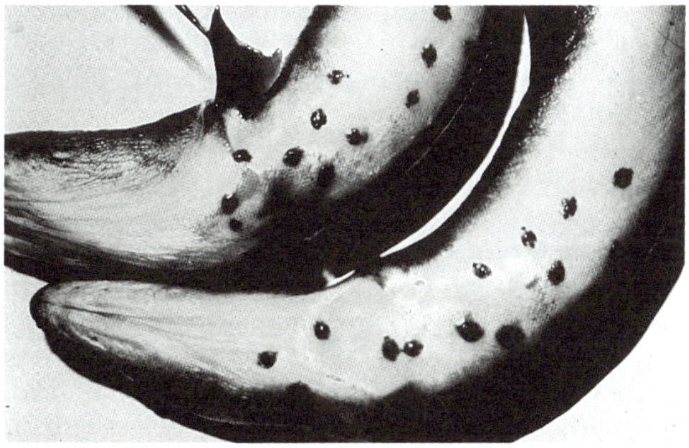

Figure 13—*Argulus giordanii* can be seen grossly on the ventrum of these fish. (Courtesy of AH Walsh, Pfizer, Inc., Groton, Connecticut)

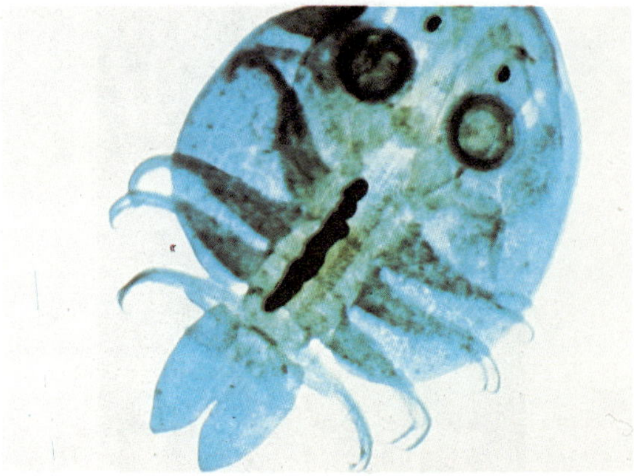

Figure 14—*Argulus* spp. are dorsoventrally flattened and have two very conspicuous sucking disks that may give the appearance of being large eyes. (Courtesy of AH Walsh, Pfizer, Inc., Groton, Connecticut)

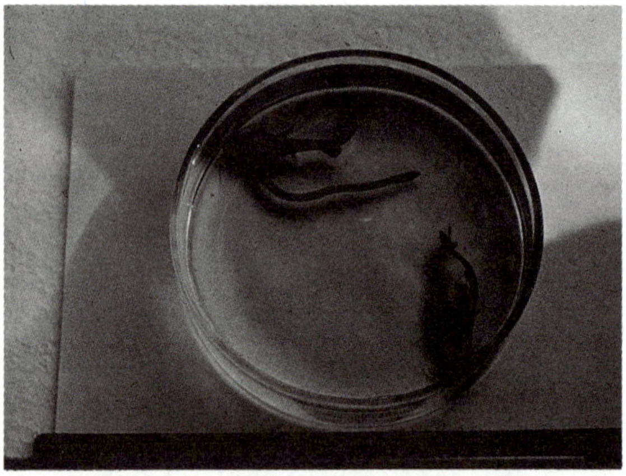

Figure 15—Leeches are grossly obvious parasites common on ornamental carp. (Courtesy of AH Walsh, Pfizer, Inc., Groton, Connecticut)

introduced into tropical freshwater aquaria with live food or plants. Leeches attach almost permanently to their fish hosts and pierce the skin to take periodic blood meals. Anemia, secondary infections in the ulcerative lesions, and transmission of blood flagellates are problems associated with leeches.[4,6,9]

Integumentary Mycoses

Many mycotic agents have been associated with skin lesions in fish, but it is not clear how many of these are primary infectors and how many are secondary invaders. Fungal spores are ever present in aquarium water. Some predisposing factor usually seems necessary to initiate fungal infection in fish. Mycotic lesions are seen following handling or trauma to the skin, with overcrowding or pollution, and secondary to viral, parasitic, or bacterial infection. Temperature also seems to play a role; most fungal epizootics occur when temperature is either much higher or lower than normal.[12]

By far the most common of the integumentary mycoses are those caused by members of the *Saprolegnia* genus. These are ubiquitous fungi found in fresh- and saltwater as well as in soil. Their growth is favored by moderately acidic pH, low temperatures, and the presence of decaying plant and animal material.[13] The typical clinical appearance of saprolegniasis is a grossly visible white cottonlike covering over the surface of affected fish (Figure 16). Initially the lesions are focal and circular. They grow progressively with radial and inward extension into the deeper subcutaneous and muscular layers. In later stages of the disease, the fungal growth is often brown or gray because of the presence of mud and melanosomes from disrupted melanophores which are tangled up with the hyphae.[12] When epizootics occur in an aquarium, an acute inflammatory skin response may occur in addition. The skin of infected fish will become edematous and reddened, produce excessive mucus, and show signs of subcutaneous hemorrhage. Fish with saprolegniasis become anorectic and inactive and seek secluded areas of the tank. Infection leads to blood loss and fluid imbalance, which result in shock. Mortality may be as high as 80% and as rapid as within 36 hours following initial infection.[12,13]

The skin and gills are the most frequently affected sites in saprolegniasis, although severe infection may occur in internal organs as well.[13] The distribution of the lesions is random in most fish species. More heavily armored thick-skinned fish are more resistant to generalized involvement than other fish are. They tend to have localized lesions confined to thinly epithelialized areas of their bodies (fins, tail, pores of the lateral line system, cornea). Fin lesions can progress to complete loss of fin membrane and exposure of the bony spines.[13] Fish eggs are also susceptible to *Saprolegnia* infection. Dead or infertile eggs will be the first to develop a mottled, opaque appearance with the typical cottony growth on their surface. From there, the infection spreads to other viable eggs.[13]

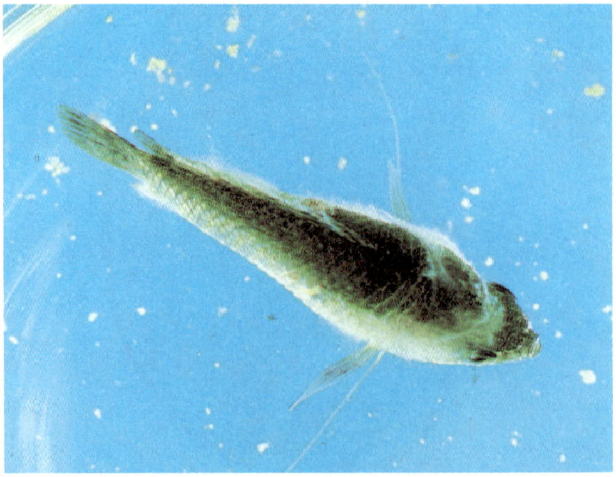

Figure 16—Saprolegniasis is characterized clinically as a grossly visible white cottonlike covering over the surface of the fish. (Courtesy of L Leibovitz, Marine Biological Laboratory, Woods Hole, Massachusetts)

On fresh direct smears, profusely branched, aseptate, hyphal elements can be seen (Figure 17). To diagnose the specific fungus causing the lesions, isolation and morphologic characterization are required. However, this is not necessary clinically since *Saprolegnia* is by far the most common and since treatment for all mycotic infections is identical.

Bacterial Skin Infections

Many pathogenic species of bacteria have been isolated from lesions in the integument of fish. Most are gram-negative organisms. However, it is probably erroneous to consider bacterial infections as primary disease entities.[14] They nearly always occur secondarily to some other primary stress such as parasites, transportation, or chemical imbalances in aquarium water. Nonetheless, at least one bacterial disease has been recognized as a specific entity. It is columnaris disease (saddleback disease, fin rot, tail rot). *Flexibacter columnaris*, a gram-negative rod, is the main causative agent. Columnaris disease is a skin infection characterized by blanched, necrotic lesions. The most distinctive lesion is a saddle-like marking behind the dorsal fin. The fins and tail of some affected fish develop whitish areas and split. Diagnosis of the disease can be made most easily by skin scrapings or cut sections of affected fins viewed as direct wet mount preparations. Long, flexible rods exhibiting typical gliding and column-forming activity are characteristic (Figure 18).

Aeromonas hydrophila is a very common cause of bacterial infection in fish. It is responsible for bacterial hemorrhagic septicemia, a disease characterized by hemorrhage around lesions on the body surface, at the bases of the fins, and internally. *Aeromonas* spp. are also associated with ulcer disease of goldfish in which large gaping ulcers develop on the sides of the body.

Mycobacterial Infection

Mycobacteriosis is a relatively uncommon systemic granulomatous disease of tropical fish and is a zoonosis.

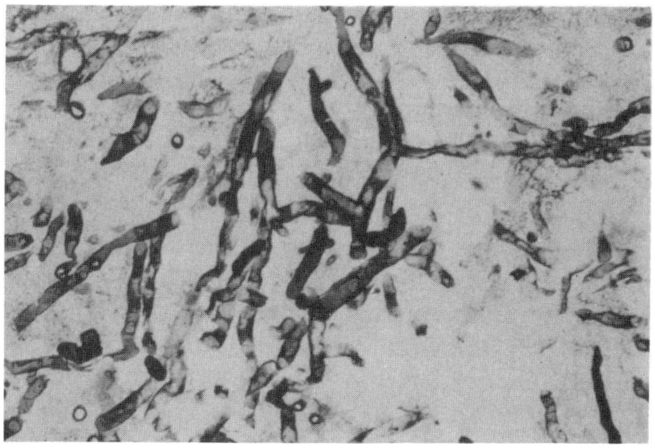

Figure 17—Profusely branched, aseptate hyphae are characteristic of *Saprolegnia*. (Courtesy of AH Walsh, Pfizer, Inc., Groton, Connecticut)

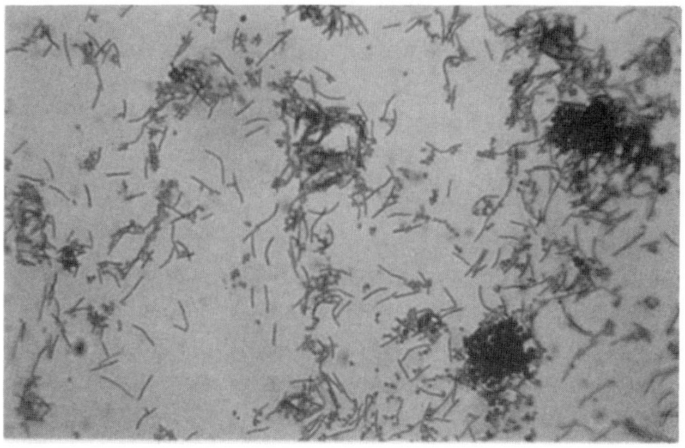

Figure 18—Gram's staining a direct smear of a skin scraping demonstrates the long, flexible, gram-negative rods of *Flexibacter columnaris*. (Courtesy of AH Walsh, Pfizer, Inc., Groton, Connecticut)

In freshwater aquarium fish it can be caused by *Mycobacterium piscium*, *M. platypoecilus*, or *M. fortuitum*. The clinical signs of the disease are variable and usually nonspecific. They include loss of coloration, lifting of scales, exophthalmos, skin ulcerations, frayed fins, ascites, listlessness, anorexia, and weight loss (Figure 19).

On necropsy, grayish white granulomatous foci can be found in the skin as well as the liver, spleen, and kidneys. Histopathological examination of these lesions identifies them as tubercles with an outer fibroblastic wall surrounding a central zone of epithelioid cells, histiocytes, pigment cells, and tissue debris.[15] Definitive diagnosis depends on the demonstration of acid-fast bacilli within the tuberculous lesions or on tissue impression smears.[1,15]

Treatment should not be considered for these fish since it cannot eliminate infection. Fish suspected of infection should be destroyed since the agent is transmissible to humans. Skin infections have been known to develop in people exposed to fish mycobacteria. *M.*

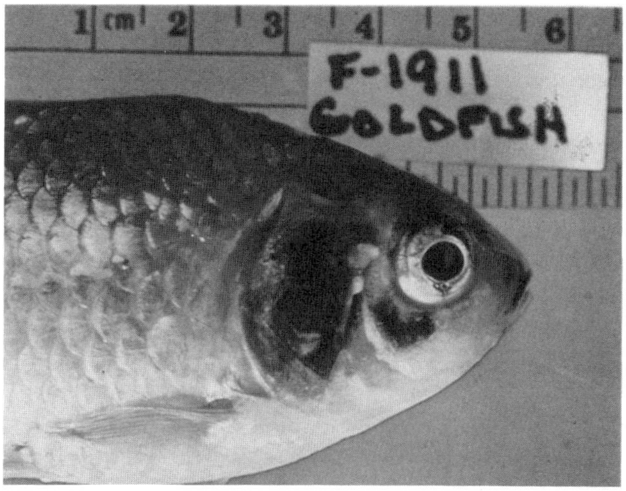

Figure 19—This ulcerative nodule on the operculum of a goldfish was later identified as mycobacterial infection. (Courtesy of L Leibovitz, Marine Biological Laboratory, Woods Hole, Massachusetts)

fortuitum is one of the species known to cause pulmonary disease resembling tuberculosis in humans. The aquarium and its contents should be totally disinfected prior to the introduction of new fish.

Tumors of Fish Integument

Tumors are known to occur in fish integument and should be included in the differential diagnosis for skin lesions. However, few of these tumors have been reported in the literature, and far fewer have been characterized histologically.[16] Melanomas are tumors of melanocytes and melanophores and are thought to be a relatively common tumor type in tropical fish. Their occurrence in platy-swordtail hybrids is being studied as a model for human melanoma.[17]

Clinical Approach to Fish

The clinical approach to the diagnosis of health problems in aquarium fish is similar to that used with any animal species. The history should include the age of the tank, acquisition dates of the fish, diet, and schedule of water changes and additions. A complete description of the current problem should be obtained and include the number of fish affected, the time course of the disease, treatments attempted, and mortality.

Physical examination should start at the whole aquarium level. Construction and location of the tank should be noted, as well as the type of filtering system and pump. Lighting, depth of aquarium substrate, and the presence or absence of living plants are all factors of importance. Fish stocking density should not exceed 2.5 to 3 in. of fish length per square foot of tank floor area.[18] The amount of dead and decaying organic material in the tank should be assessed.

Water quality is the next aspect of the aquarium to be examined. A temperature of 25°C (76 to 78°F) is good for most tropical fish species. The water should be clear and odor free. The veterinarian should measure the ammonia, nitrite, and pH levels using commercially available colorimetric water quality kits. Ammonia exists in two forms in the aquarium—toxic NH_3 and nontoxic NH_4^+. The relative percentage of each depends on the pH. The higher the pH is, the higher is the concentration of toxic un-ionized ammonia. High NH_3 levels are thought to interfere with oxygen transport in fish. Ammonia levels should not exceed 0.2 ppm in the aquarium.[14]

Nitrite concentration should be less than 0.1 ppm.[14] Levels higher than this can be lethal to fish by causing the development of methemoglobinemia. Affected fish have chocolate-colored blood on necropsy. The pH of aquarium water should range between 6 and 8. pH levels outside this range interfere with respiration and osmoregulation in fish. A pH lower than 6 interferes with *Nitrosomonas* spp., bacteria critical to the nitrogen cycle in all aquaria. With a decrease in the viability of the *Nitrosomonas* population, less NH_3 is converted to nontoxic nitrogen products, and ammonia concentration rises to toxic levels. The quality of water aeration in the tank should be assessed visually. A commercially available test kit can also be used to monitor oxygen levels in the water. Seven to eight parts per million of dissolved oxygen is recommended.[14] Abnormal values in these parameters can usually be corrected via water changes and filtering and circulation system improvements.

Next the attention of the veterinarian should be turned to the animal population. It is important to note the mixture of animals present. The keeping of mollusks and fish together cannot be recommended since they share the same digenetic trematodes and together allow these parasites to enjoy complete life cycles within the tank. Live plants, if present in the aquarium, should be carefully searched at the time of purchase and small adherent snails should be removed.

Dead fish decompose very rapidly and generally are of very little diagnostic aid, even if they have been preserved or frozen.[19] Moribund fish should be examined. Their color, condition, behavior, and locomotor abilities should be noted. Fine-mesh nets or specially designed homemade slings can be used to carefully catch individual fish for examination. Lesions should be observed grossly and the presence of any macroscopic parasites on the external surface, mouth, or opercula should be noted. Skin scrapings of affected areas in the skin can be mounted in aquarium water and examined directly. This procedure alone can be diagnostic for many infections.

For a suspected bacterial problem, several specimens from a variety of clinically affected fish (both early and late in the course of the disease) should be obtained. Gram's-stained smears of obvious lesions can be of great help in guiding therapy. If the lesions are granulomatous, the Ziehl-Neelsen staining method for acid-fast bacteria should be used. Culture of skin lesions from fish can be misleading, because of invasion by saprophytic or secondary bacteria and fungi. The isolation and interpretation of results can also be problematic. Many of the potential pathogens of fish are from genera unfamiliar to classical veterinary or human medicine. Furthermore, many bacterial species are normal flora of the aquarium environment and become pathogenic only when they are present in significant quantities. Close attention to the clinical history of the tank is critical to rational interpretation of laboratory results.[19]

When histopathology is required for diagnosis, the moribund fish is placed in a container of euthanasia solution (0.2 g of benzocaine in 5 ml of acetone, added to 8 L of water is recommended[19]) for 5 to 10 minutes. Alternatively, the fish may be quickly decapitated. The fish must be handled carefully both before and after death to avoid iatrogenic lesions. Fish tissues undergo very rapid autolysis compared with homoiotherms, so they must be handled rapidly. Excised tissues are placed in formaldehyde, 40% by weight for fixation.

Chemical Treatment of Integumentary Diseases

As is true in all animal species, it is easier to prevent disease in fish than to treat it. Quarantine of all new fish for two weeks prior to adding them to an established aquarium community is highly desirable. Most harbored disease problems will appear clinically in this amount of time. They can be treated and the disease eradicated in the quarantine tank before the fish are mixed with other healthy animals. The best way to avoid disease in the established aquarium is with good husbandry, correct feeding, and good water quality. Overcrowding of fish, anoxia, trauma, and abrupt changes in temperature should be avoided. The home aquarist should be encouraged to monitor water chemistry closely for increases in concentrations of ammonia or nitrite, and pH changes. The majority of disease outbreaks in aquaria are related to inadequate husbandry or management.[20]

When an outbreak occurs, a correction in husbandry or management may result is spontaneous clearing of the problem. Such conservative therapy is always preferable, but in some cases, chemical treatment may be required. The state of chemical therapy in fish, especially tropical fish, is still relatively unsophisticated. There are no funds available for the development of ornamental fish medicine. Most of what is known is derived from warm water culture studies of food fishes.[1] Even so, there have been few research efforts to establish drug toxicity and efficacy or methods of administration. Treatments that aquarists have found successful have been reported incidentally. The literature is fragmentary. Nevertheless, some therapeutic regimens have emerged over the years.

There are three ways in which chemicals can be applied to aquarium fish—externally, per os, and parenterally.[20] External application can be accomplished via swabbing or immersion. Swabbing involves the use of a cotton-tipped applicator and is useful in treating localized external lesions in individual fish. Immersion can be carried out in a short time by using a dip or a bath. A dip involves moving affected individuals to a small treatment tank and exposing them to high drug concentrations for one to five minutes before returning them to the aquarium. A bath also requires moving the affected fish temporarily to a small treatment tank. With this method, the fish are exposed to low drug concentrations for 30 to 60 minutes. The dissolved-oxygen levels, temperature, and other water parameters of the bath must be monitored carefully before and during treatment.

Immersion can also be prolonged by adding chemicals directly into the established aquarium. Very low drug concentrations are maintained for 12 or more hours. All fish in the tank are exposed to the chemical simultaneously. Although this method of treatment is the easiest, there are some problems associated with it. Suspended organic solids arising from poor tank hygiene can absorb the treatment chemical and decrease its efficacy.[20] Bacteria necessary to the nitrogen cycle such as *Nitrobacter* can be impaired by the chemicals. Drug dosage must be decreased when the pH of the aquarium water is low since acid pH makes therapeutic chemicals more toxic.[20]

Therapy per os requires that the diseased fish are eating. Unfortunately, anorexia is often one of the earliest signs of illness. Administration per os is accomplished by mixing the drug and a small amount of cod liver oil with the normal daily ration.[14] This method of treatment is generally used only during the early stages of systemic bacterial infection. Therapy per os has several associated disadvantages: fish may show reluctance to eat medicated food; it is impossible to achieve exact, known drug levels by this dosage method; and the antibiotics must be mixed with food immediately before feedings because some antibiotics degrade rapidly.[20]

The third method of chemical administration in fish is the parenteral route. The fish must be restrained by some atraumatic means. Injections can be made intraperitoneally in the ventral abdomen or subcutaneously just caudal to the dorsal fin. Intramuscular injections are not recommended because of the poor vascularization of fish muscle.[1] Any parenteral therapy should be regarded as experimental, however, because there is little literature on the subject.[20]

Chemicals Effective Against Ectoparasites

There are several chemicals that have been found effective in the treatment of parasitic infections in fish. The first of these is formalin (37 to 40% solution of formaldehyde in water, usually with 12 to 15% methanol as a preservative) which is usually recommended as a bath (1:6000 administered one time for one hour). Formalin is effective against most ectoparasitic protozoa as well as some monogenetic trematodes. Paraformaldehyde, a white precipitate that forms in stored formalin, causes toxicity and must be removed via filtration prior to usage. A prolonged immersion regimen of adding 15 to 25 ppm formalin to an aquarium every other day for five to seven days has also been suggested.[21]

A second chemical used in the control of protozoal parasites is malachite green ($C_{23}H_{24}N_2(C_2H_2O_4)_3$). This chemical is available in several forms—oxalate, chloride, and sulfate salts. Any of these is satisfactory for use with fish. The double salt of zinc chloride, however, contains toxic levels of zinc and should be avoided.[20] Since *Ichthyophthirius multifiliis* adults are encysted in host tissue, therapeutic dips and baths are not very effective. Prolonged immersion aimed at the destruction of the free-swimming stages of the parasite must be used. Treatment must be continued once daily for 7 to 10 days, with water temperature in the tank as close to 32°C (90°F) as the fish will tolerate. Malachite green may be used alone at a concentration of 0.1 to 0.15 ppm. Alternatively, it may be used in combination with formalin[a] (0.1 ppm malachite green + 25 ppm formalin) at three-day intervals.[22] Malachite green is an herbicide and will

[a]Quick Cure®, Aquarium Products, Glen Burnie, MD 21061.

result in some plant decay in aquaria containing live plants. Plant decay, in addition to formalin decomposition and higher water temperature, will decrease the level of dissolved oxygen in the water.[7] Fish should be observed carefully for signs of anoxia throughout the treatment period.

Copper sulfate ($CuSO_4$)[b] has been recommended by some as an alternative treatment for protozoal parasites.[1,23] A concentration of 0.15 ppm free copper ions should be maintained in the aquarium water for two weeks. This will kill mature parasites as they leave the fish host and immature forms as they emerge from cysts.[23] Invertebrate animals are very susceptible to copper toxicity; if any are present, they must be removed prior to the initiation of treatment. Copper ions bind easily to other ions in the aquarium, so the actual copper level will vary from that calculated in the dosage. Therefore, to assure therapeutic levels, it is essential for the free copper ion level to be monitored via a commercially available colorimetric test kit.

Organophosphates have been reported to be effective against monogenetic flukes, digenetic trematodes, *Lernaea,* leeches, and *Argulus.*[4,7,20,21,23] A 1% dip of o,o-dimethyl-2,2,2-trichloro-1-hydroxyethyl phosphonate[c] administered for two to three minutes has been recommended. Treatment may have to be repeated once weekly for one month.[7,20] Alternatively, this drug may be administered at a concentration of 1 ppm as a two-day-long bath. One bath is given per week for three consecutive weeks.[23] Because some of the parasites have stages in their life cycles that can survive off the host, the entire aquarium may have to be treated with a prolonged immersion of 0.25 to 1.0 ppm for five days.[4,21] Dimethyl 1,2-dibromo 2,2-dichlorethyl phosphate used at a concentration of 0.1 mg/L may be a more effective prolonged immersion treatment.[20,21] Persistent adult copepods that are not killed by these chemicals may have to be removed surgically.[4,21]

Chemicals Effective Against Fungal Infections

Treatment of saprolegniasis is aimed at eliminating the primary disease, killing the fungus growing on the fish, and restoring the integument. Fungal spores are ubiquitous and their eradication is not a treatment goal. The chemical of choice for all fungal infections is malachite green. Application of a 1% solution with a swab or of a 67 mg/L dip for one minute is effective. The chemical may also be administered as a bath, using a concentration of 1 to 2 mg/L for one hour. Prolonged immersion is also effective at a 0.15 mg/L concentration.[20] As a prophylactic treatment for fish eggs, a concentration of 2 mg/L for one hour is recommended.[20] Other chemicals that have been successfully used as locally applied swabs include 10% tincture of iodine, 1% potassium dichromate, hydrogen peroxide, and 2% Mercurochrome.[d,1,12-14,23] Fifteen-minute baths of 1000 ppm formalin have been used with good results in commercial fisheries, and so have one-hour baths with 0.5 ppm copper sulfate.[24]

Antimicrobials

When considering an antibiotic for use in treating fish disease, two factors must be considered: (1) the absorption of the drugs by the fish, and (2) the solubility of the drug in water. When treating systemic infections, the former consideration is most important because therapeutic blood levels must be achieved. Blood levels may not be important, however, when an antibiotic is being used to treat an external infection. Water solubility of the drug may be more significant in these instances.[14] It should also be borne in mind when using antibiotics that drug resistance can develop in aquatic microbes as well as it can in terrestrial species. Indiscriminate use of antibiotics should therefore be avoided.[14] However, antibiotics can be used appropriately as prophylactics against secondary infections while other primary disease problems are being treated.

Since the majority of fish pathogens are gram-negative organisms, treatment is usually with a broad-spectrum antibiotic. Gram-positive bacteria are not the significant cause of acute, fulminating infections that they are in mammals. They are usually associated with chronic disease that is not amenable to treatment.

The sulfonamides are some of the few antimicrobials that have been cleared by the FDA for use in commercial meat fish.[14] They are used per os at a dosage of 22 g/100 kg of fish per day for one day, followed by 11 g/100 kg of fish per day for 5 to 10 days. The sulfonamides have the advantage of being inexpensive, but they have been associated with renal toxicity and anorexia.[20] Mixtures of sulphadiazine and trimethoprim in a 5:1 ratio have shown increased therapeutic activity at a lower dose and without the dietary and toxicity problems. The per os dosage for this combination is 5.5 g/100 kg of fish daily for 5 to 10 days.

The nitrofurans are another broad-spectrum group of antibiotics that have been successful in the treatment of fish. Outstanding among them is nifurpirinol which is readily absorbed from water into the blood circulation of fish.[14] The nitrofurans are more expensive than the sulfonamides but have fewer toxicity and appetite problems associated with them. Nitrofurans may also be administered per os at a dosage of 11 g/100 kg of fish per day for 5 to 10 days.[20]

Oxytetracycline is another broad-spectrum antibiotic that has been used widely with fish. It also has been approved by the FDA for use in the commercial fish industry and has proven efficacy. However, because of its popular usage as a prophylactic agent in the water of transported fish, bacterial resistance is developing. The recommended dosage for prolonged immersion is 20 to

[b]Copper Sulfate Solution, Marine Enterprises, Timonium, MD 21033.
[c]Flouse®, Jungle Laboratories Corp., Sanford, FL 32771.

[d]Trademark, Becton-Dickinson, Rutherford, NJ 07070.

50 ppm. The tetracyclines are chelated in excessively hard water (more than 200 ppm as $CaCO_3$). In these conditions, the drug is not ideally used unless the dosage is increased by one-third to one-half over recommended levels.[14] If more than one dose is required, treatment should be given on alternate days with 50 to 75% water change on each of the nontreatment days. This will dilute the lactose carriers associated with many tetracycline preparations which would otherwise cloud the water and contribute to further bacterial growth.[14] Oxytetracycline can also be administered per os at a dosage of 7.5 g/100 kg of fish per day for 5 to 15 days.[20]

The aminoglycosides have been used in teleosts, but it is thought that only the water-soluble kanamycin sulfate may have application in fish medicine. The suggested dosage for prolonged immersion therapy is 50 to 100 ppm repeated every three to four days as needed. Aquarium water should be partially changed two days after each treatment.[14]

Chloramphenicol sodium succinate[c] is a water-soluble broad-spectrum antibiotic that has been used very effectively as a prolonged immersion for external bacterial infections. The dosage used is 20 to 50 ppm, repeated as necessary every third day, with a partial water change 24 hours after each treatment.[14] This drug has reportedly also been used as an intraperitoneal injection with excellent clinical results. A dosage of 25 mg/kg of body weight was injected once weekly for two weeks.[14]

Acknowledgment

The authors gratefully acknowledge the assistance of Drs. A. H. Walsh, L. Leibovitz, and G. Migaki in the preparation of this article.

[c] Chloromycetin® Sodium Succinate, Parke-Davis, Morris Plains, NJ 07950.

REFERENCES

1. Paul L: Exotic fish medicine: A new specialty field. *Auburn Vet* 36(1):17-21, 1979.
2. Durham PJK, Anderson CD: Lymphocystis disease in imported tropical fish. *NZ Vet J* 29(6):88-91, 1981.
3. Leibovitz L: Lymphocystis disease. *JAVMA* 176(3):202, 1980.
4. Sommerville C: Parasites of ornamental fish. *J Small Anim Pract* 22(6):367-376, 1981.
5. Leibovitz L: Ichthyophthiriasis. *JAVMA* 176(1):30-31, 1980.
6. Needham T, Wooten R: The parasitology of teleosts, in Ribelin WE, Migaki G (eds): *Pathology of Fishes.* Madison, WI, University of Wisconsin Press, 1975, pp 157-167.
7. Kocan AA, Landolt ML: Diseases of warm water fish. *Calif Vet* 35(5):8-13, 1981.
8. Leibovitz L: Vaccine for "white spot" in fish. *JAVMA* 178(2):103, 1981.
9. Richards R: Disease of aquarium fish—2: Skin diseases. *Vet Rec* 101:132-135, 1977.
10. Leibovitz L, Riis RC, Georgi ME: Diseases of aquarium fish: Digenetic trematode infection. *JAVMA* 177(1):40-42, 1980.
11. Hoffman GL: Argulus, *a Branchiuran Parasite of Freshwater Fishes.* Washington, DC, US Dept Interior, FDL—49, 1977.
12. Richards RH: The mycology of teleosts, in Ribelin WE, Migaki G (eds): *Pathology of Fishes.* Madison, WI, University of Wisconsin Press, 1975, pp 205-209.
13. Leibovitz L, Pinello C: Mycotic infections. *JAVMA* 177(11):1110-1112, 1980.
14. Gratzek JB: An overview of ornamental fish diseases and therapy. *J Small Anim Pract* 22(6):345-366, 1981.
15. Leibovitz L: Fish tuberculosis (mycobacteriosis). *JAVMA* 176(5):415, 1980.
16. Harshbarger JC: Neoplasms in zoo poikilotherms emphasizing cases in the registry of tumors in lower animals (fish, amphibians, reptiles), in Montali RJ, Migaki G (eds): *Comparative Pathology of Zoo Animals.* Washington, DC, Smithsonian Inst Press, 1980, pp 585-591.
17. Roberts RJ: Melanin-containing cells of teleost fish and their relation to disease, in Ribelin WE, Migaki G (eds): *Pathology of Fishes.* Madison, WI, University of Wisconsin Press, 1975, pp 399-428.
18. Carlson R: *Aquarium Medicine.* Woods Hole, MA, Aquavet, 1980.
19. Bullock AM: Laboratory methods, in Ribelin WE, Migaki G (eds): *Pathology of Fishes.* Madison, WI, University of Wisconsin Press, 1975, pp 235-267.
20. Poupard CJ: Therapy of fish diseases, in Ribelin WE, Migaki G (eds): *Pathology of Fishes.* Madison, WI, University of Wisconsin Press, 1975, pp 268-275.
21. Hoffman GL: *Control and Treatment of Parasitic Diseases of Freshwater Fishes.* Washington, DC, US Dept Interior, FDL—28, July 1970.
22. Meyer FP: *Parasites of Freshwater Fishes; II, Protozoa 3.* Ichthyophthirius multifiliis. Washington, DC, US Dept Interior, FDL—2, Aug 1974.
23. Dulin MP: Exotic fish medicine. *Mod Vet Pract* 58:31-33, 1977.
24. Hoffman GL: Parasites of freshwater fish I. Fungi. Washington, DC, US Dept Interior, FDL—21, Dec 1969.

Environmental and Disease Problems in Ornamental Marine Aquariums*

Daniel J. Oestmann, DVM†
Stone Veterinary Clinic
Moline, Illinois

With the right education, the tropical fish hobbyist in the United States could become an active part of the veterinarian's clientele. A survey sponsored by the United Nations showed that the United States was the world's largest importer of tropical fish in 1979. Americans spent $272 million buying dogs, followed closely by $234 million for pet fish. Bird owners spend $83 million, and cat owners spent $48 million.[1] Human population trends influence pet ownership. Increasing urbanization favors pets such as caged birds; however, these figures suggest that a client is more likely to have an aquarium than a bird cage in the living room.

Tropical fish come from warm water and equatorial regions, many from East Asia and the Amazon River.[1] Africa and South and Central America also are source areas. Tropical fish can be of freshwater or saltwater origin. Marine fish are from salt water, either warm (tropical) or cold (North Atlantic or North Pacific). Tropical coral reef fish are the most popular in display aquariums because of their bright colors and various forms. Cold water varieties of fish tend to be drab in appearance but hardier; they require expensive chiller units to maintain proper temperature. Veterinary services are sought more often for marine fish, which are more expensive, than for most freshwater tropical fish.

Environment of the Marine Aquarium

Management of the saltwater aquarium, more difficult than that of the freshwater one, requires constant attention and knowledge of the systems involved. The specimens in the tank live in a subtle balance between salinity, ammonia-nitrite-nitrate, pH, temperature, aeration, filtration, and waste (Table I). Most disease problems probably occur secondary to environmental changes within the aquarium.

Population Density

One of the most common environmental problems in display aquariums is population density. Because the natural fish-to-water ratio of the

---

*Kansas State University Agricultural Experimental Station Journal Series No. 84-295-J. (The research for this article was performed while the author was a student at the College of Veterinary Medicine.)

†Dr. Oestmann's present address is Berwyn Veterinary Associates, Berwyn, Illinois.

TABLE I
Parameters of a Marine Aquarium

Size	Easily maintained if over 75 L (20 gal)
Material used	No metal in contact with water; glass sealed with silicone and plastic airflow systems preferred
Filtration capacity	15–23 L (4–6 gal)/hr for each 3.8 L (1 gal) tank capacity
Aeration capacity	5.7–7.6 L (6–8 qt) of air/hr for each 3.8 L (1 gal) water
Population density	Approximately 13 L (3.5 gal)/ medium-sized fish
Temperature	21°–29.4° C (70°–85° F); 24.4° C (76° F) optimal
Water changes	One tenth to one third of capacity each 4–6 weeks
Salinity	34–35 ppt
Specific gravity	1.020–1.025, depending on temperature
pH	8.0–8.3
Ammonia	Less than 0.01 ppm un-ionized ammonia; test kits that measure total ammonium nitrogen should indicate 0.1 ppm or less
Nitrite	Less than 0.1 ppm
Nitrate	Less than 20 ppm

coral reef would be unacceptable for a home aquarium, many people overpopulate a tank without proper compensatory apparatus.

Many public aquariums overcome this problem by having a small display tank, with a high fish-to-water ratio, in circulation with huge filtration tanks that the public never sees. This system is similar to the natural reef environment, in which the surrounding ocean constantly replenishes and cleans the local fish habitat.

Few home hobbyists can afford large filtration tanks. As little as 28 L (7.5 gal) of water can be used, but at least 75 L (20 gal), and preferably more, is recommended for marine fish.[2] A safe number of fish for larger tanks can be estimated as follows: 30 fish 5 to 7.6 cm (2 to 3 inches) in length per 380 L (100 gal) of water, or approximately 13 L (3.5 gal) for one medium-sized fish. If the fish are longer than 7.6 cm, population density must be reduced. No more than 10 fish of 10 to 13 cm (4 to 5 inches) can be maintained safely in 380 L.[3] The capacity of the tank also can be estimated as a function of the surface area of the bacterial filter-bed. Approximately 7.6 cm of fish per 926 cm^2 (1 ft^2) of bed is proper, provided that the gravel is 3/16-inch grain and 7.6 cm deep and that the flow of water is at least 3.8 L (1 gal)/min/926 cm^2.[4] Species selection also must be considered because territorial aggression often is more of a limiting factor than tank volume.[a]

Aeration and Filtration

Vigorous aeration and filtration must be maintained to compensate for high fish-to-water ratios in display aquariums. As little as 3.8 to 7.6 L (1 to 2 gal) of water per medium-sized fish is sufficient if there is proper undergravel filtration and heavy aeration and if proper attention is given to species combination. A breakdown in the system can result in rapid loss of fish.[3]

Gas exchange is critical in marine aquariums because salt water, with its dissolved solids, contains approximately 20% less oxygen than fresh water.[5] Most gas exchange occurs at the water-to-atmosphere interface. A long, low tank, which provides a larger interface, is recommended.[4] Aeration is the principal means of moving water in the marine aquarium. Rising columns of air bubbles create water circulation from the bottom of the tank to the top, where gas exchange can occur. To maintain proper aeration, 5.7 to 7.6 L (6 to 8 qt) of air for each 3.8 L of water should be moving through the system.[6] An excess of air probably will do no harm in a home aquarium situation and may be required for high population densities.

With the current equipment, aeration and bacterial filtration can be accomplished with the same undergravel filtration equipment. External power filters provide the necessary mechanical and chemical filtration and rapid flow of water. In such filters, incoming water flows over Dacron™ floss, which removes large particulate matter by trapping it in the mesh.[6] The floss must be changed regularly to prevent plugging of the system and subsequent anaerobic conditions. The resulting bacteria release many by-products that are potentially toxic to the fish. The filter system should circulate approximately 15 to 23 L (4 to 6 gal) of water per 3.8 L of tank capacity per hour.[5]

The water then flows through a bed of activated charcoal. Although the charcoal does not remove ammonia, nitrite, or nitrate, it does absorb the substances that eventually turn the tank yellow.[6] These organic substances, which are in solution, are not removed mechanically by the floss. Other types of chemical filtration—such as airstripping, ozone, and ultraviolet light—are options for very large aquariums.[4]

Ammonia-Nitrite-Nitrate

The third type of filtration is invisible and takes time and expertise to develop and maintain. The biologic filter consists of various populations of bacteria that must be cultured in a new tank. These bacteria exist in and under the gravel bed of the tank as long as enough water is flowing through it to maintain aerobic conditions.

[a]Klocek R: Personal communication, John G. Shedd Aquarium, Chicago, Illinois, 1985.

The first group of bacteria, the heterotrophs, perform the process of ammonification. Heterotrophic bacteria use organic matter from excess food, dead organisms, and detritus as an energy source. They decompose this matter to form ammonia and other products.[4]

Ammonia is toxic to aquarium fish and must be removed. This removal is accomplished by nitrifying bacteria, which use ammonia as an energy source. One group of bacteria, the *Nitrosomonas* spp., convert ammonia to nitrite, which, still somewhat toxic, is in turn converted to nitrate by the *Nitrobacter* spp. bacteria.[4]

Aquarium denitrification is accomplished by bacteria that reduce nitrates to nitrous oxide and elemental nitrogen, which are used by diatoms (also called *brown algae*) and green algae.[6] The algae in turn provide oxygen and other products that contribute to the health of the fish when eaten, such as vitamin B_{12}, trace elements that apparently have a tonic effect on fish, and antibiotic substances[6] (Figure 1).

The bacterial culture-bed can be established in a new tank by placing a hardy specimen, such as a hermit crab or a clownfish, in the tank. The crab or fish will start the cycle by excreting ammonia products. Within two weeks the ammonia level should peak at approximately 6 ppm. Slightly later, the nitrite level will peak at the same mark. The nitrite level will gradually decrease as the nitrate level rises (Figure 2). It can take up to two months until the tank is ready to be populated with fish.[4] This should be done slowly to avoid overwhelming the bacterial filter and causing another ammonia spike. The process can be accelerated by as much as a month by adding gravel from a well-established aquarium or by adding a small amount of common garden soil.[6] Care must be taken to avoid adding soil and developing the culture too quickly; excessive heterotrophs will inhibit the growth of denitrifying bacteria.[b]

The tank should be monitored daily during the culturing period. After the tank has been stabilized, the nitrite level should be less than 0.1 ppm and the nitrate level less than 20 ppm.[4] Monitoring test kits are available in pet stores.

Aquarium algae are useful in proper maintenance of the nitrogen cycle, depicted in Figure 1. Fish might stay healthy longer and experience better growth rates in tanks that contain abundant algae growth or that maintain algae filters. The presence of brown or blue-green algae can indicate that the bacterial balance is upset, or that nitrates have accumulated from excess feeding.[a] These algae can survive poor light, low oxygen content, low pH, and low oxidation-reduction potentials.[6] Brown algae are usually the first evident growth, but, if a seed culture is used from an established tank, they should be replaced by green algae within three to four weeks after the tank has been stabilized.

Organic Matter

The bacterial filter can be upset easily and quickly,

[b]Herwig N: Personal communication, Houston Zoological Gardens, Houston, Texas, 1983.

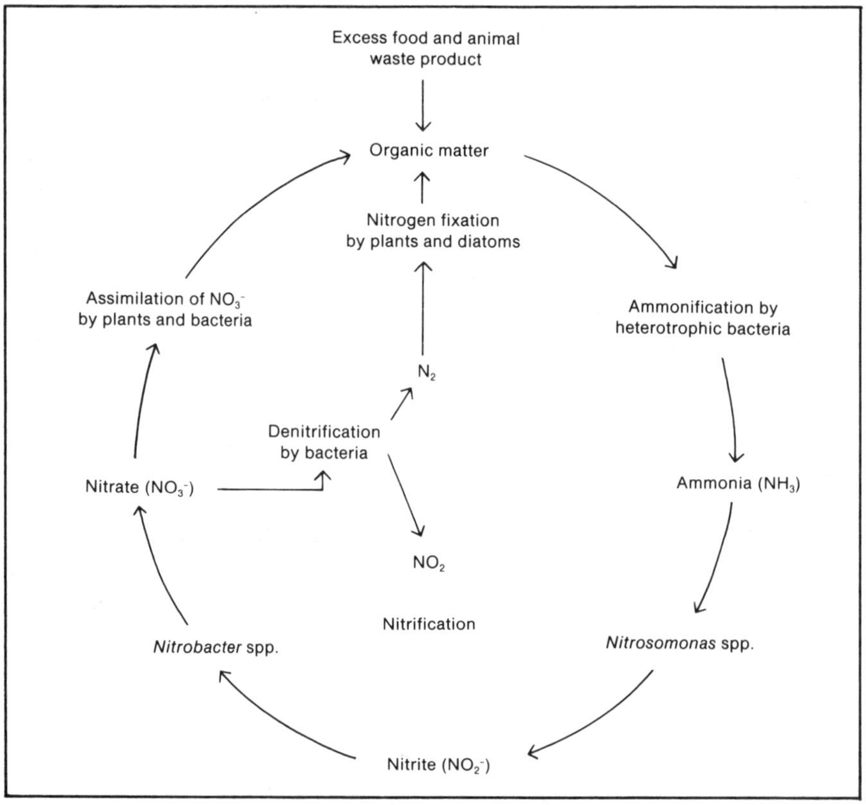

Figure 1—Ammonia-nitrite-nitrate cycle of a saltwater tank.

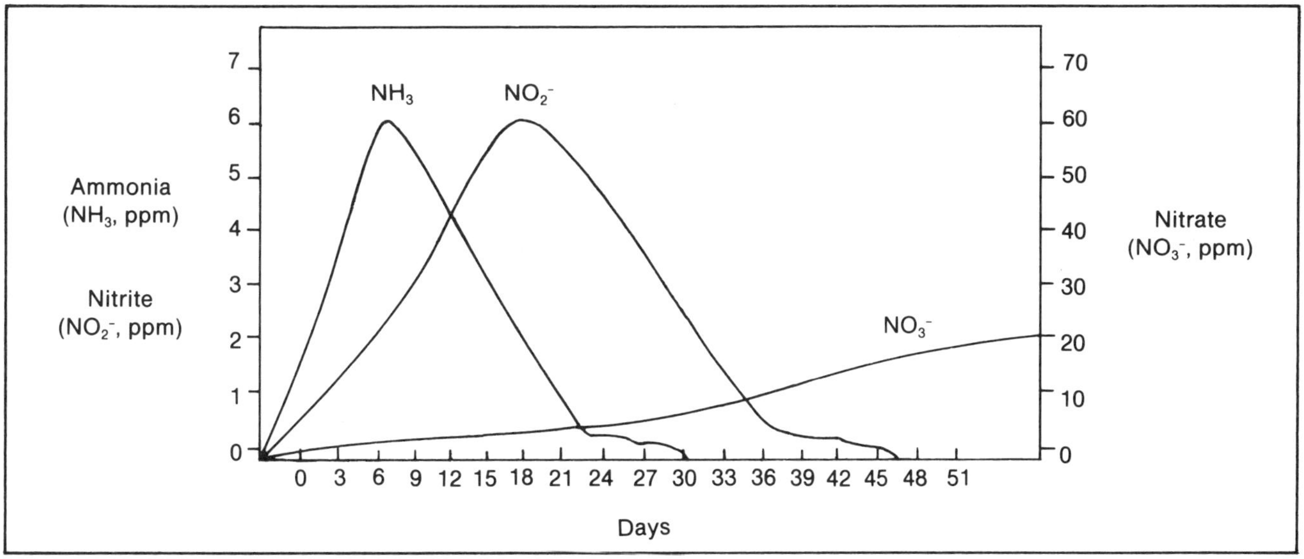

Figure 2—Ammonia, nitrite, and nitrate levels during culture period.

causing disease and death to the fish. If the fish are improperly fed and excess food settles to the bottom and decays or if a specimen dies and is not promptly removed, organic matter floods the tank. *Bacterium coli, Bacterium proteus,* and *Bacterium subtilis* begin to digest these proteins. As metabolic by-products, the bacteria release toxins that even in relatively small concentrations are dangerous to specimens.[6]

These bacteria do not live within the filter system of the aquarium. All excess food and protein should be filtered out by mechanical filtration or hand siphoning. In this way, the *Bacterium* spp. will not be able to act on the proteins because they live on the bottom soil, the stones, the corals, the glass, and the fish.[6]

Amino acids are released when excess protein floods the tank. One group, the sulfurous amino acids, lowers the oxidation-reduction potential, thus decreasing the oxygen capacity of the water. The proliferation of the *Bacterium* spp. also uses large amounts of oxygen and releases much carbon dioxide (CO_2). The release of amino acids and CO_2 into the water lowers the pH, which also contributes to a lower oxygen capacity of the water.[6]

High surface tension (the bubbles from aeration persist for an extended time) and a temporary drop in pH are clues to excess protein in the tank. Other, less dangerous bacteria degrade protein by releasing aromatic amino acids, causing the tank to emit a ripe fruit or onion odor. Still other bacteria degrade amino acids to phenols and cresols, which are dyes that accumulate in the water and turn it yellow or yellowish brown.[6]

pH

The pH of natural sea water normally is 8.0 to 8.3. The aquarium should be kept as close to this as possible; a range of 7.8 to 8.5 is acceptable. The amount of dissolved CO_2, the amounts of magnesium and calcium, and the production of acids and nitrates are major factors affecting aquarium pH.[6]

The effect of CO_2 concentration on pH is illustrated in Figure 3. A pH drop occurs in situations in which CO_2 concentration rises, such as water stagnation, too great an animal load, or bacterial (*Bacterium* spp.) overgrowth resulting from excess protein. Proper aeration can help a tank blow off excess CO_2. This accumulation of CO_2 can be avoided with proper filtration, proper tank population, and proper algae growth levels maintained by harvesting.

Normally, there is scant free CO_2 dissolved in the water. The CO_2 that is present is rapidly used by algae for photosynthesis. When the CO_2 is gone, the algae turn to hydrocarbonates for photosynthetic fuel; this causes the precipitation of carbonates and results in increased pH levels, up to 10.[6]

Phosphates accumulate in the water as an end product of the decomposition of organic matter. When phosphates reach the saturation point, they precipitate as magnesium phosphate and calcium phosphate.[6] The magnesium and the calcium come from the many dissolved seawater salts, primarily calcium sulfate ($CaSO_4$), magnesium sulfate ($MgSO_4$), calcium carbonate ($CaCO_3$), and sodium chloride (NaCl). Seawater salts provide dissolved ions, both acid and alkaline, with buffering capacity. This capacity is lost when magnesium and calcium precipitate with phosphates from organic matter decomposition.

Dolomite gravel or oyster shells and coral ornaments can be used as renewable sources of calcium and magnesium.[4] Phosphates will react with the calcium and magnesium of the shells so that the seawater salt ions are not removed from the water. Dolomite and coral sand are dissolved readily by carbonic acid to form calcium hydrocarbons. In this way, CO_2 is removed and the equation in Figure 3 is shifted to the left, keeping the pH high.[6]

The dolomite gravel, composed of magnesium and

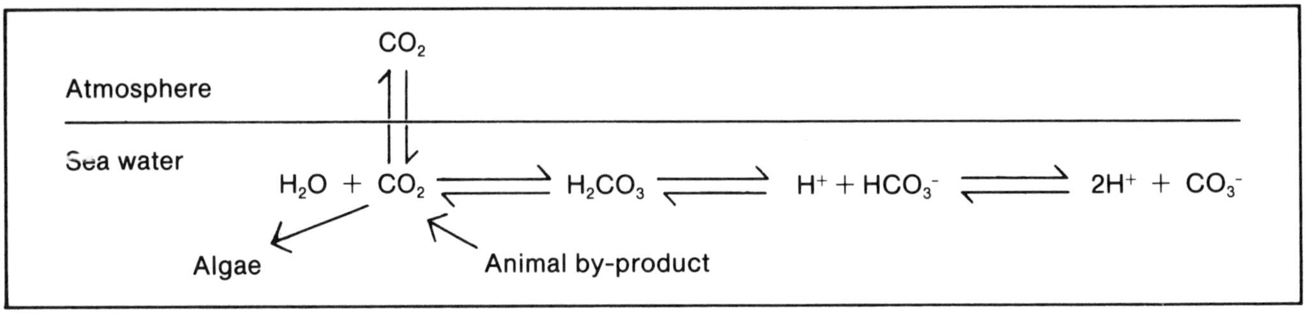

Figure 3—The effect of CO_2 concentration on pH.

calcium carbonate, will form a layer of mineral apatite on its surface resulting from its reaction with phosphates. The apatite layer renders dolomite ineffective as a buffering agent.[a] If the pH level drops for this reason, a mixture of six parts sodium bicarbonate and one part sodium carbonate can be added slowly, while the pH level is monitored until it returns to normal. An additional 5 ml (1 tsp) of the mixture then is added for every 95 L (25 gal) of water.[6] This is a temporary solution; renewal of the saltwater or the buffering gravel is essential.

Ammonia levels must be determined before the pH level is corrected. At pH 6, ammonia is all in the harmless ammonium form. Correcting the pH to 8.3 will cause slightly more than 4% of the ammonium to convert back to toxic ammonia (Table II).[6]

Accumulation of excess organic matter produces organic acids that will lower the pH level. Normally these acids are broken down rapidly and begin to go through the ammonia-nitrite-nitrate cycle; however, excess ammonia accumulation slows down this process, and the organic matter will remain longer in the organic acid form, keeping the pH level low.

Water Changes

Because a steadily falling pH is a sign of water aging, regular pH monitoring is imperative.[6] It is advisable to replace one tenth to one third of the salt water every four to six weeks. If the tank is overpopulated, it might be necessary to replace half of the water.[6] Because of the various interrelating factors, each tank will have distinct needs and care requirements. When cleaning a tank and changing its water, care must be taken to not disturb the bacterial filter-bed because the bacteria can be killed.[6] For this reason, siphoning of superficial detritus that might clog the gravel bed also should be done carefully.[a]

Aquarium cleaning should coincide with water renewal. Harvesting excess algae and scraping it from the sides of the tank should be done at this time. If excess algae are not removed, they can become a major source of excess organic matter when they die.

Water test kits for pH, ammonia, nitrite, nitrate, copper, and other indicators are available from pet stores. Liquid pH indicators are more accurate and more consistent than paper ones.

Temperature

The temperature of the marine aquarium should be as close as possible to that of the fish's natural environment; for most reef fish, this is between 21° and 29.4° C (70° to 85° F). Some sources claim that display fish thrive at 26.7° C (80° F).[3] This temperature provides adequate warmth for metabolism (most fish are cold blooded) and permits proper oxygen content of the water.

A temperature of 26.7° C might be unnecessary, however. A temperature of 23.3°C (74° F) will decrease the replication rate of microbes and will slow the life cycle of parasites. The fish's metabolism also is slowed; although they are not as active, they produce less waste products to contaminate the tank and will live longer.[b] Oxygen content actually is increased at the lower temperature.[6] Water temperature should not fluctuate more than 2.8° C (5° F) during a 24-hour period.[a]

Salinity and Specific Gravity

Because marine animals have a slightly lower salt content in their bodies than that in the water around them, they must maintain hypo-osmoregulation. Freshwater fish are hyperosmoregulatory, that is, their bodies contain *higher* salt concentrations than the surrounding water. The marine fish loses water through its skin to its environment down the osmotic gradient and must constantly drink water, at a rate of 0.2% to 0.5% of its body weight/hr.[4] The excess salts are excreted through the mucus cells in the skin, in the feces, by the kidneys, and particularly by specialized cells in the gills.[4] Because of their constant water loss through the

TABLE II
Conversion of Ammonium to Ammonia at Various pH Values

pH	*% Ammonium (NH_4OH)*	*% Ammonia (NH_3)*
6	100	0
7	99	1
8	96	4
9	75	25
10	22	78
11	4	96

skin to the environment, marine fish excrete scant urine —approximately 2 to 4 ml/kg/day. Freshwater fish can excrete 300 ml/kg/day.[6]

Marine fish can endure slight fluctuations in salinity, but abrupt changes can be harmful. The optimum salinity for tropical marine fish is 34 to 35 parts per thousand (ppt). Salinity varies with temperature changes and is directly related to specific gravity, which is measured with a hydrometer. A specific gravity range of 1.021 to 1.025 at 26.7°C is optimum for most ornamental marine fish.[6] The effect of temperature on salinity is crucial. A nomogram can be used to find the proper hydrometer reading to keep the salinity at 34 to 35 ppt at varying temperatures (Figure 4).

A salinity of 20 to 24 ppt and a specific gravity of 1.018 to 1.020 has been recommended[b]; the majority of saltwater pathogens and parasites are obligatory halophils, and reduced salinity endangers them and thus might decrease the likelihood of disease. Reduced salinity is still experimental, and stress on the pathogens also stresses the fish. Lower salinity also slows the fish's metabolism, thus decreasing waste production.

Tank Material

The marine tank itself is a vital consideration. The tank parts and the materials in the tank are subjected to the weight (salt water weighs more than fresh water) and the highly corrosive action of the salt water. Metal salts, which are toxic to the fish, can form if the tank has metal parts or if any metal from the pumps, the heater, the lighting, or the airways is in contact with the water.[5] All-glass tanks sealed with inert silicone are preferred. Even plastic tubing, air lifts, and siphon tubes can be toxic. To keep the plastic pliable, many contain mollifiers that eventually dissolve into the water and become toxic to the fish. Tygon tubing is recommended for the marine aquarium.[6]

Disease in the Marine Aquarium

Because the ocean is vast, the constant mixing of water in the reef environment causes any change to be diluted quickly. Thus, the changes are, in effect, slight and of short duration. Coral reef fish therefore might never have been exposed to oxygen shortages or various pollutants and probably never have developed adequate adaptive mechanisms to accommodate for environmental stresses.[6] Fish in the marine aquarium change the water and cause it to differ significantly from sea water. These factors are important in considering disease in a marine tank (Table III).

Environmental poisoning can cause signs that resemble those of other diseases. Metal (copper or zinc) poisoning accelerates respiration because of the coagulation of slime on the gills.[6] Rapid respiration is a common sign of protozoal disease, gill flukes, and a lowering pH because of poor water quality. Phenol and ammonia poisoning manifest as sudden, uncoordinated bursts of swimming. A significant water change must be performed to correct the poisoning.[6] This sign, however, also can indicate irritation from crustaceans or protozoa.

There is scant information available about treatment

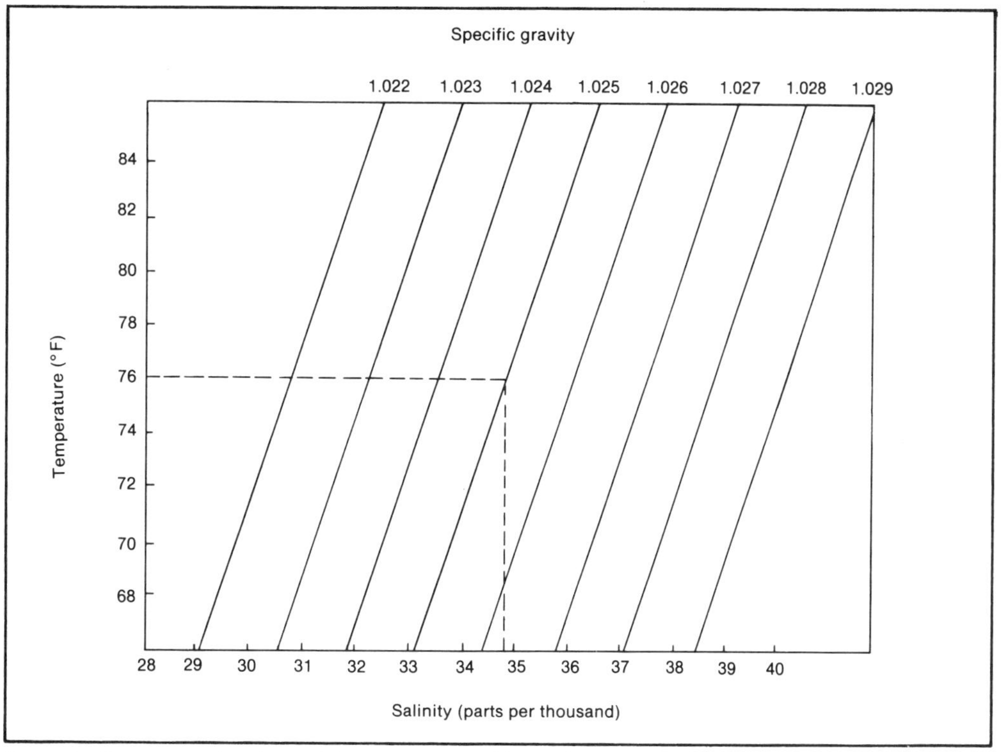

Figure 4—Nomogram for determining proper specific gravity at varying temperatures. (From de Graff F, Spiekman J [trans]: *Marine Aquarium Guide*. Harrison, NJ, Pet Library Ltd, 1973. Modified with permission.)

of specific diseases in marine aquariums. Treatments advocated for tropical freshwater fish often are inadequate and unsuccessful in the marine tank; this is especially true of the use of antibiotics. Penicillin can cause blindness in clownfish, and high doses of broad-spectrum antibiotics, such as chlortetracycline or chloramphenicol, are relatively ineffective in the tank.[3] Sulfa drugs and oxytetracycline also are not recommended because long-term use has created resistance in some bacteria.[7]

Most diseases can be treated and controlled by applying the following principles. A "sick tank" should be established. This tank also can serve to quarantine new arrivals. The tank should be kept in semidarkness and should have some hiding places—clay flowerpots are suitable for this. The temperature must be constant. Biologic and chemical filtration should not be maintained in the sick tank because it will absorb or destroy many of the antibiotics used to treat the fish. The display tank never should be treated with antibiotics, which are nonspecific in their action and can damage the bacterial filter-bed of the tank. Vigorous aeration of the sick tank should be maintained, and ammonia levels should be controlled by water changes, which are required daily for most antibiotics to maintain effective levels.[4]

One theory suggests that the sick tank should be

TABLE III
Disease Problems in a Marine Tank

Disease Condition	*Signs*	*Treatment*
Low pH	Sudden darting movements, heavy respiration, milky-white clouding of the skin (sometimes with pinpoint hemorrhages), decreased appetite	Slowly add a mixture of six parts sodium bicarbonate to one part sodium carbonate until pH is normal, then add 5 ml/95 L more; change water or gravel
Metal or ammonia poisoning	Abnormal swimming, darting, heavy or irregular respiration	Control with water changes and proper filtration
Salinity changes	Fish lies on bottom, heavy breathing after transfer to new tank, shock	Prevent with gradual water changes
Viral lymphocystis	Small, cauliflowerlike, white tubercles on fin edges or skin	Heals spontaneously; ozone or ultraviolet light might speed cure
Tuberculosis, *Mycobacterium* spp.	Exophthalmos, fading colors, emaciation, loss of appetite, skin and scale defects with ulceration, fin destruction	Streptomycin, 80 mg/3.8 L (1 gal) for 1 week (usually diagnosed too late to cure)
Red disease, *Vibrio parahaemolyticus*	Inactivity, loss of appetite, skin hemorrhages, discolored skin patches, fin degeneration, cloudy eyes, red cloaca, internal organ distention and congestion	Gentamicin or kanamycin baths, 66 mg/L; or nitrofurazone baths, 25 mg/3.8 L (1 gal)
Fin rot, *Vibrio* or *Pseudomonas ichthyodermis*	Whitening and deterioration of fin tissue	Check water quality; touch area with copper sulfate; nitrofurazone baths, 25 mg/3.8 L (1 gal)
White spot disease, *Cryptocaryon irritans*	Coarse, white to grayish dots on skin, especially fins, cloudy eyes, heavy respiration, some tissue sloughing	Copper sulfate solution in treatment tank, 0.15-0.25 ppm for 2 weeks
Coral fish disease, *Oodinium ocellatum*	Small, white to yellowish dots on skin, especially gills, heavy respiration, cloudy eyes, erratic swimming and rubbing	Copper sulfate solution in treatment tank, 0.15–0.20 ppm for 2 weeks
Brooklynella hostilis and *Uronema marinum*	Lethargy, loss of appetite, excess mucus production and progressive boillike body lesions with skin sloughing	Copper sulfate bath, 0.25 ppm; malachite green bath, 0.15 ppm; 50-min bath of 1 ml of 37% formalin per gal of water
Fungus (external)	Cottonlike growth on skin or wounds; very rare	Touch with copper sulfate, check water quality
Ichthyophonus hoferi	Same as tuberculosis	No known cure
Crustaceans or worms	Immobile or mobile skin parasites, visible to the naked eye, usually oblong	Pull with tweezers; for worms, 15-min bath of 1 ml of 37% formalin per gal of water

maintained at a higher temperature[6] to speed up the life cycle of the pathogen and thus force it into a vulnerable stage in which chemotherapy will be effective against it. This effect might be achieved, but the higher temperature also places additional stress on the already stressed patient; care and close observation therefore are indicated.

Viral Disease

Although there are numerous viral diseases of saltwater fish, only lymphocystis disease has been observed in marine aquarium fish. This wartlike lesion can be removed surgically, but a spontaneous cure usually occurs within approximately two months.[7] Ozone or ultraviolet light can hasten resolution in the sick tank (Figures 5 and 6).[4]

Bacterial Disease

Most bacterial pathogens that affect fish are gram-negative. Fish can be given antibiotics orally in food or parenterally (subcutaneously or intraperitoneally). Intramuscular injections are inappropriate in fish; because fish muscle is poorly vascularized, absorption is slow and sterile abscesses can develop around the injection site.

Piscine tuberculosis caused by *Mycobacterium* spp. is a common bacterial disease of captive marine aquarium fish.[4] Usually, the disease is slowly progressive. External signs include listlessness, rapid respiration, lack of appetite, emaciation, skin and scale defects, exophthalmos if the bacteria infect the eye socket (Figure 7),[6] skin ulceration, and fin destruction.[8] Necropsy findings include grayish, knoblike lesions in and on the internal organs, especially the liver, the spleen, and the intestine.[6] The organism can be isolated from a swab of an infected organ or nodule and is microscopically visible (Figure 8).

If the disease is recognized early, a streptomycin bath at 80 mg/3.8 L (1 gal) for one or more weeks can be beneficial.[6] Isoniazid (Rifamate®—Merrell Dow Pharmaceuticals) and rifampin (Rifadin®—Merrell Dow Pharmaceuticals) also have been recommended.[6] If piscine tuberculosis is diagnosed on necropsy by the presence of acid-fast bacteria in lesions, the patient should be burned or buried with quicklime at a site far from water drainage because this mycobacterium can spread to humans. Most reported cases have occurred in aquarists, who contracted localized, open, papulopustular lesions on the hands and the arms after cleaning a contaminated tank; therapy is required for 12 to 24 months.[8] Sick or dead fish probably are best left in the garbage rather than flushed down the toilet—this disease occurs in freshwater and saltwater fish.

Vibrio infection, also called *red disease*, is most often caused by *Vibrio parahaemolyticus*. It occurs commonly in winter months in newly imported fish and new additions to tanks. Fish under stress during transport are more susceptible.[9]

Vibrio parahaemolyticus is closely related to the human pathogen *Vibrio cholerae*. *V. parahaemolyticus* is responsible for the human disease known as *seafood poisoning*, which is mostly limited to the Orient because of dietary preference. Like red disease in fish, seafood poisoning is a gastrointestinal disease in humans.[9] *V. parahaemolyticus* spreads from fish to fish in the same way that seafood poisoning is disseminated, through ingestion. The disease usually spreads during holding and transport in small amounts of water, which is also a high-stress period.

The bacteria replicate in the gastrointestinal tract and spread to other organs. Feces are often a pure culture of the bacteria, causing a bloody discharge and reddening of the cloaca. Distention and congestion of the liver, the spleen, and the intestine are common. Congestion and necrosis of the kidneys often complicate recovery even if bacterial replication can be halted.[9] The most noticeable lesions are bloody ulcerations on the skin, with loss of scales and muscular necrosis, surrounded by light-colored areas of freshly infected tissue. These lesions begin as small petechial hemorrhages and grow into lumps or boillike lesions (Figure 9). A tentative diagnosis can be made by examining the curved or S-shaped *Vibrio* organisms in fecal material or in a swab of a skin lesion (Figure 10).[9]

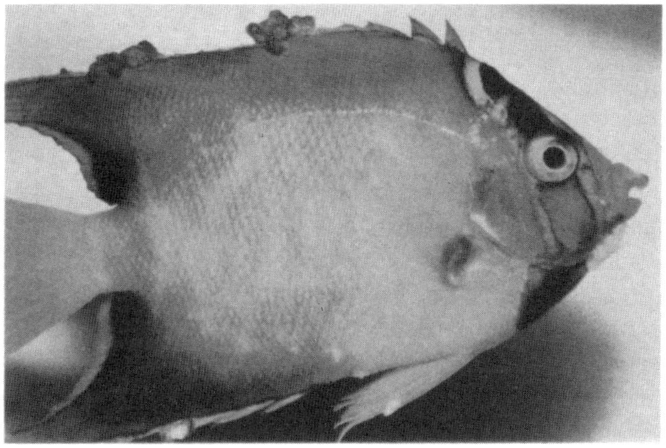

Figure 5—Queen angelfish with lymphocystis.

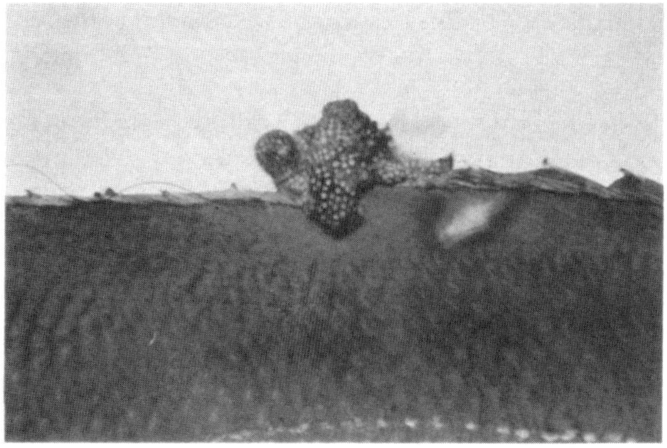

Figure 6—Close-up of Figure 5.

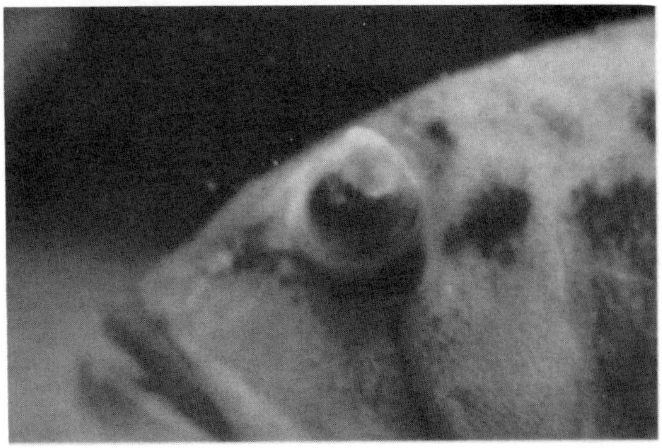

Figure 7—California rockfish with exophthalmos. The patient responded to tuberculosis therapy.

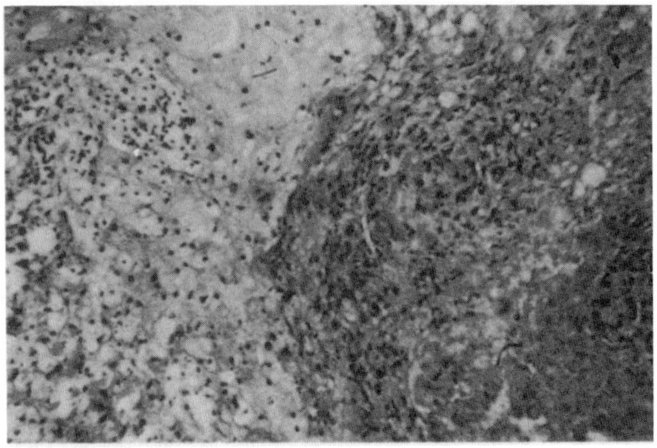

Figure 8—Piscine tuberculosis organisms.

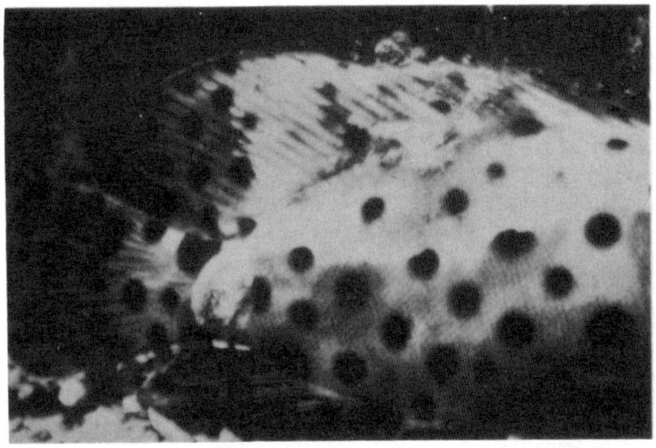

Figure 9—Panther grouper with *Vibrio parahaemolyticus* infection.

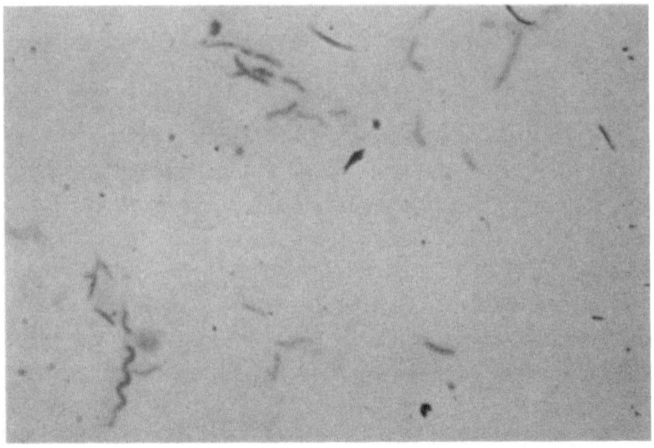

Figure 10—*Vibrio parahaemolyticus* organisms.

The condition is treated with antibiotics. Gentamicin or kanamycin used at a dose of 66 mg/L (250 mg/gal) probably is most effective. Nitrofurazone, at 25 mg/3.8L, or water also can be used.[9] Chloramphenicol has been recommended at a dosage of 13 mg/L (50 mg/gal) for seven days with a 50% water change each day.[4] Chloramphenicol is pH sensitive; it must be used at a pH of 8.0 or higher. Its effectiveness as a water bath treatment therefore is limited, but it might be helpful as an intraperitoneal injection.[9]

Vibrio anguillarum often is considered to be the cause of red disease.[6,10] This bacterium is a prevalent pathogen in marine food fish but rarely, if ever, occurs in marine hobbyist tanks.[6]

Fin rot is a disease the primary cause of which can be poor water quality, lack of oxygen, or poor circulation in extremities. Usually there are bacteria present that might play a primary role also. The bacterium involved is *Vibrio ichthyodermis* or *Pseudomonas ichthyodermis*—the classification is being debated.[11] An early sign is the fins and the tail turning white and cloudy. The affected areas eventually die and become torn and frayed. The skin mucus on the body is affected next, showing bloodshot epidermal patches.[6] These patches eventually ulcerate and lead to other serious secondary invasions.[11] The frayed appearance of the tail and the fins must be differentiated from that caused by aggression or territorial fighting.

Acute fin rot rarely can be cured. Touching the affected area with copper sulfate can help in the early stages.[5] A streptomycin-penicillin combination given parenterally or oxytetracycline given in food also can be effective.[11] Tetracycline baths at a dose of 250 mg/3.8 L for one to two hours given for seven consecutive days also might effect a cure.[a] A nitrofurazone bath at a dose of 25 mg/3.8 L might be the preferred drug for this and all *Vibrio* spp. infections.[9]

Protozoal Disease

White spot disease, the marine counterpart to freshwater *Ichthyophthirius* (also called *Ich*), is caused by the ciliate protozoan *Cryptocaryon irritans* (Figure 11). The protozoan has a wide host range and a complex life cycle.[12]

Initial signs include loss of appetite, bizarre swimming behavior, and minor respiratory distress. The first lesions appear on the skin rather than the gills, as in oodinosis. The skin lesions are pinhead-sized, white to gray nodules caused by the trophonts burrowing into the epidermis (Figure 12). This burrowing causes severe irritation, excess mucus production, and hyperplasia of the epithelium. Large areas of the epithelium can fall off, exposing the fish to secondary bacterial invasion. If the eyes are affected, exophthalmos can be present; the eyes will turn cloudy, and blindness can result.[12] Death can occur with few or no gross disease signs.[a]

Diagnosis is made by scraping off a nodule and examining it for trophonts. This should be done early because the disease is highly contagious and fatal in three to five days.[12] The diseased fish should be removed to a sick tank immediately.

The encysted tomites are difficult to eliminate from an aquarium. An endless cycle will continue until all the fish die or develop acquired immunity. The water quality, the population density, and the stress level will determine which fish will prevail.[4]

Several treatments are available for white spot disease. Copper sulfate is used widely with moderate results. The treatment water should contain no invertebrates, which are highly susceptible to copper toxicity. A copper sulfate solution of 0.15 ppm (± 0.1 ppm) should be prepared in the treatment tank. The copper sulfate level, which never should rise above 0.3 ppm, can be tested with a colometric kit purchased from a pet store. The copper will kill the trophonts and the free-swimming tomites but not the encysted tomites, which emerge in two to eight days at 26.7°C (80° F). A copper sulfate bath lasting 14 days therefore will kill all infectious stages. Recurrence is not uncommon,[12] but new infections also can be introduced from unquarantined new arrivals.[a]

Coral fish disease, also called *marine oodinosis,* is a flagellate protozoal disease caused by *Oodinium ocellatum.* The early signs are rapid respiration, erratic swimming, and rubbing on gravel and coral. Initially the gills are parasitized heavily with small, dustlike, white nodules. A swab of the gills should reveal the organism (Figures 13 and 14). After respiratory signs are observed, the lesions can spread over the skin and are most visible on the fins and the tail.[13]

The disease has a rapid onset, and death occurs within two days after respiratory distress is noted. Death can be within 12 hours at higher water temperatures. Avoiding the pathogen by using ozone filters or ultraviolet light is recommended.[4] All incoming fish should be quarantined for two weeks. During this period, several freshwater baths, lasting a minimum of three minutes and as long as 15 minutes, should be given. Ten minutes is suitable for most species.[a] These baths cause the *Oodinium* organisms to rupture.[13] If the disease does occur, treatment with copper sulfate is effective. The regimen used for white spot disease can be followed.[4]

Brooklynella hostilis and *Uronema marinum* are look-alike ciliate protozoa that are gaining prevalence as severe, rapidly fatal diseases in marine aquariums.[a,b] *Uronema marinum* probably occurs more frequently than *Brooklynella hostilis.*[a] The majority of *Brooklynella hostilis* cases have been confirmed in the Philippine clownfish and in seahorses, but other fish are not immune.[14] Skin lesions on recent arrivals should be checked because they can be misdiagnosed as bacterial infections. The diseases are contagious, and fish can die within 12 hours from metabolic exotoxins produced by the organisms.

In both protozoa, infection initially is confined to the gills. Although the parasites do not burrow into the skin, they cause significant tissue irritation and damage. Infected fish demonstrate lethargy, lack of appetite, and excess mucus secretion that causes respiratory distress. Body lesions eventually appear as small, diffuse, discolored foci. The epithelium ultimately can slough, an important diagnostic sign[a,14] (Figure 15).

The parasites are confirmed by gill or skin smears; gill smears are necessary to confirm suspected fish not yet showing skin lesions. The living parasite is heart-shaped or kidney-shaped and has an oval macronucleus, several micronuclei, and numerous food vacuoles. The most recognizable structure of *Brooklynella hostilis* is a caudoventral adhesion organ used to attach to the host.[14] *Uronema marinum* is recognized by elongated caudomedial cilia.[a]

Copper sulfate solution used at 0.15 to 0.20 ppm has not been successful in eradicating the parasite,[14] but the

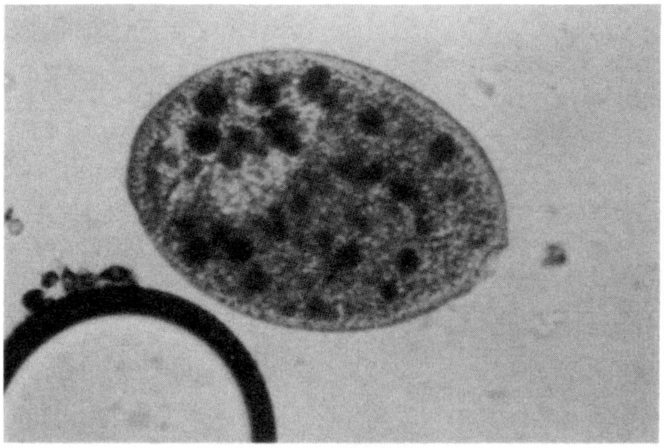

Figure 11—Ganbaldi skin scrape, demonstrating *Cryptocaryon irritans* ciliated tomite measuring 56 × 42 μ. (vital red stain, × 400)

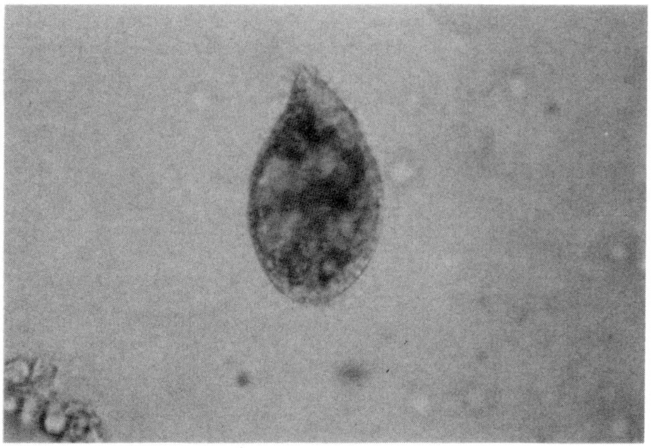

Figure 12—Skin smear from a Stoplite parrot, demonstrating *Cryptocaryon* trophont measuring 400 × 80 μ. (methylene blue stain)

solution has been effective at 0.25 ppm.[a] The infection can be controlled by using 50-minute baths of 1 ml of 37% formalin per 3.8 L. A single formalin treatment usually is required for *Brooklynella hostilis*[14]; *Uronema marinum* can necessitate more than one bath.[a] Freshwater dips lasting 10 minutes also are safe and effective. Malachite green baths at 0.13 to 0.15 ppm for 50 minutes can be useful. Patients with severe body lesions should be placed on antibiotic therapy to prevent secondary bacterial infections.[14]

Fungal Disease

Undetermined external fungi can grow filamentous projections from sites of external injury. Faulty environmental conditions, such as dissolved organic matter, low pH, or accumulation of organic substances, contribute to their occurrence. These fungi are rare and are much less common in marine aquariums than in freshwater tanks.[5]

Treatment is simple and effective: copper sulfate is touched to the site. In severe cases, a griseofulvin freshwater bath of 25 mg/L might be necessary.[5]

Ichthyophonus hoferi, a more common external fungus, also is rare. It infects vital organs, and the spores spread to other organs via the bloodstream (Figure 16). The fungus usually is not discovered until it has disseminated and the fish are dying. *Ichthyophonus hoferi* is found most often in the liver and the kidneys. Clinical signs can include exophthalmos, emaciation, abnormal swimming, abdominal swelling, fin decay, and blackish skin discoloration.[6] There is no known cure.

Some patients can survive by encapsulating the parasite. Raising the water temperature to 28° to 30°C (82° to 86°F), feeding vitamins A and B_{12}, and feeding food soaked in 1% solutions of phenoxyethanol or parachlorophenoxetol might overcome an acute crisis. The disease is likely to break out of encapsulation when the fish are stressed again. The fungus probably is introduced into a tank most often through feeder fish. It might be preventable by feeding frozen fish.[6] Because of its presenting signs, *Ichthyophonus hoferi* frequently is misdiagnosed as piscine tuberculosis.

Crustaceans and Worms

Most crustaceans that infest fish, such as copepods, are visible near the eyes or the gills. These crustaceans usually cannot reproduce in the aquarium and will eventually die off and disappear. A 15-minute bath of 1 ml of 37% formalin per L can be used if necessary.

The fish lice *Argulida,* which can reproduce in the tank, can cause serious problems. They can reach several millimeters in length and have a sucking disk. The mandibles sting the victim, and venom (which can kill a small fish) is released; the lice then live off of the wound's blood and mucus. The wound is a potential site for secondary bacterial infection.

The lice are hardy, and all treatments also are stressful and potentially fatal to the fish. The lice therefore should be pulled with tweezers.[4] Pet stores sell products that claim success in treating lice, but care must be exercised because such products probably will stress the fish.

Trematode worms of the genera *Gyrodactylus* and *Benedinia* can be observed near the eyes or the gills of fish. They are grayish white parasites up to 1.5 mm in

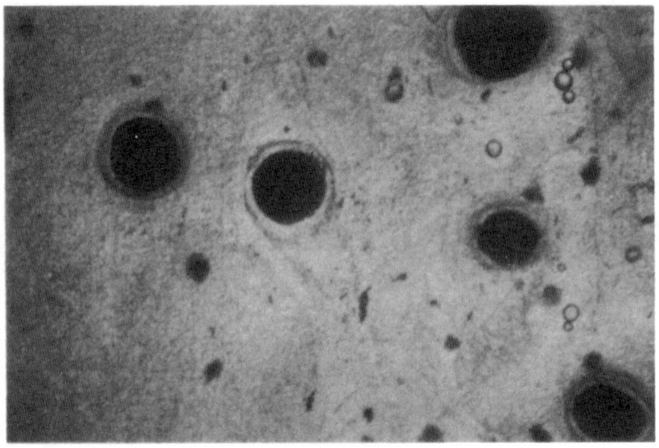

Figure 13—Swab from a Green sunfish gill, demonstrating *Oodinium limnetic* organisms. (× 1000)

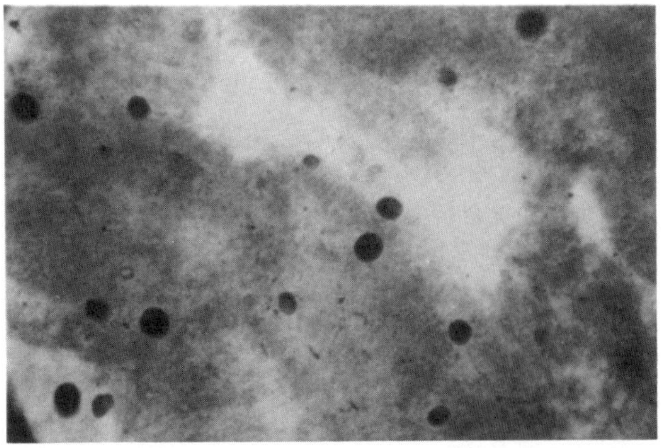

Figure 14—Sample of mucus from gills, demonstrating *Oodinium* organisms.

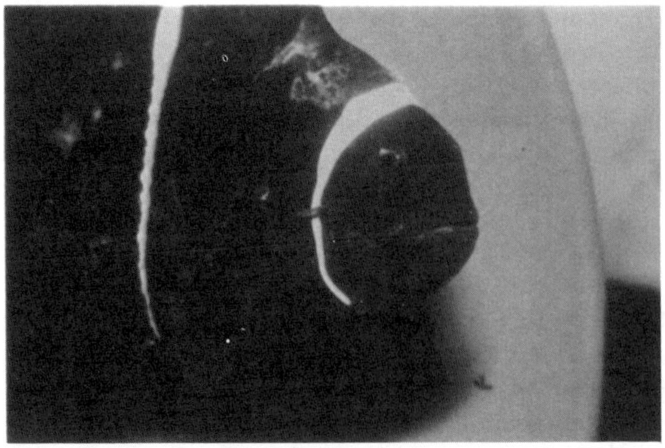

Figure 15—Maroon clownfish with *Brooklynella hostilis* infection.

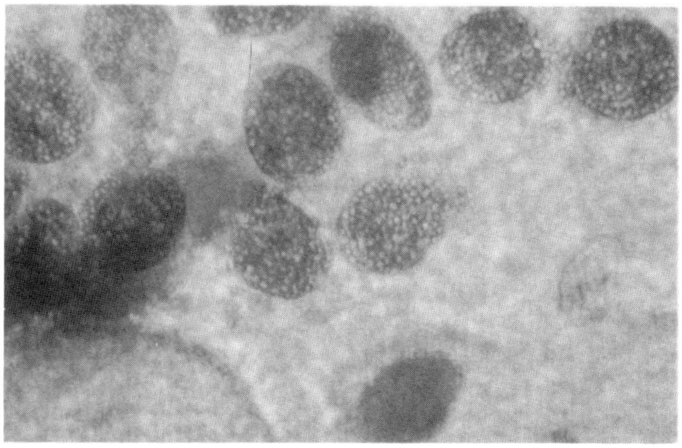

Figure 16—Liver squash smear from a Snook, demonstrating *Ichthyophonus hoferi* organisms. (unstained, × 100)

length. Infected fish demonstrate signs of heavy respiration and rubbing against rocks and gravel; their eyes might become inflamed, and they might hover in the water with fins clamped against the body. The condition is highly contagious and must be treated.[6]

Treatment is the same as that for crustaceans: a 15-minute bath of 1 ml of 37% formalin per L of salt water. A copper sulfate bath at 0.20 ppm also can be used until the parasite is no longer visible on the patient's gills.[6]

Summary

Management of a marine aquarium is not difficult but does require an understanding of the interaction of fish, waste, and water. Most general principles of medicine can be extended to aquarium fish. Veterinarians armed with medical knowledge, an awareness of aquarium management, and access to information on specific diseases can adequately diagnose and treat sick fish and unhealthy tank environments.

As with any medical problem, a proper history is essential. A data base consisting of water samples, microscopic examination (of skin or gill swabs, feces, or necropsy lesions), and keen observation is vital in treating specific diseases or avoiding potential problems.

Acknowledgments

The author thanks Dr. Roger Klocek at the John G. Shedd Aquarium in Chicago and Dr. Nelson Herwig, Curator of Fishes at the Houston Zoological Gardens, for supplying information and photographs and for making important corrections. Figures 5, 6, 8-10, 14, and 15 appear through the courtesy of Dr. Herwig; Figures 7, 11-13, and 16 appear through the courtesy of Dr. Klocek. Dr. Nathan Gabbert and Dr. James Coffman at Kansas State University also provided help and guidance in the writing of this article.

REFERENCES

1. Ford DM: Ornamental fish keeping and the veterinary profession. *Proc Kal Kan Symp Treatment Small Anim Dis*: 20, 1980.
2. Wickler W: *The Marine Aquarium*. Neptune City, NJ, Tropical Fish Hobbyist Publications, 1973, pp 23-24.
3. Axelrod HR, Burgess WE, Emmens CW: *Exotic Marine Fishes*, ed 4. Neptune City, NJ, Tropical Fish Hobbyist Publications, 1975, pp 26, 53-55.
4. Spotte S: *Marine Aquarium Keeping: The Science, Animals, and Art*. New York, John Wiley & Sons, 1973, pp 27, 28, 55-57.
5. Curry C: Management of salt water fish. *Iowa State Univ Vet* 38(2):76-79, 1976.
6. de Graff F, Spiekman J (trans): *Marine Aquarium Guide*. Harrison, NJ, Pet Library Ltd, 1973.
7. Dulin MP: An overview of the more prevalent marine and fresh water aquarium fish diseases. Unpublished paper, Kansas State University, Manhattan, KS, April 20, 1982.
8. Dulin MP: A review of tuberculosis (mycobacteriosis) in fish. *VM SAC* 74(5):731-735, 1979.
9. Herwig N: Disease prevention and control. *Fresh Water and Marine Aquarium* 2(3):38-39, 83-86, 1979.
10. Sinderman CJ: *Principal Diseases of Marine Fish and Shellfish*. New York, Academic Press, 1973, pp 18-19.
11. Curry C: Diseases of salt water fish. *Iowa State Univ Vet* 39(1):26-30, 1977.
12. Dulin MP: White spot disease (cryptocaryoniasis) of marine fish. Unpublished paper, Kansas State University, Manhattan, KS, April 20, 1982, pp 1-3.
13. Dulin MP: Marine oodinosis. Unpublished paper, Kansas State University, Manhattan, KS, April 20, 1982, pp 1-3.
14. Blasiola GC: Disease prevention and control. *Fresh Water and Marine Aquarium* 3(3):18-19, 82-83, 1980.

Selected Diseases of the Head and Face in Caged Birds

Robert D. Zenoble, DVM, MS*
Diplomate, ACVIM
College of Veterinary Medicine
Iowa State University
Ames, Iowa

Avian Pox

Avian pox is a viral infection of birds characterized by discrete, proliferative lesions on the skin of the face and feet and/or mucous membrane of the upper digestive and respiratory tracts. Avian pox is caused by a DNA-containing, enveloped virus which develops in the cytoplasm of the infected epithelial cell. The various strains have adapted to different avian hosts yet retain the basic characteristics of *Poxvirus avium*.[1]

Poxvirus avium is transmitted by direct contact and by mechanical insect vectors (e.g., mosquitoes). Poxvirus is unable to penetrate unbroken skin, but small abrasions are sufficient to permit infection. Poxvirus infections have been found in many wild bird species, domestic ducks, geese, chickens, and certain exotic caged birds.[2,3] Canaries and lovebirds are highly susceptible to pox infection. Psittacines (except lovebirds) are more resistant to poxvirus infection than are canaries. Poxvirus infection has been confirmed in Amazon parrots[4,5] and is suspected in macaws, pionus, Australian parakeets, South American parakeets, and conures.[6]

The clinical signs of poxvirus infection are anorexia, weight loss, and pox lesions. Poxvirus infection occurs in one of two forms or a combination of both. The cutaneous form is characterized by discrete proliferative lesions that develop on the nonfeathered parts of the body (eyelids, beak, legs, and feet). In the diphtheritic form, extensive fibronecrotic lesions occur in the mucous membranes of the oropharynx, upper respiratory tract, and esophagus. Bacteria and yeast organisms are commonly isolated from diphtheritic lesions. Eye diseases secondary to pox infection include scarring of lids, chronic lacrimal discharge, and corneal opacities (Figure 1). Effects of chronic pox infection also include beak and cere distortion, chronic sinusitis, and scarring of the choanal cleft and surrounding respiratory epithelium.[2,3,5] Lesion distribution is variable and depends on the clinical form of the pox disease, the strain of virus, and the host affected. Canaries and lovebirds can show dry pox lesions on the face, feet, and legs; however, diphtheritic lesions are also common in the oropharynx and upper respiratory tract.[2] Psittacines can show cutaneous

*Dr. Zenoble's present address is Auburn University, Auburn, Alabama.

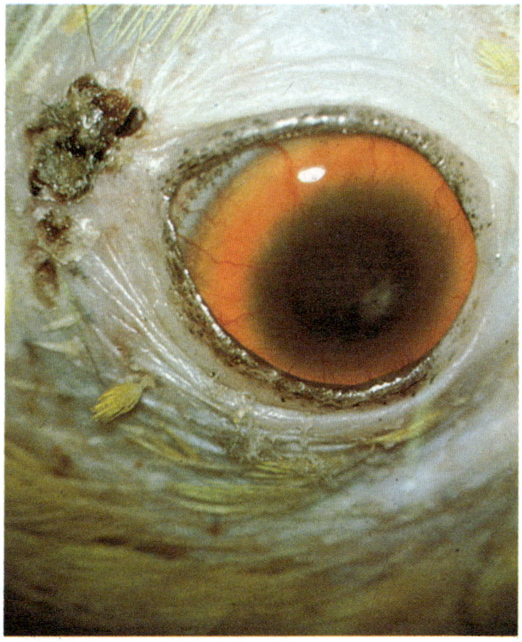

Figure 1—Amazon parrot with typical cutaneous pox lesions near the eye. Associated ocular disease is shown by the abnormally smooth lid borders and blood vessels on the cornea.

and diphtheritic lesions. The choanal cleft is a common site for diphtheritic lesions in psittacines. Macaws usually have only the dry form with face lesions.[6]

Epithelial cells affected by the poxvirus become hyperplastic and hypertrophic. Large granular acidophilic intracytoplasmic inclusions appear in cells above the stratum germinativum. The piling up of infected epithelial cells to form *pocks* occurs at variable rates, and the lesions may persist for different lengths of time in the different avian species. The inflamed lesions desiccate and a scab results which eventually sloughs off and is replaced by normal skin. Elevated pox lesions are easily traumatized by resulting bacterial infection. The poxvirus is species specific with a variable clinical course. In certain species, the virus is retained for months with little mortality, whereas in other species (canaries) there is characteristically higher mortality.[2,3,5]

A diagnosis is suggested by clinical appearance and confirmed by histopathologic demonstration of typical intracytoplasmic inclusions. The majority of wild bird pox infections are mild and self-limiting. Infections of the dry form of pox in psittacines and canaries are generally self-limiting, with occasional mortality. However, acute death may occur in the diphtheritic form without cutaneous lesions. The cause of death from the diphtheritic form of pox is usually from septicemia (bacterial or fungal), starvation due to painful oral lesions, and/or diphtheritic plugs in the tracheobronchial system.

Treatment of poxvirus infection is directed toward supportive nutrition (especially vitamin A) and preventing secondary bacterial infection. Systemic antibiotics such as gentamicin and cephalexin are commonly used along with local treatment (gentle cleaning and topical Mercurochrome). These antibiotics include gentamicin IM 5 mg/kg twice a day; ampicillin PO 200 mg/kg three times per day; cephalothin IM 100 mg/kg four times per day; and cephalexin PO 35 to 50 mg/kg four times per day.

An experimental live-virus, embryo-propagated canary pox vaccine has been developed which is safe and effective in canaries.[7] It is administered by a single-needle wing-web stab. At present, there is no commercial vaccine available in the United States.

Respiratory Infection

Respiratory infection in caged birds is common. Some of the clinical findings, such as nasal discharge, periorbital sinus abscess, and sinusitis, involve the head. Systemic clinical signs are anorexia, depression, dyspnea, and abnormal respiratory sounds. Respiratory infections can be rapidly fatal; however, in many instances evidence of chronic infection is found without dyspnea and other systemic symptoms.

Chronic nasal discharge and/or sneezing may be the only signs seen (Figure 2). In such a case, culture and sensitivity testing of the exudate will identify the bacterial organism and suggest the appropriate antibiotic treatment. Parenteral, nebulized, and intranasal antibiotics may be beneficial. Increasing the humidity in the bird's environment may soothe chronically inflamed and/or infected sinuses. Birds that sneeze chronically may be healthy in other aspects and poorly responsive to therapy. Signs may worsen during winter months due to dry heat and low humidity in homes. Spontaneous recovery may occur during the higher-humidity summer months even without antibiotic therapy.[3,8-10]

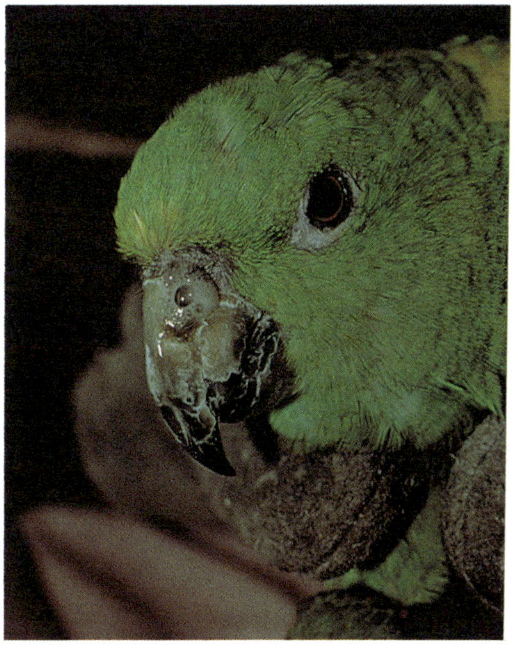

Figure 2—Amazon parrot showing copious nasal discharge. The bird was not systemically ill and eventually became asymptomatic.

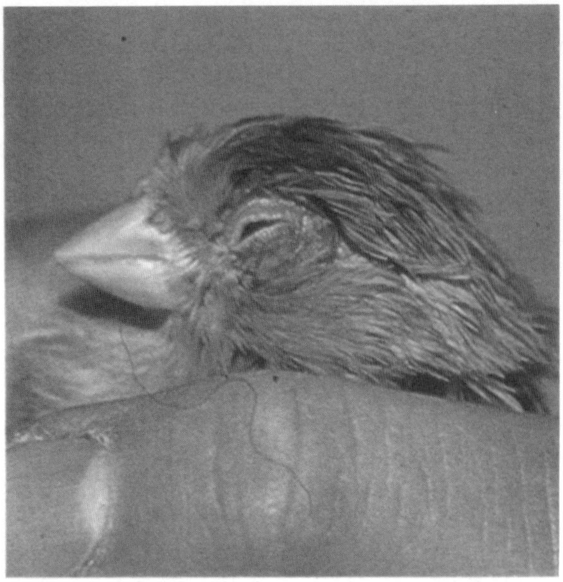

Figure 3—Canary showing periorbital swelling typical of sinusitis.

Sinusitis may be found with respiratory infections and may be the presenting complaint. Sinuses are freely communicating, membrane-lined compartments within the bird's skull. Evidence of sinusitis may be a ring of swollen tissue around the eye or a focal swelling between the eye and the cere (Figure 3). Infected material can be aspirated from the sinuses and cultured for bacteria. Treatment can include systemic antibiotics (gentamicin or cephalexin), nebulization with gentamicin or cephalothin, and local instillation of gentamicin or cephalothin into the sinuses. Sinuses can be flushed by injection with saline and antibiotics. During the flushing procedure, the bird should be held in an upright position to prevent aspiration of the infused material. Flushing can be performed without anesthesia. The sinus is entered and the solution instilled by opening the bird's beak and carefully inserting a 25- to 26-gauge × ⅜- or ½-inch needle through the skin to a depth of 2 to 4 mm. The site of injection is midway between the commissure of the mouth and the medial canthus of the eye. Excess fluid injected into the sinuses will drain through the nares or back into the pharynx. Tissue surrounding the eye will bulge as the sinuses are filled with the injected fluid. The swollen tissue will return to normal as the fluid is absorbed. Since the sinuses communicate freely, only one side need be injected with fluid. Injections should be daily when the disease is at its worst; the frequency can be reduced to every other day with clinical improvement.[3,8]

Signs of chronic sinusitis may not be observed by the owner, and the presenting complaint may be a mass lesion above or below the eye (Figure 4). This mass is inspissated pus and requires opening and curettage.

Diseases of the Cere

The cere is a specialized structure from the stratum corneum. The cere is thinner and more flexible than the beak, and the external nares exit through it. It shows marked sensory innervation, in contrast to the relatively insensitive beak.[11,12]

Chronic rhinitis and sinusitis can result in inspissated pus which can cause a bulge of the cere. This may be seen even without specific respiratory signs. Exudate occasionally can be expressed from the nares by gentle pressure of the cere. A chronic discharge from the nares may result in an enlarged and misshapened opening. Treatment of chronic sinusitis was discussed in the section on respiratory infection.

Tumors of the cere occur infrequently and require surgical biopsy for diagnosis. The prognosis is usually poor because of the difficulty in excising the entire tumor.[13,14]

Knemidokoptic Infestation

Parakeets are frequently presented with dry, proliferative lesions of the cere and around the eyes. Clients often suggest that the bird has fungus on the face. Close

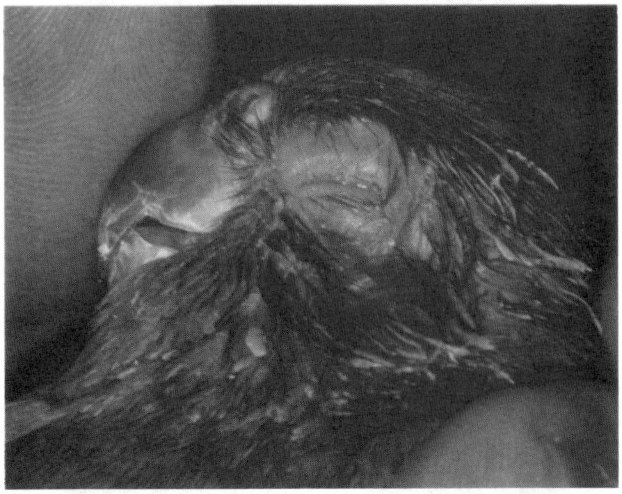

Figure 4A

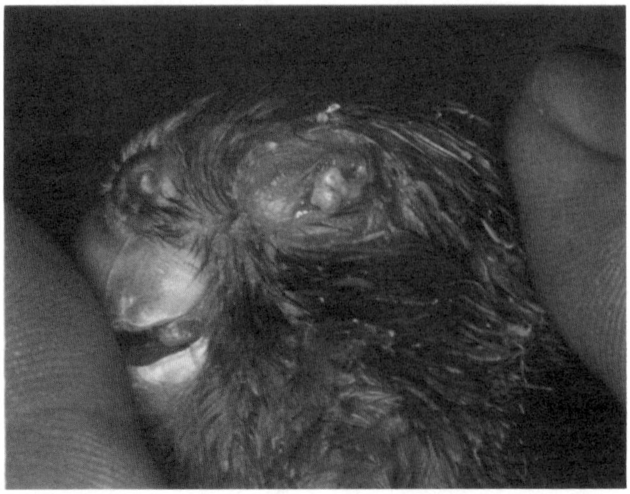

Figure 4B

Figure 4—Cockatiel showing swelling above the eye (**A**). The skin was incised, and inspissated pus was removed (**B**). The condition is associated with sinusitis.

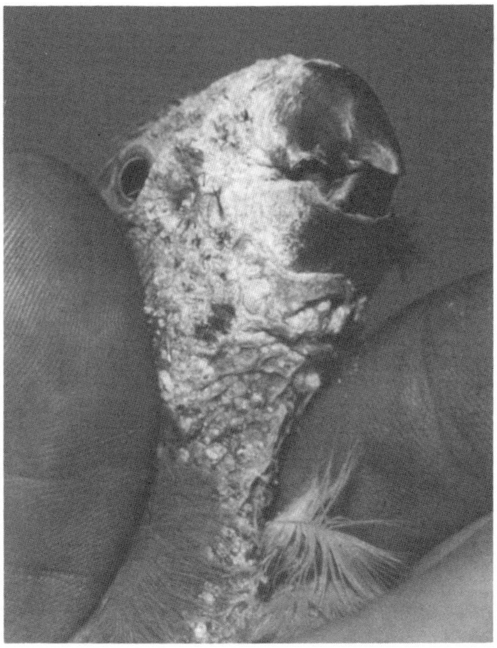

Figure 5—Ring-necked parakeet showing extensive cutaneous involvement of *Knemidokoptes* mite infection.

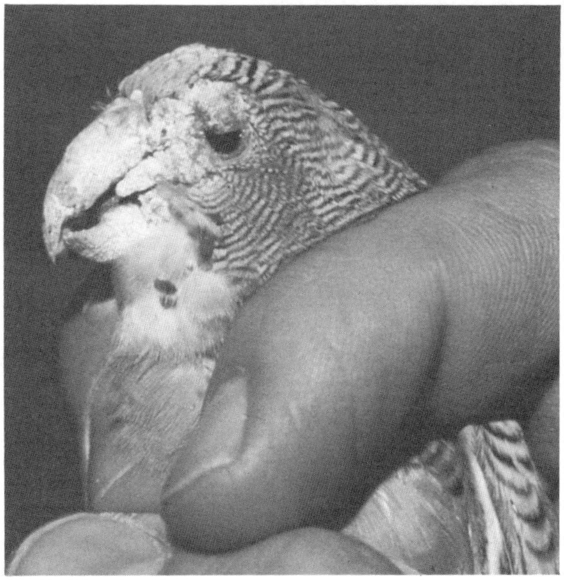

Figure 6A

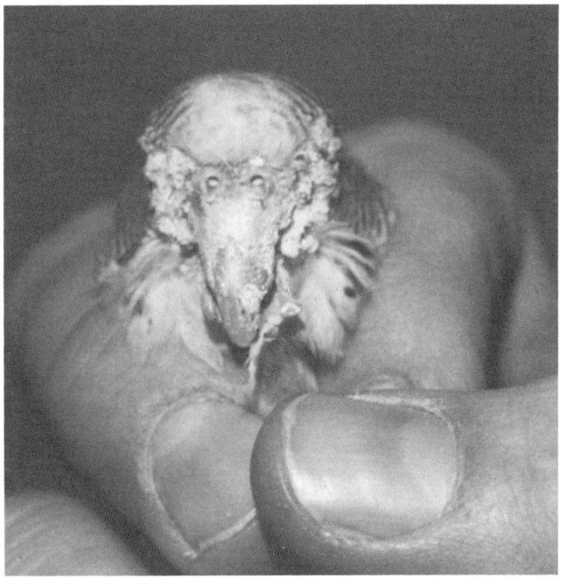

Figure 6B

Figure 6—Parakeet affected with *Knemidokoptes* mites (**A** and **B**). The involvement includes the beak, cere, and skin around the eyes. Note the large keratotic masses at the commissures of the beak.

examination reveals a fine, honeycombed appearance due to numerous tiny pits caused by *Knemidokoptes* mites. Lesions from *Knemidokoptes* mites can be found on the beak, cere, eyelids, vent, legs, and feet. Occasionally, they extend to the feathered areas of the bird (Figure 5). The lesions often begin on the cere or at the commissures of the mouth. The extent of the lesions varies, and the entire bird should be examined if lesions are found at one location.

The earliest knemidokoptic lesions are tiny pits in the nonfeathered area with little or no hyperkeratosis. Advanced lesions can show extreme hyperkeratosis, which the client may think is fungus or neoplasia (Figure 6). Infestations can be so severe that they cause beak deformities and sloughing of toes.[3,8,15]

Knemidokoptes mites spend their entire life cycle on the host, burrowing into the epidermis. The mites can apparently be carried without causing visible lesions, because unnoticed infestations have been found in birds that have not been exposed to other birds for several months. The disease is seen sporadically in parakeets kept in aviaries, suggesting that the mites are not highly communicable. Parakeets are the most susceptible hosts, but infestations are also common in canaries. Infestations are uncommon in other caged birds.

The diagnosis can be made by direct observation of lesions and confirmed by identifying the mite from a skin scraping. Treatment of knemidokoptic infestation requires topical application of almost any mild acaricidal lotion or oil, including plain mineral oil. Certain substances are potentially toxic (such as benzyl benzoate and lindane) and should be used with extreme caution or totally avoided. The hyperkeratotic lesions will quickly absorb moisture from the topical ointments and should be gradually removed as they loosen. Killing of mites should be begun early to prevent beak growth deformities. Excessive oiling of lesions must be avoided. If the bird wipes its wings on the oily lesions, the feathers lose their insulating value and the bird can become chilled. The lotion or oil is applied twice weekly until lesions disappear. Treatment should be continued weekly for several weeks after clearing to ensure that all mites are dead. Cage mates without lesions need not be treated, but the owner should periodically examine all birds for new lesions.[15-17]

The cere color of a mature male parakeet is blue, and that of a female is brown or tan. This can change, though: occasionally, a parakeet's cere will initially show the blue color of a male and then gradually turn brownish. This bird may be a true female. Usually a

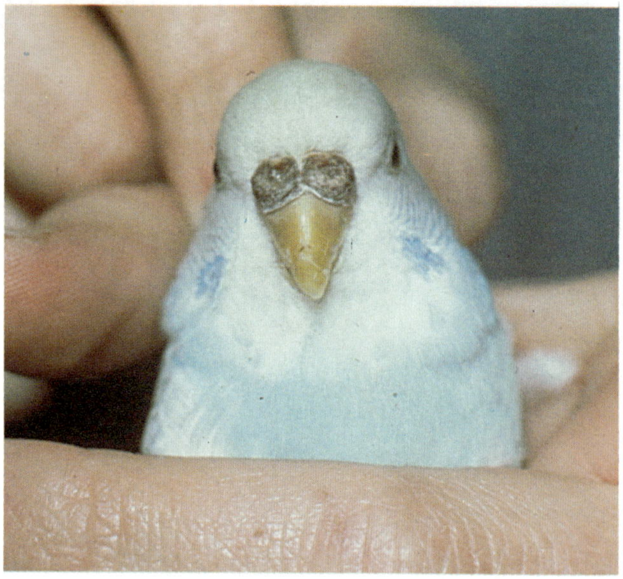

Figure 7—Female parakeet showing brown hypertrophy of the cere.

color change of the cere is a benign condition. However, cere color change has occurred in parakeets with serious disease, including cancer. The association between cere color change and specific diseases is too variable to be used as a good clinical aid.

Brown hypertrophy of the cere occurs in female parakeets and is characterized by thick brown keratin adhered to the cere (Figure 7). The keratin does not slough off as it normally should, and the cere becomes thickened with keratin. Treatment is aimed at softening the keratin with topical application of a lanolin-base ointment or small amounts of mineral oil and gently flaking the softened keratin away. The cause of this problem is unknown. It does not affect the general health of the bird.[12]

Diseases of the Beak

The beak is a thickened, hardened region of the stratum corneum epidermis. A healthy beak is shiny on its outer surface and impervious to most substances. It grows constantly and is worn down by feeding, grooming, climbing, and purposeful rubbing on a cage. The size and shape of the beak vary greatly in birds and are correlated with feeding habits. The cutting edges may be serrate, ridged, or smooth.[11,12]

The veterinarian must recognize two types of beaks. Passerines, the nonpsittacine, seed-eating species have a relatively straight bill of varying length. Psittacines have the other type—the hooked, heavy bill. In parrots, the upper beak is massive and curved, whereas the lower is smaller and U shaped. The upper beak of the parakeet is sharp tipped and closes over the lower beak, hiding most of the latter from view. Both the upper and lower beak act as extensions of the jaw.[12,18]

Malocclusion causes deformity of the beak because of the beak's continuous growth. In passerines (e.g., canaries), the overgrowth occurs at the tip and along the nonoccluding edges of the upper mandible. This can be trimmed with cuticle nippers. Malocclusion problems occur more frequently in psittacines than in passerines. Both the point of the bill and lateral edges may need trimming. The corresponding margins of the lower bill, which no longer have an occlusal surface and grow unevenly, must also be trimmed. In parrots and parakeets, the line of demarcation between the vascular and nonvascular parts of the beak can be seen if the bird is held between the examiner's eye and a bright light source (transillumination). Trimming should be done as frequently as necessary. Ferric subsulfate solution is used to control hemorrhage.[12]

Overgrown beaks in parakeets are most commonly the result of *Knemidokoptes* mite infestation (Figure 8). Beaks may be injured traumatically, causing malocclusion. Even with extensive beak deformity, birds are able to hull seeds and survive surprisingly well (Figure 9).

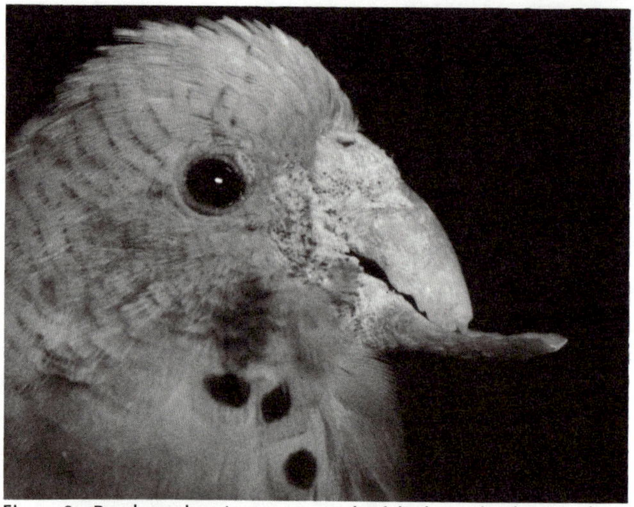

Figure 8—Parakeet showing overgrowth of the lower beak secondary to *Knemidokoptes* mite infection.

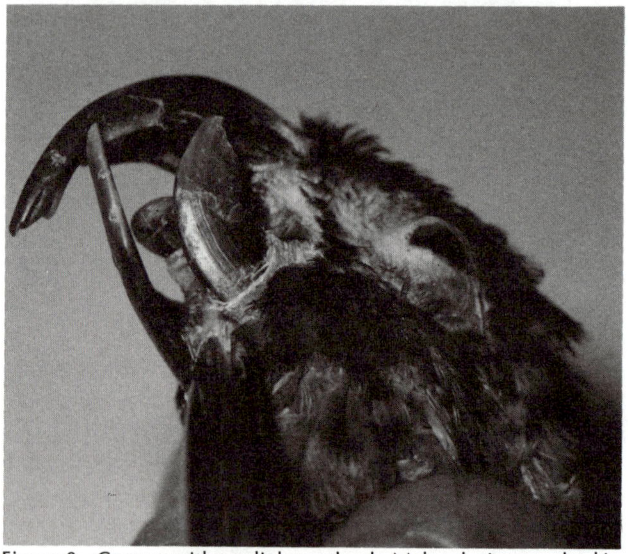

Figure 9—Conure with a split lower beak. Malocclusion resulted in marked overgrowth of both segments of the lower and upper beaks. The bird survived well for two years with this injury.

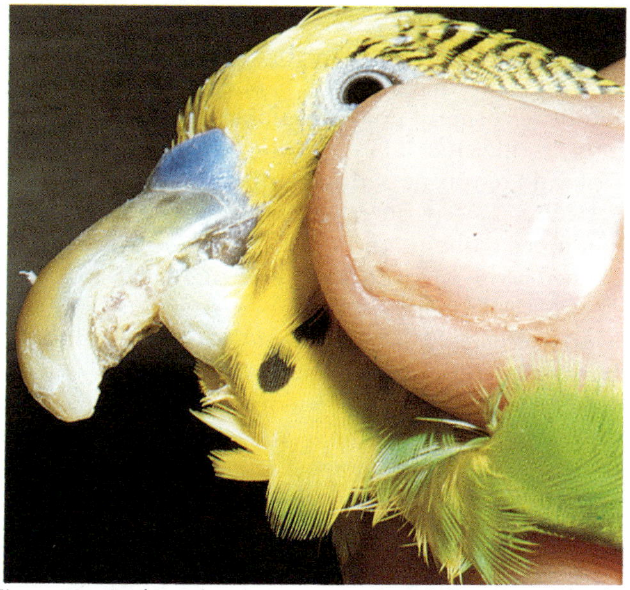

Figure 10—Parakeet showing overgrowth and distortion of beak from fibrosarcoma.

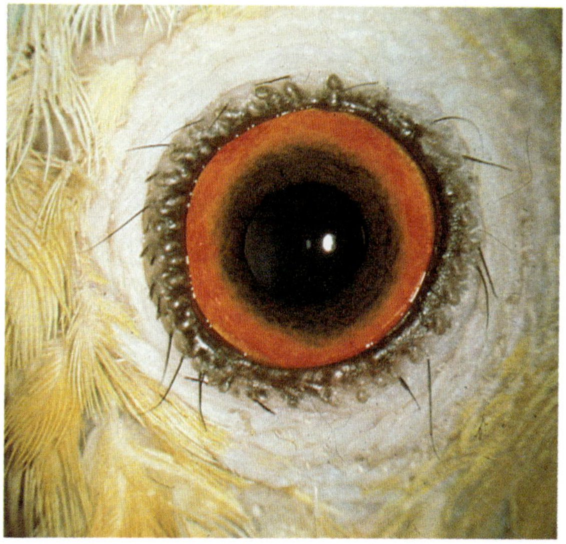

Figure 12—The eye of a normal Amazon parrot. Note the ruffled border of the eyelids, the numerous bristle feathers, the round eye opening, the two colors of the iris, and the round pupil.

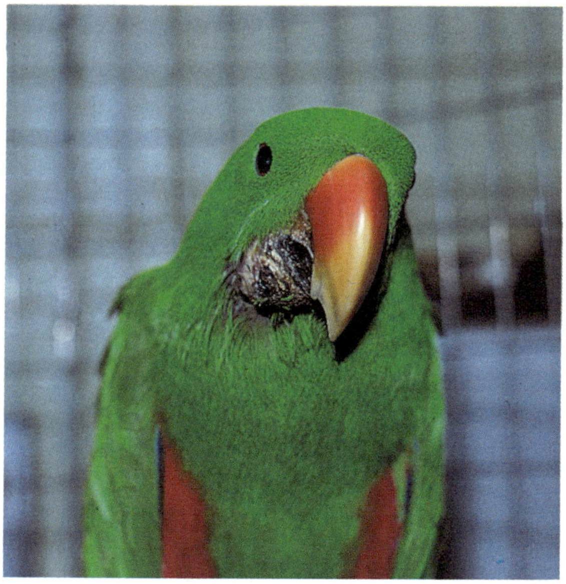

Figure 11—Eclectus parrot with a squamous cell carcinoma near its mandible.

Metabolic causes of beak deformity have been suggested such as mycoses, liver disease, malnutrition, specific nutritional deficiencies, and rickets.[12] Cancer occurs in the beak infrequently and almost exclusively in the parakeet. Fibrosarcoma is the most common tumor, and it eventually causes the death of the bird (Figure 10).[12,19,20] Adenocarcinomas and squamous cell carcinomas also occur in the beak region of caged birds (Figure 11).

Diseases of the Eye

Eye diseases of caged birds have been infrequently described in the literature. Periorbital diseases, such as pox, *Knemidokoptes* infestation, and sinus abscess, are commonly seen, but ocular diseases are uncommon. Since the eye is small, owners often fail to recognize abnormalities when they do occur and fail to seek veterinary care.

In the normal psittacine bird, the palpebral fissure is nearly round, and its border is usually pigmented with a finely ruffled edge (Figure 12). There are numerous fine, bristle feathers at the upper and lower border of the lids. The iris coloration varies. The iris normally shows hippus, which is a rapid, cyclic dilation and constriction of the iris. The pupil is round. Pressure on the cornea during examination will partially collapse the anterior chamber; upon release of the pressure, fluid gradually refills the globe without harm to the eye. The nictitating membrane moves from the upper medial area downward across the cornea. The avian retina is avascular.[21-25]

There are two major differences between the avian and mammalian eye: (1) The iris and ciliary body musculature are different, and (2) birds have a pecten, and mammals do not.

The musculature of the iris and ciliary body is striated in birds rather than smooth, thus apparently providing them with voluntary control over pupil size. Topical administration of drugs that act on the autonomic nervous system (e.g., atropine and tropicamide) will not create pupillary dilatation for ophthalmoscopy; rather, skeletal muscle–paralyzing agents must be used. A solution of d-tubocurarine chloride can be prepared for retinal examination. The effectiveness varies, depending on the species being examined.[22,23]

The avian eye contains a pecten, which is a heavily pigmented, highly vascular pleated structure extending from atop the optic disk into the vitreous. The pecten may be a producer of intraocular fluid.[21,23]

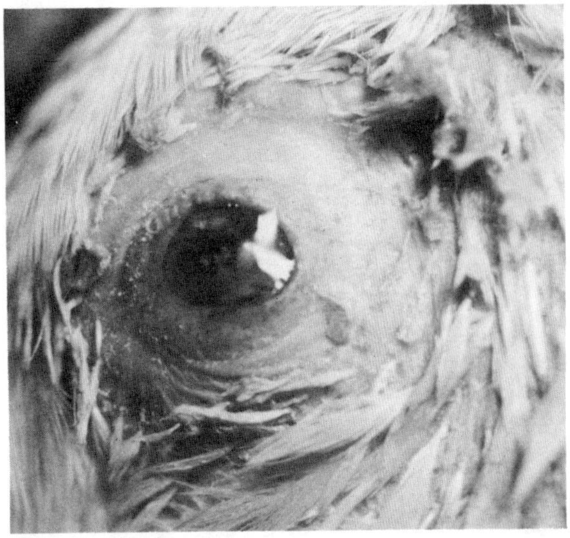

Figure 13—Amazon parrot from a group of birds believed to have poxvirus infection. The ocular abnormalities are loss of the normal ruffled lid margins, reduction of the palpebral opening, and chronic keratitis. *Escherichia coli* was isolated from the corneal surface.

The eyelids can reflect generalized systemic disease or local eye disease. A depressed and sick bird will sit quietly with its eyelids partially closed. When disturbed, it will open the lids to their normal position. A unilateral narrowing of the palpebral fissure suggests eye disease. Conjunctivitis is indicated by inflamed conjunctival membranes and may be due to concurrent sinusitis. Severe, chronic eye disease can result in an abnormal appearance of the lids.[5] The lid edge will lose its pigmented, corrugated appearance and become smooth. The palpebral fissure may become smaller (Figure 13) and asymmetrical, losing its round shape. Excessive lacrimation is a sign of eye disease in birds. Corneal opacities and blood vessels on the cornea are signs of chronic keratitis. Corneal ulcers will stain with fluorescein dye as in mammals. Panophthalmitis is a severe condition usually due to perforation of the eye and massive infection. The condition is usually uncontrollable and results in phthisis bulbi.

Cataracts occur in caged birds and are most often diagnosed without other eye disease present. Senility is blamed because cataracts are most commonly found in aged birds. In canaries, though, cataracts are not confined to old birds and there is evidence that they may be inherited in certain varieties. Congenital cataracts have been found in canaries. In domestic fowl, numerous infections and nutritional and other noninfectious causes of cataract are known. In caged birds, the specific cause of cataracts is generally unknown.[24-26]

Bulging of the eye and periorbital tissue can be due to sinusitis or pressure from behind the eye. In both instances, the eye normally shows no inflammation. The diagnosis of a mass lesion behind the eye (such as a tumor) can be suspected but is difficult to confirm antemortem.[27] Uni- or bilateral proptosis was present in 9 of 50 parakeets with chromophobe pituitary tumors in one report.[28] Intracranial tumors are uncommon in caged birds.[20] Enucleation is required for severe ocular diseases such as tumors, abscesses, and panophthalmitis. The avian eye lies tightly in the orbit, and access behind the eye is more difficult than in most mammalian species. The surgical procedure has been described.[13]

Little is specifically known about the treatment of avian eye diseases, and they should be approached with the same fundamental knowledge and care as with other animals.[22-25]

REFERENCES

1. Giddens WE Jr, Swango LG, Henderson JD Jr, Lewis RA, Farner DS, Carlos A, Dolowry WC: Canary pox in sparrows and canaries (*Fringillidae*) and in weavers (*Ploceidae*): Pathology and host specificity of the virus. *Vet Pathol* 8:260, 1971.
2. Cavill JP: Viral diseases, in Petrak ML (ed): *Diseases of Cage and Aviary Birds*. Philadelphia, Lea & Febiger, 1982.
3. Fowler ME: Infections and zoonotic diseases, in Fowler ME (ed): *Zoo and Wild Animal Medicine*. Philadelphia, WB Saunders Co, 1978.
4. Graham CLG: Pox virus infection in a spectacled Amazon parrot. *Avian Dis* 22:340, 1978.
5. McDonald SE, Lowenstine LJ, Ardans AA: Avian pox in blue-fronted Amazon parrots. *JAVMA* 179:1218, 1981.
6. Clubb SL: Personal communication, FL, 1981.
7. Hitchner SB: Canary pox vaccination with live embryo-attenuated virus. *Avian Dis* 25:874, 1981.
8. McDonald SE: Respiratory diseases in psittacine birds, in Kirk RW (ed): *Current Veterinary Therapy*. Philadelphia, WB Saunders Co, 1980.
9. Steiner CV Jr, Davis RB: Diseases of the respiratory system, in *Caged Bird Medicine*. Ames, IA, The Iowa State University Press, 1981, pp 59-74.
10. Soifer FK: Infectious respiratory diseases of psittacine birds. *VM SAC*, 74:1307, 1979.
11. Arnall L: Conditions of the beak and claw in the budgerigar. *J Small Anim Pract* 6:135, 1965.
12. Altman RB: Conditions involving the integumentary system, in Petrak ML (ed): *Diseases of Cage and Aviary Birds*. Philadelphia, Lea & Febiger, 1982.
13. Altman RB: General principles of avian surgery. *Compend Contin Educ Pract Vet* 3:177, 1981.
14. Crane SW, Jacobson E, Shields RP: Cryosurgical removal of an intranasal granuloma from an African Gray parrot. *VM SAC* 75:499, 1980.
15. Greve JH: Parasitic diseases, in Fowler ME (ed): *Zoo and Wild Animal Medicine*. Philadelphia, WB Saunders Co, 1978.
16. Richards DA: Cnemidocoptic mange in parakeets. *VM SAC* 70:729, 1975.
17. Spira A: Parasitic diseases of cage and aviary birds. *Annu Sci AAHA Proc*:15, 1981.
18. Altman R: Noninfectious diseases, in Fowler ME (ed): *Zoo and Wild Animal Medicine*. Philadelphia, WB Saunders Co, 1978.
19. Steiner CV Jr, Davis RB: Tumors and egg binding, in *Caged Bird Medicine*. Ames, IA, The Iowa State University Press, 1981, pp 105-113.
20. Arnall L, Keymer IF: Tumours, cysts and similar structures, in *Bird Diseases*. Neptune City, NJ, THF Publications, Inc, 1975, pp 345-366.
21. McLelland J: Eye, in Getty R (ed): *The Anatomy of the Domestic Animals*, vol 2. Philadelphia, WB Saunders Co, 1975.
22. Bellhorn RW: Ophthalmologic disorders of exotic and laboratory animals. *Vet Clin North Am* 3:345, 1973.
23. Bellhorn RW: Laboratory animal ophthalmology, in Gelatt KN (ed): *Veterinary Ophthalmology*. Philadelphia, Lea & Febiger, 1981.
24. Arnall L, Keymer IF: The organs of special senses, in *Bird Diseases*. Neptune City, NJ, THF Publications, 1975, pp 64-67.
25. Small E, Burke TJ: Diseases of the organs of special sense, in Petrak ML (ed): *Diseases of Cage and Aviary Birds*. Philadelphia, Lea & Febiger, 1982.
26. Keymer IF: Cataracts in birds. *Avian Pathol* 6:335, 1977.
27. Rambow VJ, Murphy JC, Fox JG: Malignant lymphoma in a pigeon. *JAVMA* 179: 1266, 1981.
28. Schlumberger HG: Neoplasia in parakeets: Spontaneous chromophobe pituitary tumors. *Cancer Res* 14:237, 1954.

Clinical Manifestations of Cervicocephalic Air Sacs of Psittacines

Michael T. Walsh, DVM
Department of Special Clinical Sciences

Maron Calderwood Mays, VMD, PhD
Department of Comparative and Experimental Pathology

College of Veterinary Medicine
University of Florida
Gainesville, Florida

An increase in ownership of psittacine birds as companion animals has led to much interest in improving their medical care. Upper respiratory tract problems, such as rhinitis, rhinorrhea, and sinusitis, are common reasons for presentation to the veterinarian. Psittacines have features of the upper respiratory system that may be overlooked. For example, the cervicocephalic air sacs of psittacines are not recognized by many veterinarians, and there are clinical problems associated with this portion of the upper respiratory system that are important in managing upper respiratory diseases.

Regional Anatomy of the Upper Respiratory System

Some terms that are used in reference to the upper respiratory system and the relationship of the nasal cavities to the sinuses are reviewed in Table I.

The two major divisions of the upper respiratory system in birds are the rhinal cavities and the infraorbital sinuses. In many species, air from the external nares first encounters the operculum protruding just inside the cere. It then travels down the rhinal cavity, which is sometimes tubular in shape, past the chonchae. The chonchae, by projecting into the passageway, give the rhinal cavity a greater surface area, which allows the cavity to act as a site for heat exchange, heat conservation, olfaction, filtration of airborne debris, and water conservation.

The right and left nasal cavities are separated by a nasal septum. They communicate at the choanae, which in turn communicate with the glottis of the trachea. The lateral walls of the rhinal cavities separate them from the sinus cavities.

The infraorbital sinus (paranasal sinus) is a fairly spacious cavity located laterally to the nasal area and rostroventrad to the eyes. The lateral borders of the sinus are the facial musculature, though there are portions caudad to the upper beak that are fairly superficial. These are the most commonly noted sites of swellings in extreme cases of sinusitis. Many diverticula of the infraorbital sinus from the main body surround the eye. Figure 1 shows the extent of this sinus in the head of a conure that has been injected with latex. Portions of the sinus may extend into the upper beak and mandible and may communicate with extensive pneumatized sections of the skull. Through small openings in its medial

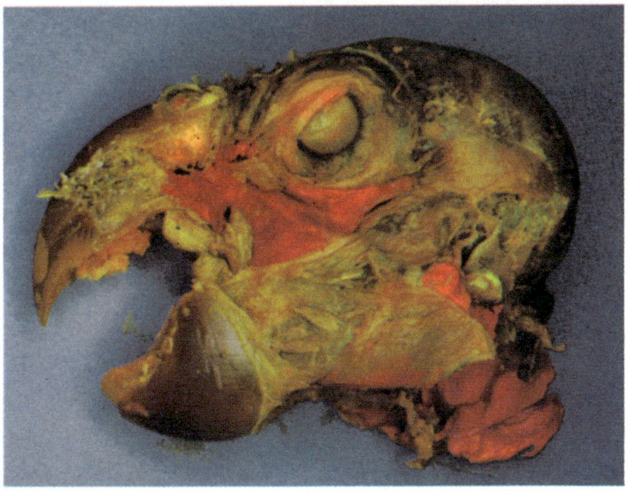

Figure 1A

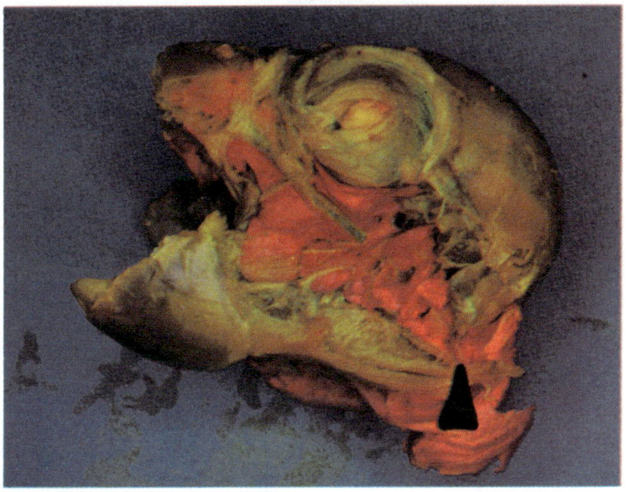

Figure 1B

Figure 1—(**A**) The skin has been removed on the head of this conure after latex injection of the infraorbital sinus. The red area at the commissure of the oral cavity is a common site of swelling associated with sinusitis. (**B**) The facial musculature and portions of the upper and lower beaks have been removed to show the extent of the infraorbital sinus cranially into the beak and caudally, exiting at the tympanic area (*arrow*) to communicate with the cervicocephalic system.

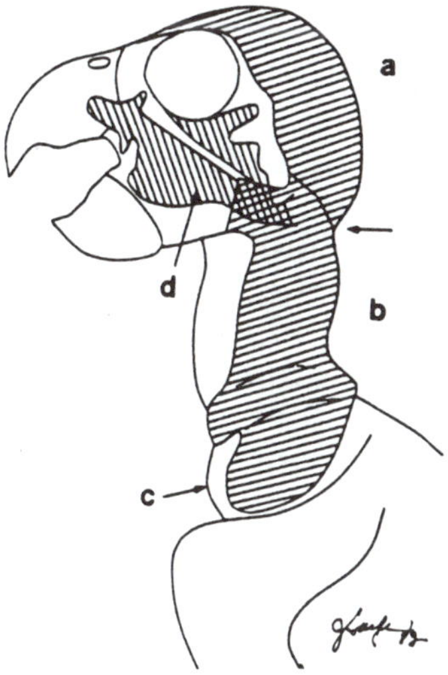

Figure 2A

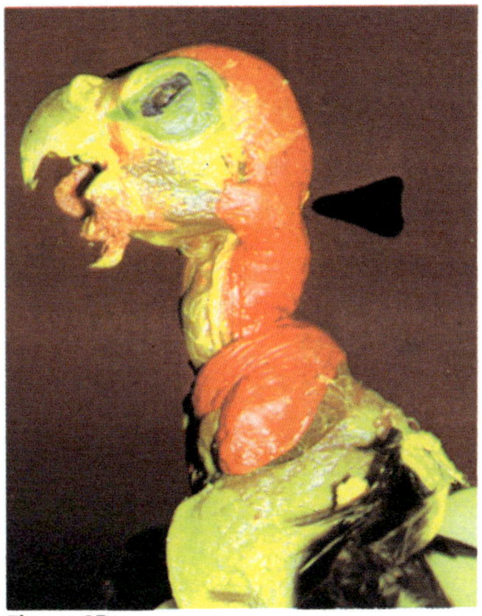

Figure 2B

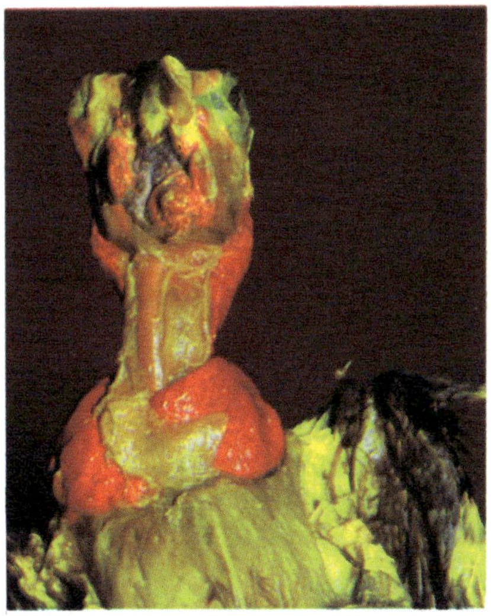

Figure 2C

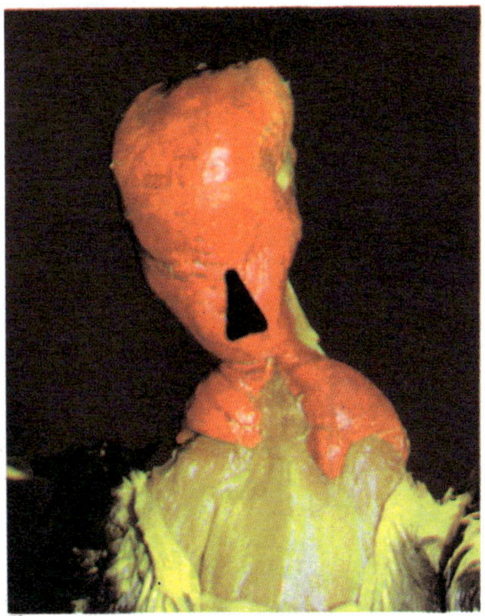

Figure 2D

Figure 2—(**A** through **D**) Illustration of the relationship of the sinus to the cerviocephalic air sacs. (**A**) *Unlettered arrow* indicates the division between the cephalic portion (*a*) and the cervical portion (*b*). *c* = crop; *d* = infraorbital sinus. The caudal aspect of the infraorbital sinus connects to the cerviocephalic air sacs. (**B**) Lateral view of a cockatiel. The cerviocephalic air sacs have been injected with red latex, and the skin is removed. Note the caplike cephalic portion over the head and the distal extent of the cervical portion to the shoulders. The *arrowhead* denotes the division between the cervical and cephalic portions. (**C**) Anterior view of the cockatiel in **B**. Note the latex filling the air sacs that surround the crop. (**D**) Posterior view of the cockatiel in **B** and **C**. *Arrowhead* indicates the point of division between the cervical and cephalic portions.

TABLE I
Some Anatomic and Pathologic Terms Relating to the Upper Respiratory System

Air sacculitis	Inflammation of the air sacs
Cere	Area surrounding the external nares; in psittacines, often ovoid and consisting of raised keratinized tissue
Choanae	Slit-like opening in the maxillary portion of the pharynx (internal nares)
Chonchae	Bony scroll-like protrusions (usually 2 to 3) into the rhinal area; consist of epithelial-lined tissue
Infundibular cleft (sphenopalatine cleft)	Small oval opening, located posterior to the choanae; connects the pharynx to the infraorbital sinus
Operculum	Flat rounded bony protrusion into the area of the external nasal opening
Rhinitis	Inflammation of the mucous membranes of the nasal passages
Rhinopathy	Any disease of the nasal passages
Rhinorrhea	Free discharge of a thin nasal mucus
Sinusitis	Inflammation of a sinus; may be acute or chronic, purulent or nonpurulent

wall, the infraorbital sinus also communicates with the corresponding nasal cavity. Ventrally, the sinus is in contact with the oral pharyngeal area through the infundibular slit. Caudally, the sinus communicates through channels in the tympanic area with the cervicocephalic air sac system, as shown by the arrow in Figure 1B.

Avian Air Sac Systems

The term *air sac* is usually used in reference to the pulmonary air sac system in birds. William Harvey gave the first detailed description of the air sacs in 1651, and it has been said that Aristotle knew of them 2000 years before. In fact there are three systems of air sacs: the pulmonary system, the pharyngeal tracheal system, and the cervicocephalic system.

The pulmonary system is the most familiar. It is widely recognized that there are nine air sacs present in the adult psittacine. The embryonic fusion of one pair forms the clavicular sac,[1] and the remainder are the cervical,[2] anterior thoracic,[2] posterior thoracic,[2] and abdominal air sacs.[2]

The pharyngeal tracheal system is used mainly in courtship in some species. This system consists of saclike diverticula that extend from the oral cavity or trachea and are inflated during display behaviors, such as those seen in the frigate bird *(Fragata magnificens)*.

The third system, the cervicocephalic air system, was first well described by Bignon in 1889. Though present in at least six avian orders, the system is absent in diving birds, such as penguins and grebes. Ratites (emu, rhea), pigeons, and chickens have only a partially developed cervicocephalic system. This system is most extensively developed in strong flyers (e.g., stork, albatross) and in birds with large heads and beaks (psittacines). Within the psittacine family there is a great deal of variability in the sacular development.

There are two main divisions of the cervicocephalic system: a cranial cephalic portion and a cervical, or neck, portion. As seen in Figure 2A (arrow), the system is connected by bilateral channels that travel below the ear to the infraorbital sinuses. The relationship is best visualized by injecting latex into the system through the infundibular cleft, to fill the sinuses and then the cervicocephalic system. The cephalic portion is extensive in some species, such as the conures and parakeets. This caplike portion (Figures 2A through C) is connected to the cervical portion by a small median communication. The cephalic portion of the system may extend from the occipital region to just caudad to the cere rostrally and dorsad to the eyes laterally. The cervical portion, which originates in the tympanic area, extends in two columns bilaterally down the neck to rest in a saddlelike fashion over the shoulders (Figure 2D). In some species, e.g., macaws, there may be discrete communications between the two columns at various intervals. The crop is flanked on each side by the distal cervical portions. When viewed externally, the inflated air cells appear nearly to encase the vertebral column. This development is extensive in parakeets, cockatiels, conures, amazons, macaws, and some members of the cockatoo family.

Histology of the Cervicocephalic Air Sac

In amazon parrots, the epithelial lining of the lateral wall of the cervical air sac is apparent histologically (Figure 3). These cervical air sacs are thin-walled extensions of the upper respiratory system and are completely lined by a single layer of very low cuboidal or flat squamous cells. Beneath the epithelial lining of the air sac is a thin layer of loosely arranged collagen and elastic fibers, which attaches the walls of the air sacs to adjacent tissues. Because the cervicocephalic air sacs are not used for oxygen exchange, the vasculature beneath the epithelial lining is not prominent.

Clinical Implications

Because of the direct connection between the cervicocephalic air sacs and the infraorbital sinuses, diseases can involve both the sinuses and the cervicocephalic air sac system. Many clinicians are not aware of the existence

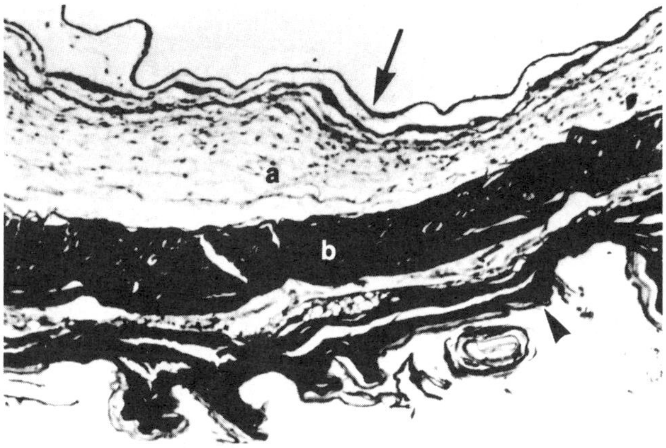

Figure 3—Histologically, the lining of a cervicocephalic air sac is a single layer of flattened cells (*arrow*). Underlying the sac are layers of loose connective tissue (a), skeletal muscle (*b*), and the skin of the neck (*arrowhead*). (H&E, ×56)

of the cervicocephalic air sacs, thus they may be overlooked in examination of a bird with a respiratory problem.

Three case histories are presented to illustrate problems that involve the cervicocephalic air sacs.

Case 1

A 12-year-old amazon parrot presented with an eight-month history of having "an enlarged neck area" (Figure 4A). The problem had been previously diagnosed as a

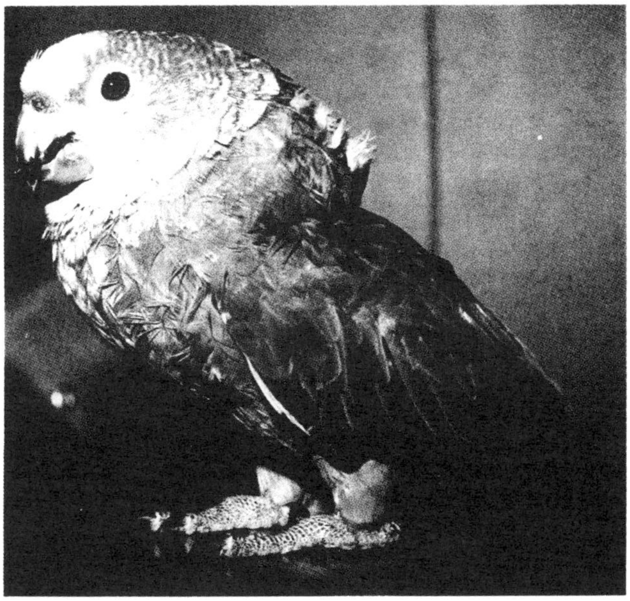

Figure 4A

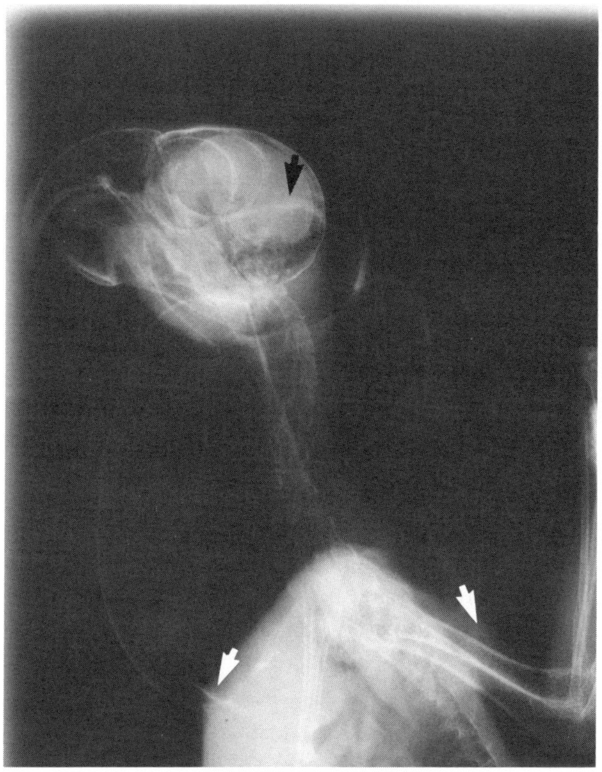

Figure 4B

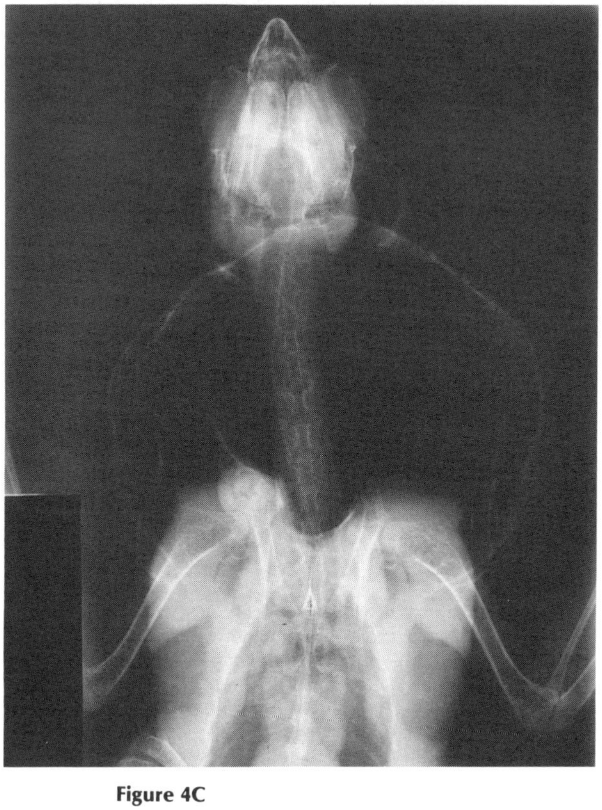

Figure 4C

Figure 4—(**A**) An amazon parrot with cervicocephalic air sac involvement showing a neck area that is distended to be two to three times normal size. (**B**) Lateral radiograph of the amazon parrot seen in **A**. The borders of the trapped air from the tympanic area to the shoulder (*arrows*) are shown. (**C**) Anterior-posterior view of the same amazon parrot. Because it can be seen that the air is limited to the cervical area, subcutaneous emphysema can be ruled out as a diagnosis. The crop and trachea are made very evident by the trapped air.

ruptured pulmonary air sac. It was noted in the history that the bird was being offered a poor diet and had clinical signs of respiratory disease (sneezing, nasal discharge) before development of swelling. There was no history of trauma. Physical examination revealed air distention from the occipital area to the shoulders. After brushing away the feathers on the back of the neck with an alcohol swab, an extra layer of tissue below the skin was revealed. The orientation of the vasculature in this layer suggested that the layer was not associated with the dermis. Radiographs were taken (Figures 4B and C), which showed trapped air that had definitive borders and did not extend below the shoulder area or above the tympanic area.

Three hundred milliliters of air were aspirated from the distended air sac; the air was replaced within 12 hours. This indicated that the connection between the infundibular cleft and the tympanic area might be obstructed in such a way as to allow air to enter the air sacs and not allow it to escape.

Case 2

A mature albino cockatiel presented with a swelling of the head and neck, which had been noted when the bird was first given to the owners 15 months previously (Figure 5A). The bird did not appear to be in any discomfort and it ate well and acted normally. There

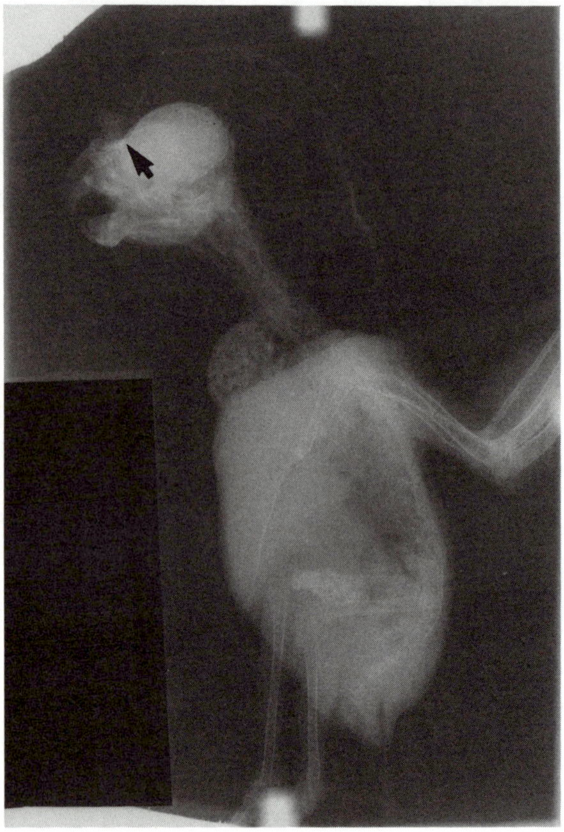

Figure 5B

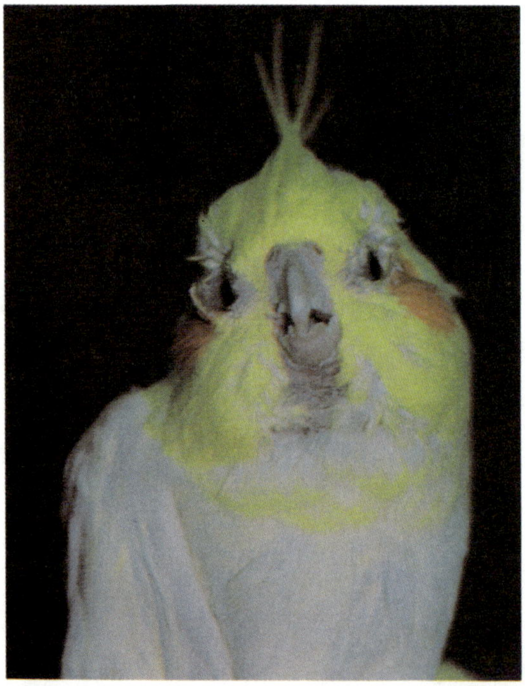

Figure 5A

Figure 5—(**A**) A cockatiel with chronic cerviocephalic air sac inflation. This case differs from the one illustrated in **4A** in that the cephalic portion is more prominent. (**B**) Lateral radiograph of the cockatiel shown in **A**. The film has been lightened to show the distention of the soft tissue. Note the cephalic involvement caudal to the cere (*arrow*). (**C**) Anterior-posterior view of the cockatiel in **A** and **B**. *Arrows* indicate distention of the air sac. The cervical portion does not extend beyond the shoulders caudally.

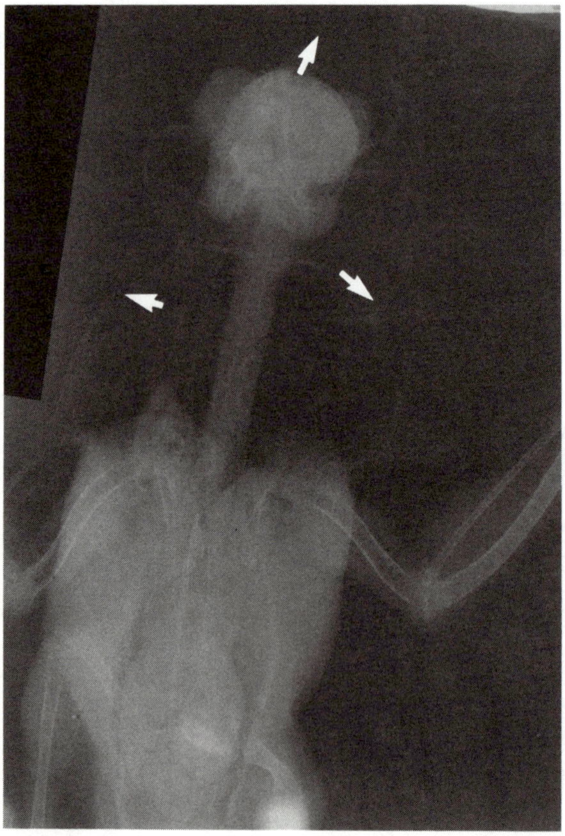

Figure 5C

had been episodes of respiratory disease that had been treated with antibiotics. Physical examination revealed a very pliable air-filled swelling that extended the length of the neck and involved the head. Determination of the extent of the swelling was facilitated by clearing away feathers with an alcohol swab. As in Case 1, there was a second layer of tissue present in close proximity to the skin. No other abnormalities were detected. Radiographs were taken to verify cervicocephalic air sac involvement and as part of a routine workup (Figures 5B and C). These showed that the air did not extend beyond the shoulder and that there was more cephalic involvement than there was in Case 1.

Case 3

A three-year-old male sulfur-crested cockatoo presented with a history of collapsing in its cage. The bird had been purchased three months previously and was on an all-seed diet. Though the appetite was good, the bird had lost weight over the preceding two weeks. Antibiotics were prescribed by a veterinarian for a "lameness problem."

Physical examination revealed an emaciated bird weighing 280 g with anemia and hypoproteinemia. Supportive therapy strengthened the bird adequately for radiographic evaluation the next day. Endostosis of the left femur as well as multiple circular densities in the soft tissue of the cervical area were noted on radiographs. The significance of the neck opacities was not appreciated at that time.

After some improvement, the bird again collapsed and died on the third day of hospitalization. Lesions found at necropsy consisted of granulomas in the medullary space of the left femur, left tibia, liver, and the soft tissue of the neck. Bacteria in these lesions were determined histologically to be acid-fast and thus consistent with mycobacteria. The reason for the multiple lesions in the soft tissue at the neck was not determined. The slides were reviewed at a later date when the possibility of cervicocephalic air sac involvement was being considered. Review of the radiographs showed that the location of the granulomas was compatible with the normal anatomic location of the air sacs (Figure 6A). Subsequent examination of the histologic sections from the neck area revealed that the granuloma was within the air sac (Figure 6B).

Diagnosis

The absence of inflated air sacs does not rule out a pathologic process in the cervicocephalic air sac system. Any bird with a history of upper respiratory disease should be examined closely for cervicocephalic air sac involvement. The first step is to examine the oral cavity visually and give particular attention to the infundibular cleft and choanae. Swelling, discoloration, obstruction, and discharge should be noted, and bacterial and fungal cultures should be taken when indicated. Visual and otoscopic examination of the ears should be routinely performed to detect signs of otitis, which may interfere with the passage of air through the tympanic area. Palpation of the cervical region from the tympanic area to the shoulders to detect focal granulomas or debris lying within the air sac should also be performed as part of a complete examination. The feathers behind the ears, along the right and left jugular area, and over the shoulders can be brushed away with an alcohol swab to aid in visualization. The skin is best seen when feathers are parted over the apterylae, the tracts of skin relatively devoid of feather follicles. These featherless tracts are the tracts used when attempting to locate the jugular vein for obtaining a blood sample.

Whole-body radiographs can help confirm a diagnosis of cervicocephalic air sac distention and detect granulomas. The most common differential diagnosis of subcutaneous emphysema can usually be ruled out on the basis of the location of the distention and a history of

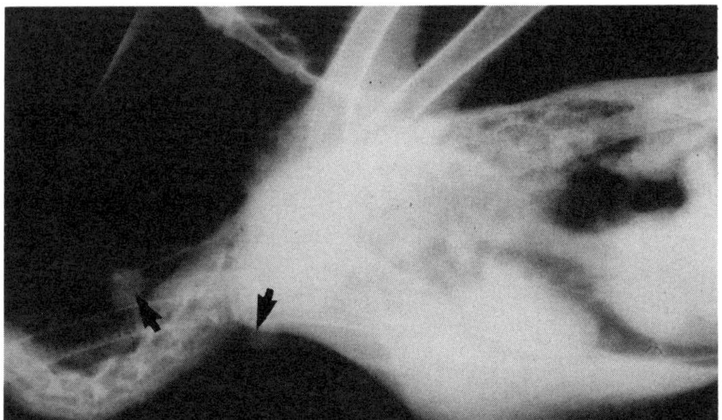

Figure 6A

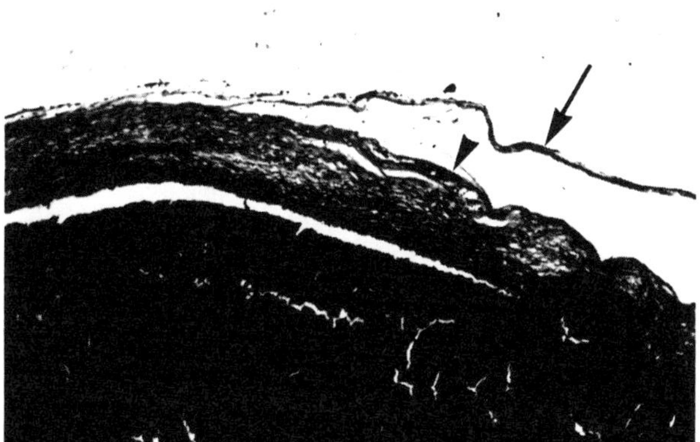

Figure 6B

Figure 6—(**A**) Lateral radiograph of a three-year-old cockatoo. The *arrows* show the positions of the granulomas in the region of the cervical air sacs of the neck. (**B**) Histologic appearance of a granuloma within a cerviocephalic air sac. The granuloma has been "peeled out." Surrounding it is a thin membrane of flattened cells, which are remnants of the air sac lining (*arrow*). Within this membrane is a band of fibrous connective tissue (*arrowhead*) and a central mass of epithelioid macrophages and necrotic debris. (H&E, ×56) trauma. Subcutaneous emphysema, as a result of tracheal trauma or air sac rupture, results in air dissecting in a diffuse irregular pattern that commonly spreads to other portions of the body.

The air sacs can be filled voluntarily on expiration. Bacteria, fungi, and other airborne pathogens may thereby be deposited in these air cells. As a result, air sacculitis and granuloma formation are probably fairly common problems but may not be easily detected. The presence of lesions, such as the granuloma detected in the neck area of the bird in Case 3, necessitates aspiration or surgical removal. Culture, cytology, and histopathology help to pinpoint the cause and aid in determining therapy.

To determine the frequency of cervicocephalic disease in birds accurately, necropsy techniques should be adapted to include a close examination of the cervicocephalic area following removal of the skin.

Therapy

Because pathology involving the cervicocephalic air sacs is not well documented or understood, definitive therapeutic principles have not been formulated. The most common problems that have been noted by the authors are granulomatous air sacculitis[2] and chronically distended air sacs.[3]

Treatment for chronically distended air sacs is mainly symptomatic. Simply aspirating the trapped air may only give short-term relief. Chronic deflation is more successful, but there is no information that can be used to compare results with known causes or to determine the recurrence rate. Basically, the treatment technique for chronic deflation involves creating a *sacculostomy*, or stoma of the air sac. The stoma is created and the skin and air sac are sutured together or are sutured to an O-ring made of silicone or Teflon® (DuPont) to maintain the opening. It appears that one opening is sufficient to relieve the distention in many species. The site for placement of the stoma can be verified by first aspirating the air to determine if bilateral drainage is achieved.

More consideration should be given to determining the initial cause of chronically distended air sacs; the cause may be related to concurrent or previous upper respiratory disease, such as chronic sinusitus. It is probable that inflammation and debris between the infundibular cleft and the tympanic area may be creating a one-way valve effect so that air is pumped in with pressure but cannot escape. The chronic release of this pressure with the air sacculostomy may be providing symptomatic relief or simply giving the involved area adequate time to heal.

Antibiotic therapy based on culture and sensitivity testing may be helpful in treatment of air sacculitis, granulomas, and the early stages of the distended air sac.

Discussion

Bignon believed that the air sacs have three functions.[1] The first is heat retention, which is important during cold periods. Birds inflate the sacs to produce an insulating layer of air to aid in heat conservation. In high-flying birds, the sacs may be inflated to decrease heat loss during flight. The second function is buoyancy control, a function exemplified in such birds as the pelican and albatross that spend long periods in the water. The third function of the air sacs is supporting the head during sleep. Other possible functions include inflation during flight for head support and reducing the force of impact during free-fall fishing (another function of the pelican).

For the most part, the results of the authors' study agreed with those of Bignon's. Bignon found that of the species she investigated, the Carolina parakeet and Ledbetters cockatoo had the most extensive development of both portions of the cervicocephalic air sac system.It is also evident that cockatiels and small conures have well-developed cervical and cephalic portions. Amazon parrots have a well-developed cervical portion and a reduced cranial portion. The macaw also has a well-defined cervical portion but no cephalic portion. It appears that both portions of the cervicocephalic system are well developed in smaller species. Development of the cervical portions of the system seems generally more advanced than that of the cephalic portion in larger birds. No direct connection has yet been found between the cervicocephalic air sac system and the pulmonary air sac system.

The veterinarian should be aware of certain problems associated with the cervicocephalic air sac system. As previously noted, this system has differences in form, function, and distribution between the species. Keeping the variations in mind will help to explain some of the subtle differences in presentation and lesion location. Although pathology of the cervicocephalic system seems rare when compared with that of other upper respiratory conditions, such as sinusitis, it is also likely that pathology in this area is overlooked by the clinicians and pathologists. It would be interesting to examine every necropsied bird for cervicocephalic air sac involvement because pathologic processes in this system may play a role in the development of other airway diseases.

Acknowledgments

The authors thank Marisa Mitchell for her translation of Bignon's article; Dr. Claus Buergelt for his translation of the Groebbels article; Jody Sayle for her artwork; Mark Hoffenberg for the photographs; and Dr. George Kollias and Lisa Biles for their help with the manuscript.

REFERENCES

1. Bignon, F: Contribution to the study of pneumacity of birds—The cervicocephalic air cells of the birds and their relation with the bones of the head. *Mem Soc Zool Franc* 2:260-318, 1889.
2. Groebbels F: *Der Vogel*, vol 1. Berlin, Borntrager, 1932.
3. King AS: Structural and functional aspects of the avian lungs and air sacs. *Int Rev Gen Exp Zool*:171-267. 1966.
4. Coe MJ: Letter. *Nature* 188:598, 1960.

The Clinical Significance of Abdominal Enlargement in the Budgerigar (*Melopsittacus undulatus*)

Marjorie C. McMillan, DVM
The Windhover Bird Clinic
Walpole, Massachusetts

Margaret L. Petrak, VMD
Angell Memorial Animal Hospital
Boston, Massachusetts

Abdominal enlargement is a common physical finding in domestic middle-aged and older budgerigars (three years and older). Many veterinarians believe that this finding indicates a tumor and they recommend euthanasia without further consideration. Although budgerigars have a high incidence of neoplasia,[1] other more treatable causes of abdominal distention should not be disregarded in making a diagnosis. The definitive diagnosis should be based on age, sex, history, physical examination, significant clinical findings, and ancillary diagnostic testing.

It is helpful to divide the causes of abdominal enlargement into nonpathologic and pathologic entities (Table I).

Depending on whether the cause is nonpathologic or pathologic, and whether the duration is acute or chronic, the bird may present with *sick bird syndrome* (fluffing, anorexia, and lethargy) or it may be asymptomatic except for an observable abdominal swelling.

History and Causes of Illness

Since many causes of abdominal enlargement are related to the female genital tract, it is important to determine the bird's sex. This is easy with many budgerigars. The cere in birds over six months of age is usually blue in males and tan to brown in females. However, a small percentage of female budgerigars have blue ceres. This can cause problems when speculating whether an abdominal enlargement in a bird with a blue cere is pathological or due to physiological hypertrophy of the oviduct (Figure 1).

Knowing the bird's age may be helpful in limiting the differential diagnosis. Since the average life expectancy of the budgerigar in captivity is about six years, birds over age three are past middle age and are at high risk for neoplasia. Liver disease with hepatomegaly also tends to occur in middle-aged and older birds, although neoplasia and liver disease have been observed in budgerigars as young as six months of age. Liver disease from a variety of causes is a common clinical finding in budgerigars; however, certain breeds may have an inherited predisposition to lipidosis[2] resulting in fatty degeneration of the liver and other organs (Figure 2). Recognizing these breeds may help in diagnosing the abdominal problem.

TABLE I

Causes of Abdominal Enlargement

Nonpathologic
1. Laying female (hen)
2. Obesity—subcutaneous lipomas and intra-abdominal fat
3. Pseudocoprostasis
4. Aerophagia

Pathologic
1. Neoplasia
2. Hepatomegaly
3. Egg binding
4. Cysts—oviduct, ovarian, and renal
5. Hernia
6. Peritonitis—egg and other causes
7. Ascites

Liver Disease

Liver disease is one of the commonest clinical problems encountered in budgerigars. The causes are categorized as either viral, bacterial, chlamydial, toxic, metabolic, or neoplastic.

Pacheco's parrot disease, caused by a herpesvirus, can be induced in budgerigars by IM inoculation of the virus, but it has not been reported in the literature as a naturally occurring disease. A parrot adenovirus and a chicken strain of adenovirus[11] have both produced hepatitis in budgerigars inoculated IM. Lymphoid leukosis, which is known to be caused by a virus in chickens, has been seen in budgerigars, but it has not yet been proven to be viral in origin.

Toxic material from the intestines passes into the liver and can cause liver damage. Because the liver functions as a filter for the intestine, it is subjected to toxic assault. The percentage of liver disease in budgerigars due to toxins is unknown. Contaminated seeds are conjectured to be a source of toxins. Mycotoxins are known to have produced liver disease in budgerigars, causing the liver to have a *hobnailed* appearance. The possibility of fungicides contaminating seed supplies should not be overlooked.

Lipidosis almost always affects the liver. Cholesterol occurs in the liver, as well as in other organs, in abnormal amounts and histiocytes attempt to remove it. The liver is often moderately enlarged and pale.

Fatty degeneration of the liver occurs commonly in obese birds and produces an enlarged yellow or yellow brown liver. Diet and abnormal metabolism of fat may both be involved in its occurrence.

Adenocarcinomas of the bile ducts and liver cells have been seen in budgerigars, including one only four months old. It is not uncommon for fibrosarcomas and malignant kidney tumors to metastasize to the liver.

Depending on the acuteness or chronicity, the liver may be larger or smaller than normal in almost any of the aforementioned diseases.

Historical information regarding diet may yield some clues as to the source of the problem. Hypocalcemia is implicated in egg binding. Many budgerigars are fed an all-seed diet with no vitamin or mineral supplementation. Seed mixtures are low in calcium and vitamin D_3, resulting in low blood calcium levels. There are also hypotheses that certain types of liver disease may be diet related. Information concerning past egg binding, recent clutches, and soft-shelled eggs may also be useful when considering egg binding and egg peritonitis problems.

Past episodes of illness with fluffing, anorexia, lethargy, and abnormal dark brown droppings, followed by spontaneous recovery are often reported in budgerigars with liver disease. Many of these birds develop epistaxis or hemorrhagic droppings. Overgrown beaks and toenails with brown streaking usually indicate liver problems.

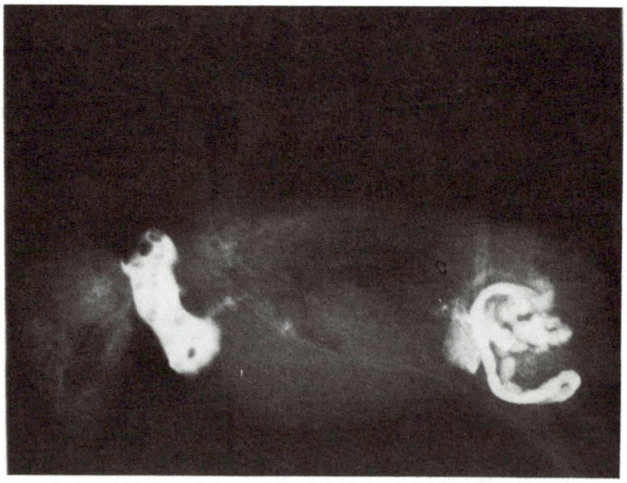

Figure 1—Lateral abdominal radiograph showing ventral and caudal displacement of barium-filled intestinal loops by enlarged oviduct *(arrow)*.

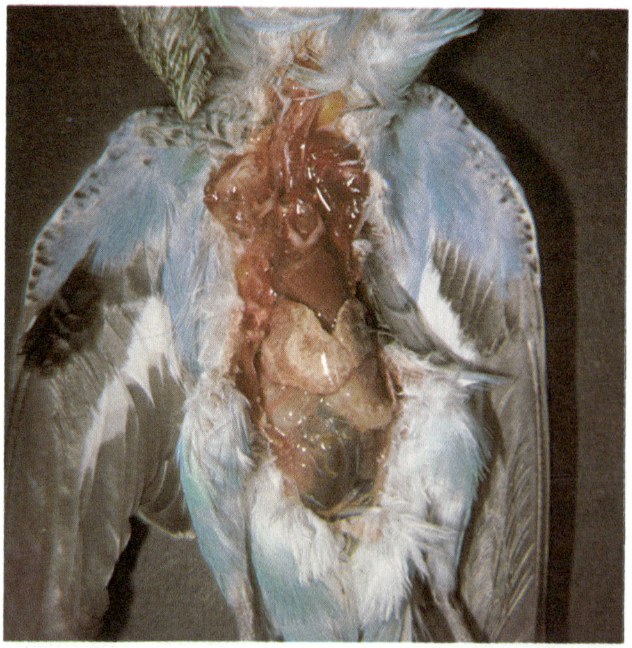

Figure 2—Gross autopsy specimen with enlarged, pale liver from lipidosis.

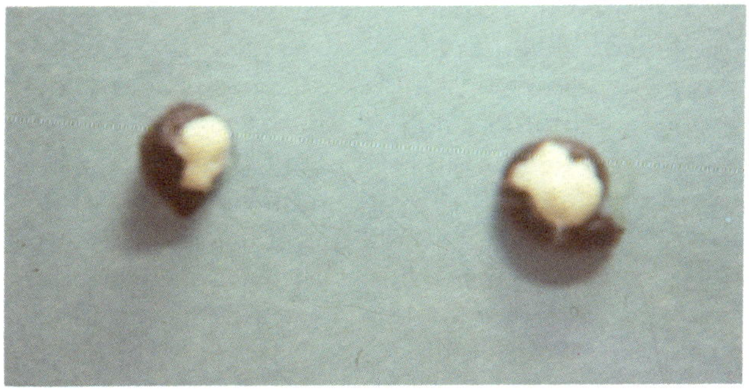

Figure 3A

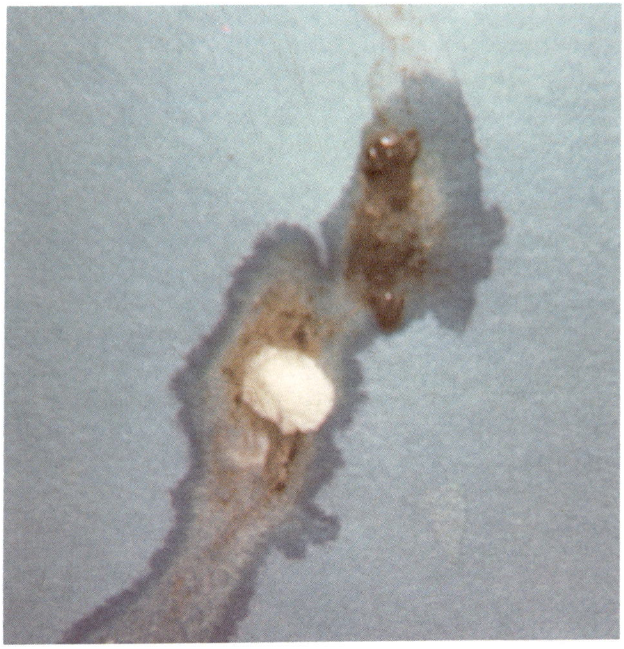

Figure 3B

Figure 3 (A and B)—Normal droppings (A) and loose gray droppings from budgerigar with lipidosis (B).

Birds with voracious appetites and weight loss usually have neoplasia or liver disease.

Physical Examination and Clinical Signs

Observation of the bird in the cage prior to handling may reveal subtle abnormalities that are not obvious when restraining the animal. *Tail bobbing,* often associated with respiratory problems, is common in abdominal disorders. Since birds lack a true diaphragm, masses often result in organ displacement, causing pressure on the lungs, air sacs, or heart. Abdominal fluid can also accumulate around the heart and lungs and cause respiratory distress. Changes in posture such as a *penguinlike* stance are often the result of egg binding. Unilateral paresis or paralysis is associated with renal tumors involving the sciatic nerve.

Regurgitation movements may be observed, or there may be regurgitated material on the cage floor. Regurgitation occasionally occurs in birds with liver disease and kidney neoplasia.

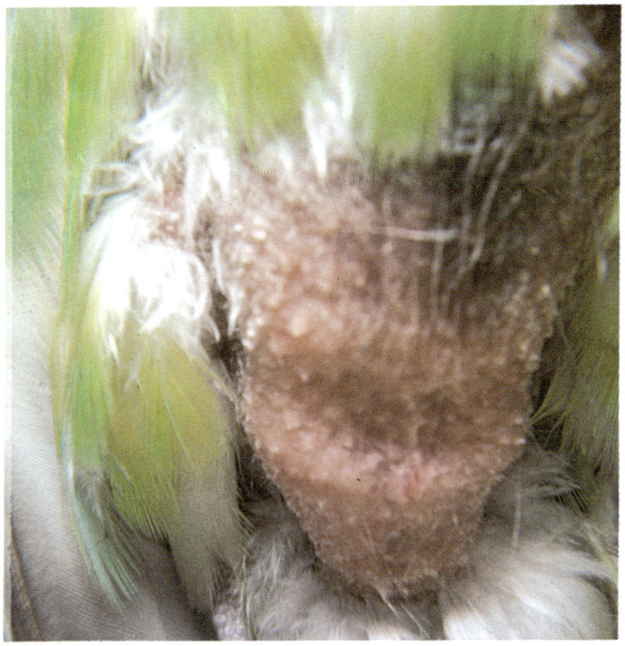

Figure 4A

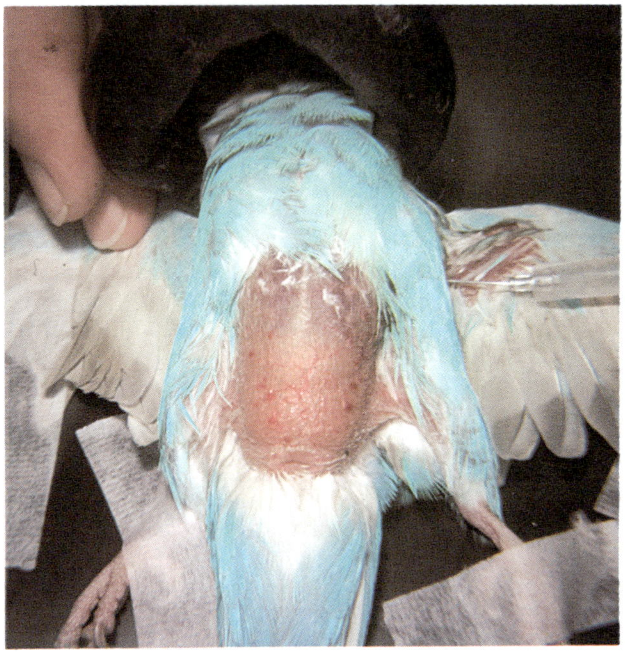

Figure 4B

Figure 4 (A and B)—Normal abdominal space measuring about 5 mm (A). Enlarged abdomen in budgerigar with abdominal mass (B).

The droppings should be evaluated for change in size, color, and consistency (Figure 3). Laying hens will normally develop large, bulky, slightly loose droppings. Dilute, voluminous urate may be seen with renal tumors, and occasionally a hemorrhagic urate portion occurs. There may be a dark brown fecal portion due to upper gastrointestinal hemorrhage or a lime green dropping with yellow urate in liver disease. Bright red blood around the droppings or streaked within the droppings

TABLE II

SUMMARY OF CLINICAL SIGNS

1. Abdominal enlargement—firm or fluctuating abdomen
2. *Tail bobbing*
3. Change in droppings—size, color, consistency
4. Postural change
5. Tenesmus
6. Unilateral paresis or paralysis
7. Regurgitation
8. Weight change

may occur with egg binding. Tenesmus and difficulty passing droppings may be the result of a lesion in the abdominal cavity. Extremely obese birds may have difficulty passing droppings or may have pasting around the vent due to accumulation of large amounts of subcutaneous adipose tissue around the cloaca.

A complete physical examination[a] should be performed unless the bird cannot tolerate the stress incurred because of its weakened condition.[b] The sternum and pectoral muscles should be palpated to determine weight loss. The normal abdominal space between the terminal portion of the sternum and pubic bones is about 5 mm (Figure 4). An increase in this distance or a lack of compressibility indicates the possibility of an abdominal problem. The consistency of the abdominal enlargement should be considered. A firm, hard swelling is usually due to organ enlargement, a displaced gizzard, a tumor, or an egg, whereas soft, fluctuant swelling is often the result of fluid, a cyst, or a hernia. If physical findings confirm an abdominal problem, additional diagnostic tests should be performed to more specifically localize the lesion.

[a]Since the scope of this paper is abdominal disease, emphasis is placed on this region and description of abnormal physical findings referable to abdominal problems. Discussion of a complete physical examination can be found elsewhere.[3]

[b]If the bird cannot tolerate a physical examination, supportive treatment such as fluids and oxygen should be started prior to examination.

Diagnosis

When an abdominal disorder is suspected, radiography often provides additional diagnostic information. Proper positioning and technique are essential for diagnostic radiographs.[4,12] Radiographic signs suggestive of abdominal disease include gizzard displacement, loss of abdominal air sac space, homogeneous abdominal density, and a mass. The grit-filled gizzard normally lies between the acetabula and to the left of the midline in the ventrodorsal radiograph. Hepatomegaly tends to cause caudal and dorsal gizzard displacement. Renal masses cause ventral displacement of the gizzard and, depending on in which pole the mass is located, they can cause cranial or caudal displacement as well. Kidney tumors are the abdominal neoplasm most commonly seen in The Windhover Bird Clinic. Because of the location of the kidneys, the tumors are not amenable to surgical removal. Oviduct enlargement usually causes ventral and caudal dislocation of the gizzard. Masses and/or fluid can cause loss of normal symmetry to the abdominal air sacs. Because the abdominal cavity is surrounded by the vertebrae, sternum, and pubic bones, there is little room for expansion, so abdominal organs tend to be compressed when a space-occupying lesion is present. This results in loss of distinction between organs and impingement on normal air sac space, making the abdomen appear to be a homogeneous density (Figure 5). In small birds it is difficult to distinguish between fluid and a mass. In larger birds this distinction is easier.

Egg peritonitis can cause loss of contrast and a functional ileus with stagnant, gas-filled loops. Normally calcified eggs are easily visualized, but soft-shelled eggs can be difficult to diagnose. Abnormal attempts at egg production can be seen and increased bone density suggestive of polyostotic hyperostosis[5] can be recognized (Figure 6).

A barium study helps demonstrate displacement of the intestinal tract and draping of the intestines over a mass when the exact location cannot be determined from survey radiography (Figure 1). Other contrast

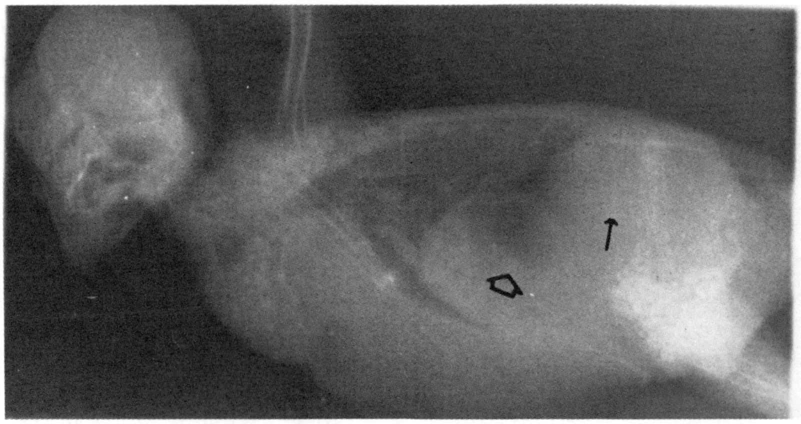

Figure 5—Lateral abdominal radiograph showing homogeneous abdominal density and displacement of gizzard ventral and caudal by renal cyst *(closed arrow)*. Air is present in the proventriculus *(open arrow)* from partial obstruction.

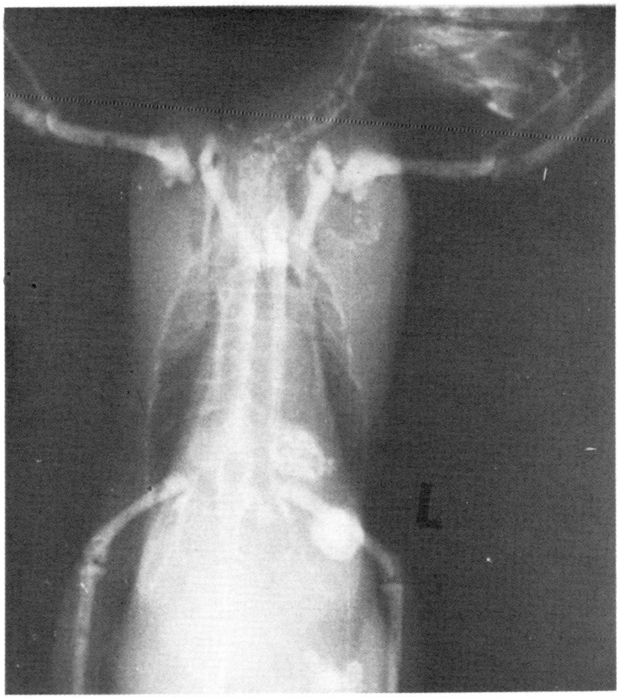

Figure 6—Polyostotic hyperostosis, abnormal calcific densities in oviduct, abdominal fluid, and cranial gizzard displacement are present in the ventrodorsal radiograph.

examinations have not proved useful in the budgerigar, and additional clinical research must be performed to determine their value.

If fluid is present, abdominocentesis and fluid analysis should be performed. The abdominal skin, from the sternum to vent, is prepared aseptically, and a 25-gauge needle is gently inserted into the abdominal cavity about 2 mm cranial to the vent and off the midline. Obvious subcutaneous blood vessels are avoided. As much fluid as possible is aspirated since this will alleviate any dyspnea associated with the fluid accumulation. The type of fluid most commonly aspirated is a clear yellow hypocellular, modified transudate that is often associated with cystic oviduct enlargement and possibly hyperestrogenism.

Yellow floccular fluid or dark brown fluid has been seen in cases of egg peritonitis. A hemorrhagic fluid is associated with bleeding secondary to liver rupture from liver disease. A clear, watery transudate is suggestive of cirrhosis or heart failure. These fluid descriptions are just guidelines, though; all fluids must be submitted for analysis and culture and correlated with clinical and radiographic findings.

Much research is currently being conducted on serum microchemistries and their clinical significance in cage birds. It appears that LDH, SGOT, GGTP, and SGPT are present in high levels in the liver of larger psittacines and they become elevated in liver disease.[6] In the authors' experience, budgerigars have shown significant elevation in SGPT correlated with serious liver disease on autopsy; however, other authors believe that SGOT and GGTP are more reliable indicators of liver problems. Uric acid levels rise in renal disease, and values greater than 15 mg/dl are considered significant.[7] The significance of hematocrits and serum total protein levels has been reported by Lafeber.[8] Changes in blood glucose levels may be useful in monitoring response to treatment. Many ill birds quickly become hypoglycemic. Chronic illness, liver problems, and starvation can result in hypoglycemia. Hyperglycemia can occur with stress, diabetes mellitus, and renal disease. Normal blood glucose values range from 210 to 520 mg/dl with a mean of 390 mg/dl.[9]

Treatment[c]

Once the cause of abdominal enlargement is determined, appropriate treatment can be recommended. In some instances exploratory surgery may be necessary to confirm what is suspected from the clinical workup or to remove a neoplasm. However, since budgerigars do not tolerate extensive surgery well and abdominal exposure is difficult, exploratory procedures are only considered after more conservative methods have been exhausted. If surgery is to be done, care must be taken to prepare the bird for the procedure to increase the chances of success. Supportive fluid therapy should be started 24 hours prior to surgery. A dose of 0.25 to 0.30 ml 2.5% dextrose and 0.45% sodium chloride/30 g body weight IM every 8 to 12 hours is helpful. If there is liver disease, 0.01 ml vitamin K can be injected IM 24 hours prior to surgery and on the day of surgery—this seems to aid in hemostasis. Food is not withheld before surgery. Halothane anesthesia is used,[10] and heat must be supplied to maintain body temperature. After induction, a 25-gauge needle is inserted into the brachial vein so that fluids and/or blood can be administered as needed during the surgery (Figure 7). If extensive blood loss is anticipated either because of underlying liver problems or because of the extent of the procedure, fresh blood for transfusion is taken from a donor colony. An ophthalmic cautery[d] is useful for maintaining hemostatis during the procedure. The bird is placed in an incubator for recovery, and fluids and oxygen are administered as necessary.

Egg and Oviduct

Egg-bound birds can usually be treated fairly easily by manually removing the egg. This can often be done in the exam room. One squeezes gently just cranial to the egg with the thumb and first finger, gradually working the egg out of the cloaca. If the egg cannot be easily extruded, placing the bird in an incubator to provide heat, administering 10% calcium gluconate orally, and injecting warm mineral oil or another lubricant around the egg with a lacrimal cannula may help in removing it or may allow the bird to pass the egg naturally. Since hypocalcemia is linked to egg binding, 10% calcium

---

[c]Dosages are based on empirical use until blood and tissue levels of drugs used in pet birds are determined.
[d]Comcept ACCU-TEMP Cautery®, Concept Inc., Clearwater, FL 33516.

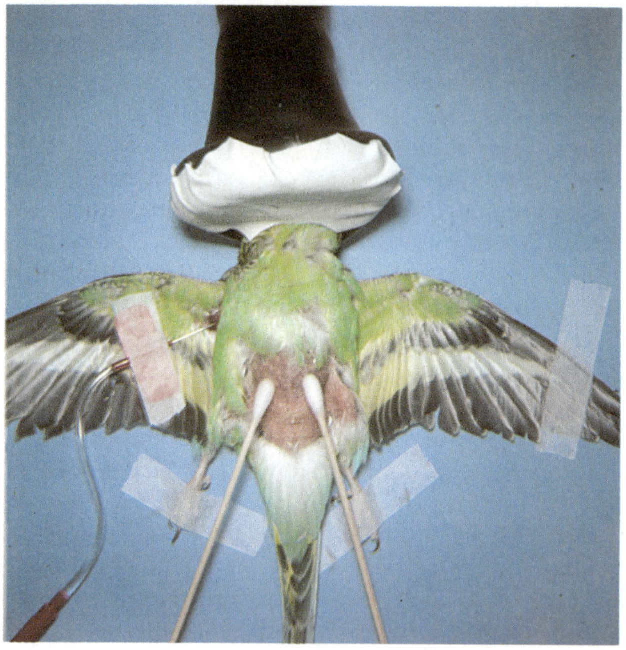

Figure 7—Administration of blood and fluid during surgery improves the chances for success.

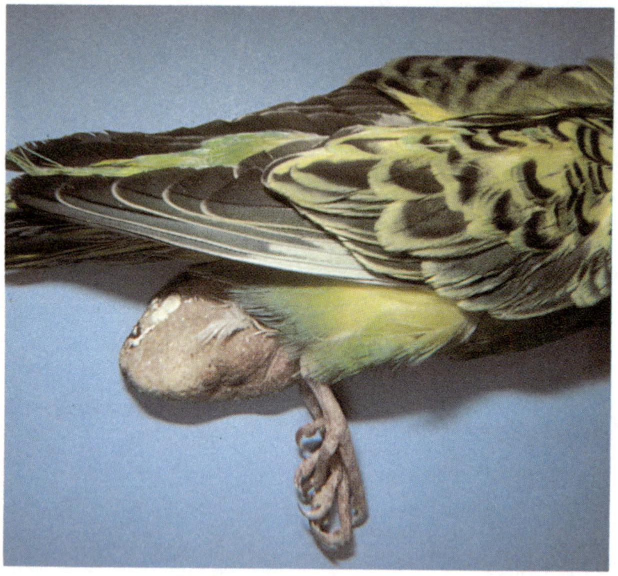

Figure 8—Abdominal hernia associated with hyperestrogenism.

gluconate is given orally at a rate of 2 drops/30 minutes for up to one to two hours or until the egg is passed. The bird's condition is carefully monitored and if it worsens, more invasive procedures should be instituted. In some instances anesthesia may be necessary to facilitate the procedure, especially if the egg is unusually large. In rare instances, surgical opening of the oviduct may be indicated. If the bird is in shock because of the egg binding, its condition should be stabilized by administering fluids and keeping the bird warm prior to any manipulation.

If the egg is broken during the procedure, the abdomen is gently massaged cranially to caudally so that the egg shell and contents can be extruded through the cloaca. If the egg shell does not pass, 48 hours are allowed for the broken shell to pass naturally before considering surgical removal. If much manipulation is necessary and the procedure is prolonged, antibiotics and fluids are indicated.

Egg peritonitis, often a chronic debilitating illness, carries a guarded prognosis. The diagnosis can be elusive and, perhaps because many cases are advanced by the time a definitive diagnosis is reached, the treatment is rarely successful. The selection of antibiotic should be based on culture results of abdominal fluid (if obtainable) and on any bacterial growth. In some instances there is only minimal fluid or a thick, tenacious exudate which defies aspiration and coats the abdominal organs. Systemic antibiotics, intraperitoneal infusion with antibiotics in small volume so as not to drown the bird, supportive fluid therapy, and gavage feeding are recommended. Despite intensive therapy, though, results are frequently unrewarding. If the bird recovers, hormone therapy (methyltestosterone 5 mg/oz drinking water daily for 7 to 10 days) is recommended to suppress ovarian activity.

Oviduct enlargement with a secondary abdominal hernia and fluid in the abdominal cavity and oviduct can be reduced with diuretics and methyltestosterone. Methyltestosterone 5 mg is given in 1 oz drinking water daily for 7 to 10 days and is gradually decreased to administration once or twice a week to control fluid and hernia size. The dosage is titrated to the individual bird's need, so recommendations may vary in different circumstances. Mibolerone[c] has not been as useful as methyltestosterone in the authors' experience. Furosemide syrup, one drop orally every other day, may aid in controlling fluid accumulation if methyltestosterone alone is not successful.

Hernias are difficult to surgically repair because of birds' scanty abdominal muscles. Birds that chronically bind eggs or that are excessive egg layers can also be controlled with methyltestosterone.

Liver Disease

Psittacosis was the great scourge of budgerigar breeders until chlortetracycline was discovered. Feeding of medicated seed has helped control this disease, but it is wise to bear in mind that budgerigars are susceptible. Psittacosis is a systemic disease, and the liver is seriously involved. Diagnosis is made by elementary bodies seen by electron microscopy in the liver, spleen, or air sacs or by injection of infective material into mice.

Since there are many causes of liver disease, a biopsy is necessary to make a sure diagnosis as a basis for proper therapy. Although the authors have sometimes done biopsies through laparotomies or surgery, as discussed previously, these are critical procedures in smaller birds. Therapy also depends on the clinical severity of

[c]Cheque®, The Upjohn Co., Kalamazoo, MI 49001.

the problem. Antibiotics, fluid therapy, and glucose are frequently given for liver problems. If there is hemorrhaging, injectable vitamin K is given IM. For neurologic manifestations, neomycin given at a rate of 1 drop twice a day has been clinically helpful. Glucocorticoids have also been administered (in critically ill birds that are not responding to other therapy), but this is a questionable procedure when the exact type of liver disease is not known, since steroids exacerbate some liver problems. Dietary changes, lipotrophic agents, and glucose can be given to aid management in chronic cases.

Conclusion

Abdominal enlargement in the budgerigar can be the result of many disease processes. Neoplasia and liver problems are common and are responsible for the majority of abdominal problems. Egg binding and cystic oviducts are easily diagnosed and are usually amenable to conservative medical management. Only through physical examination, radiography, and laboratory testing can a diagnosis be reached and appropriate therapy instituted. A rational approach to avian patients will result in better, more successful treatment.

REFERENCES

1. Petrak ML, Gilmore CE: Neoplasms, in Metrak ML (ed): *Diseases of Cage and Aviary Birds.* Philadelphia, Lea & Febiger, 1969, pp 459-489.
2. Leav I, et al: A naturally occurring lipidosis in shell parakeets, *Melopsittacus undulatus. Lab Invest* 18(4):433-437, 1968.
3. Soifer FK: Physical examination and medication of cage birds. *Vet Clin North Am* 3(2):143-158, 1973.
4. Silverman S: Avian radiographic technique and interpretation, in Kirk RW (ed): *Current Veterinary Therapy VI.* Philadelphia, WB Saunders Co, 1977, pp 671-674.
5. Schlumberger HG: Polyostotic hyperostosis in the female parakeet. *Am J Pathol* 35(1):1-23, 1959.
6. Galvin C: Laboratory diagnostic aids in pet bird practice. *1980 Scientific Proceedings of the 47th Annual Meeting of American Animal Hospital Association,* pp 41-52.
7. Altman RB: Diseases of the avian urinary system, in Kirk RW (ed): *Current Veterinary Therapy VI.* Philadelphia, WB Saunders Co, 1977, pp 703-705.
8. Lafeber TJ: Respiratory diseases. *Vet Clin North Am* 3(2):199-227, 1973.
9. Altman RB, Kirmayer AH: Diabetes mellitus in the avian species. *JAAHA* 12(4):531-537, 1976.
10. Altman RB: Avian anesthesia. *Compend Contin Educ Pract Vet* II(1):38-43, 1980.
11. Hirsch AS: Report of research in progress: a three part study. *Systemic Pathology Produced in the Budgerigar (Melopsittacus undulatus) following Virus Inoculation.* Dept. of Microbiology, Pathology and Public Health, School of Veterinary Medicine, Purdue University, West Lafayette, IN.
12. Evans SM: Avian radiographic diagnosis. *Compend Contin Educ Pract Vet* 3:660-666, 1981.

Heavy-Metal Intoxication in Caged Birds—Part I

Richard W. Woerpel, MS, DVM
Walter J. Rosskopf, Jr., BS, DVM

Animal Medical Centre of Lawndale
Hawthorne, California

Heavy-metal intoxication, resulting primarily from the ingestion of lead substances, is surprisingly common among caged birds, but it is often misdiagnosed. This article will familiarize the veterinarian with the clinical features of plumbism and prompt the practitioner to maintain a high index of suspicion for this disease.

This article represents a compilation of 10 cases of heavy-metal intoxication in caged birds that have been diagnosed in the authors' clinic and two cases on which the authors were consulted within the last three years (1979–1982). The study includes eight Amazon parrots (*Amazona* spp.), one African grey parrot (*Psittacus erithacus erithacus*), one green-winged macaw (*Ara chloroptera*), and two cockatiels (*Nymphicus hollandicus*). During the time of this study, one case of probable inhalation lead poisoning in a blue-fronted Amazon parrot (*Amazona aestiva aestiva*) and one case of zinc toxicosis in a green-winged macaw were also treated at the authors' clinic. All except four of the patients discussed are alive and well at this time. One of the deceased parrots suffered heavy-metal toxicosis twice.

In Part I of this article, a literature summary and the results of the authors' survey are presented. This is followed by a discussion of these data. In Part II, the discussion continues, focusing on treatment and pathology, and three case reports are presented.

Literature Summary

Accidental lead poisoning has been reported in the following mammals: dogs,[1-4] cats,[5] cattle,[6,7] horses,[1,6,7] sheep,[6,8] swine,[6,7] mink,[7] primates,[9] and humans.[1,2,10] Among avian species, the most well-known lead poisoning syndrome occurs in waterfowl,[1,7,11-18] resulting from their inadvertent ingestion of spent lead shot from the bottoms of ponds and other waterways in heavily hunted areas. It has been estimated that at least 2 to 3% of the U.S. waterfowl population dies each year from this cause.[13] Consequently, a tremendous amount of research has been carried out to better understand this cause of waterfowl mortality.[11-19]

Much less research has been done on lead poisoning in nonwaterfowl avian species. Locke and Bagley reported on plumbism in mourning doves resulting from the ingestion of spent lead shot taken from the ground in areas of concentrated dove hunting.[20] Plumbism resulting from the ingestion of lead shot that was embedded in the tissues of prey (either captured by raptors in the wild,[21-23] or shot and offered for con-

TABLE I

SOURCES OF INGESTED HEAVY METAL (14 CASES)

Leaded windows (stained glass, etc.)	4
Toy containing lead	2
Toy containing zinc/aluminum alloy	1
Costume jewelry	1
Curtain weight	1
Lead pellet from pellet gun	1
Lead fishing weight	1
Unknown	3

sumption to captive raptors[24,25]) has been documented in raptors by a number of authors.

Comparatively little has been written on the subject of heavy-metal intoxication in captive avian species from causes other than ingestion of lead ammunition. A relatively common cause of lead poisoning among poultry is the consumption of lead-based paint or orchard spray material (containing lead arsenate).[7] Janssen et al. presented a concise summary of lead poisoning in birds.[26] Kennedy et al. provided an account of plumbism in captive sandhill cranes resulting from the ingestion of lead-based paint.[27] Zook et al. reported on a similar occurrence in a zoological collection which caused the demise of 11 psittacines over a 2½-year period.[28] Comparatively few papers have been published on the subject of plumbism in caged (pet) birds.[29-33]

Clinical Cases

To simplify presentation of the information, some of the data has been summarized in tables that appear throughout the text. Results of the case studies are reported under specific headings and a discussion of each topic follows in the next section.

Source of Ingested Heavy Metal

Table I is a list of the sources of ingested heavy metal in the 14 cases (in 13 birds, one poisoned twice) studied. Lead-based paint was not implicated in this study. The lead-containing toy noted in two of the cases involving Amazon parrots was a lead-weighted plastic penguin commonly sold in pet stores.

Clinical Signs

In Table II, the relative frequency of the typical presenting signs is given for 13 heavy-metal intoxication cases studied. It should be noted that this table is based on a retrospective examination of the case records and that a minimum of four veterinarians were involved in the acquisition of the histories and recording of the physical examination findings. In some cases, thorough histories were not received or recorded. Furthermore, the thoroughness of the physical examinations of the

TABLE II

RELATIVE FREQUENCY OF SALIENT CLINICAL SIGNS (13 CASES)

Depression/lethargy/weakness	8
Vomiting	5
Polyuria and polydipsia	5
Central nervous system signs (incoordination, head tilt, circling, seizures)	4
Hemoglobinuria	4
Diarrhea	2

patients and interpretation of information received undoubtedly varied between veterinarians.

Radiographic Findings

Of the 13 typical cases of heavy-metal intoxication (one parrot was poisoned twice) included in this study, five had heavy-metal–dense particles located within the ventriculus (gizzard) only at the time of first x-ray; three had similar particles within the ventriculus and intestines; two had heavy-metal–dense particles within the crop and ventriculus; two had similar particles within the ventriculus and cloaca; and one patient had heavy-metal–dense particles within the crop, ventriculus, and cloaca at the time of first x-ray. The dynamics of these particles as they resided in and passed through the gastrointestinal tract of the patients are detailed in Table III.

Clinical Pathology

Hematology and blood chemistry evaluations were conducted on all but one of the cases in this survey. In Table IV, the ranges of values from hemograms of nine Amazon parrots suffering from lead poisoning are listed. This table also provides normal ranges for each test category.

Toxicology

Only one blood lead determination was made. The patient was a yellow-naped Amazon parrot (*Amazona ochrocephala auropalliata*) and its blood lead concentration was reported to be 70 mg/dl. The source of the heavy metal ingested in this case was never determined; therefore, the significance of this value is questionable.

Pathology

Of the four cases of heavy-metal intoxication that did not survive treatment, three were confirmed to be the result of ingestion of lead. In the remaining case, the source and type of heavy metal were never positively determined, although clinical signs and radiography strongly suggested plumbism. A necropsy was performed on this bird, and the histopathological report revealed significant pathology within the spleen only.[34] Severe lymphoid follicular necrosis was noted and attributed to a probable acute viral infection rather than to heavy-

TABLE III

NUMBER OF HEAVY-METAL–DENSE PARTICLES DETECTABLE RADIOGRAPHICALLY

Case	*First X-ray*	*Second X-ray*	*Third X-ray*	*Fourth X-ray*
Amazon 1	15 particles within gizzard	1 particle within gut, 7 days after first x-ray	-	-
Amazon 2	~ 35 particles within gizzard and 5 within gut	1 particle within gut 2 days after first x-ray	-	-
Amazon 3	2 particles within gizzard and 2 within gut	No particles seen 5 days after first x-ray	-	-
Amazon 4	> 50 particles within gizzard	~ 20 particles within gizzard and gut 9 days after first x-ray	3 particles within gut 12 days after first x-ray	No particles seen 14 days after first x-ray
Amazon 5	~ 50 particles within gizzard	~ 20 particles within gizzard 3 days after first x-ray	-	-
Amazon 6	2 large particles within gizzard	Both particles present; no appreciable change in size of either 5 days after first x-ray	Both particles present; each ~ $^1/_3$ original size 16 days after first x-ray	-
Green-winged macaw	1 177-caliber air gun pellet within gizzard	Pellet still present; ~ ½ original size 5 days after first x-ray	-	-
Cockatiel 1	Multiple particles within crop and gizzard	4 particles within gizzard 8 days after first x-ray	-	-
Cockatiel 2	4 particles within gizzard, 1 within proventriculus, and 1 within esophagus	No particles seen 7 days after first x-ray	-	-

metal intoxication. Sections of lung, liver, kidney, and intestine were found to be normal.

The only other necropsy performed, on a case of confirmed plumbism (ingestion of lead costume jewelry), revealed significant renal and hepatic pathology.[35] The kidney revealed granular hemoglobin casts within many convoluted tubules (Figure 1). Many tubular epithelial cells contained pyknotic nuclei and were sloughing into the tubular lumina. Other tubular cells exhibited vacuolar degeneration. Acid-fast stains failed to reveal inclusions within the tubular epithelial cells. The liver exhibited multiple large foci of hepatocellular dissociation and pyknosis, with dropout and necrosis of individual hepatocytes (Figure 2). The brain revealed numerous pale neurons, suggesting degenerative changes. The submitted bone marrow and ventriculus were normal.

TABLE IV

RANGE OF CLINICAL PATHOLOGY VALUES FOR NINE AMAZON PARROTS SUFFERING FROM PLUMBISM

*Test**	*Range of Values*	*Normal Values*[33,40]
WBCs (× 10^3/mm^3)	10.9–30.0	6–11
PCV (%)	31–58	45–55
Total protein (g/dl)	3.0–8.7	3.0–5.0
Glucose (mg/dl)	156–298	220–350
SAST (IU/L)	151–824	130–350
Creatinine (mg/dl)	<0.2–0.8	0.1–0.4
Uric acid (mg/dl)	2.7–18.9	2.0–10.0
Polychromasia	slight to marked	slight
Hemolysis	+ or –	–
Basophilic stippling	–	–

*WBCs = white blood cells; PCV = packed-cell volume; SAST = serum aspartate aminotransferase (formerly SGOT).

Discussion

Source of Ingested Heavy Metal

Of the 13 cases of heavy-metal toxicosis studied, six were presented with the clients' knowledge of the birds' having ingested lead prior to the onset of signs. In these cases, the source of the lead could be confirmed.

Table I indicates that all the known sources of ingested heavy metal (either determined prior to presentation of the patient or subsequently) are commonly found in homes. A pet bird would have access to many of these sources if allowed unsupervised freedom outside its cage or off its perch. The avian practitioner would be well advised when taking a medical history to bear in mind that allowing caged birds such freedom is common among bird owners. Caged birds have a need to chew and an unhealthy affinity toward objects made of lead as well as curiosity about this very soft metal, and frequently lead poisoning is the result. Clients must be warned of this potential problem.

Ingestion of lead paint or lead-impregnated plaster used on cages or on walls of enclosures was not impli-

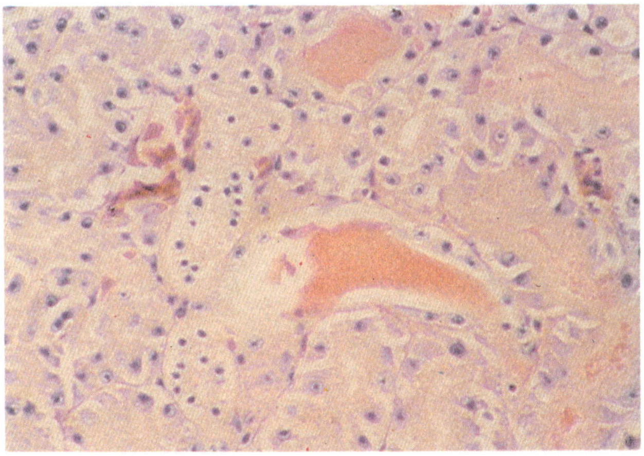

Figure 1—Histopathological appearance of kidney exhibiting granular hemoglobin casts within convoluted tubules and tubular nephrosis. No acid-fast intranuclear inclusion bodies were found within tubular epithelial cells.

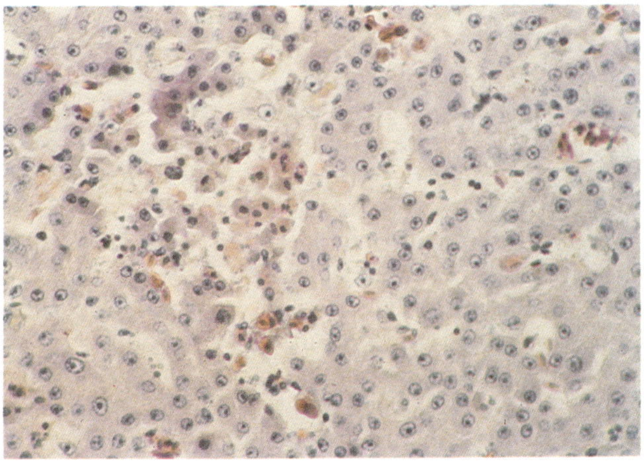

Figure 2—Histopathological appearance of liver exhibiting foci of hepatocellular dissociation and necrosis.

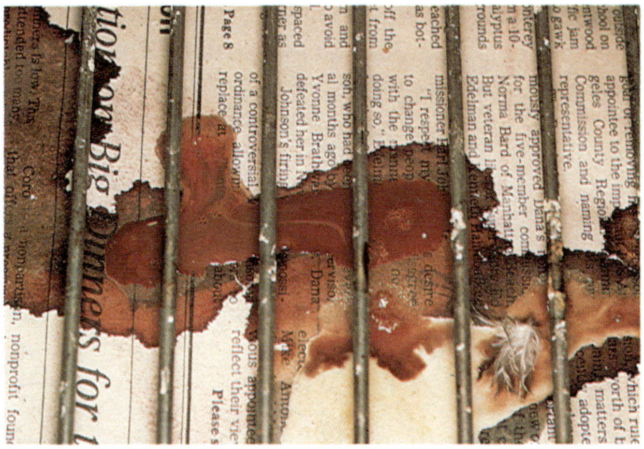

Figure 3—Hemoglobinuria in an Amazon parrot with plumbism.

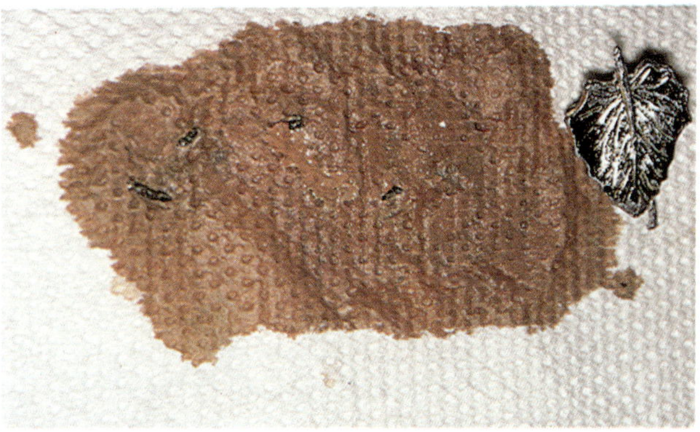

Figure 4—Hemoglobinuria often has a chocolate-milk color. Note the four small bits of relatively normal-appearing feces in the midst of the abnormal urine.

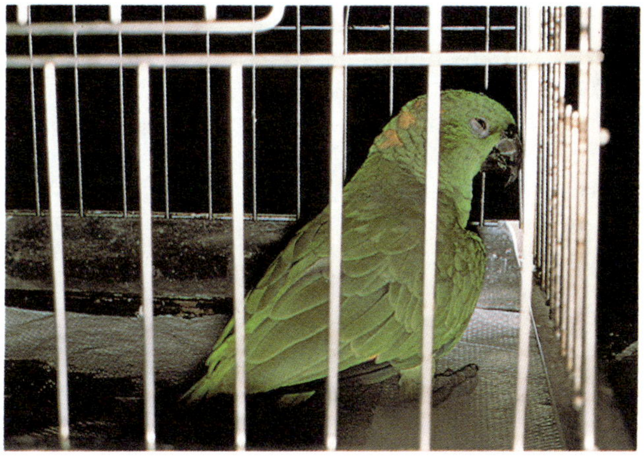

Figure 5—Yellow-naped Amazon parrot suffering from plumbism. Photo was taken within three hours of its death. Note the bird's location on cage bottom, the closed eyes, the depression, and droopy wings.

cated in this study, although it has been reported to be a common source of plumbism among captive birds.[27-29,36] The toy penguins implicated in the authors' study are intended for cockatiel-sized or smaller caged birds but often end up as toys for parrots. Buyers must be warned that such toys are potentially hazardous to birds larger than cockatiels, because the labels offer no warning or precautions. It is also important to note that psittacines have been known to chew on and swallow the lead clapper from bells that were suspended in their cages, and this also has resulted in clinical plumbism.[37]

Clinical Signs

The clinical signs result from the absorption of heavy-metal ions from the gastrointestinal tract and their subsequent effects on all tissues. No consistent correlation could be found between the severity of clinical signs and the number of heavy-metal–dense particles subsequently discovered within the gut. Even in cases in which the client knew of heavy-metal ingestion prior to presentation, it was not possible to accurately ascertain the amount of time elapsed between ingestion of the heavy metal and the onset of clinical signs. In only one case (that of a green-winged macaw ingesting a single lead pellet from a pellet gun[32]) was the illness chronic. That the onset of signs in this case was relatively gradual (one week) may be because only a single lead particle was ingested; usually in cases of plumbism, many small flakes or pieces of lead are ingested. The relative surface area for loss of lead ions into the gut would be proportionately smaller in this single-particle case than that provided in the commoner situation and would result in slower absorption of the metal into systemic circulation.

No single sign or group of signs was consistently noted in this survey. The clinical signs are those suggesting gastrointestinal, renal, and/or neurologic dysfunction. Polyuria and polydipsia and vomiting were more often recorded than the central nervous system signs (incoordination, head tilt, circling, and seizures were the most frequently noted). Diarrhea was an inconsistent clinical sign. This might be due in part to the confusion that often exists in the interpretation of polyuria versus true diarrhea. The hemoglobinuria, which is perhaps the most dramatic of the presenting signs (Figures 3 and 4), was only noted in Amazon parrots. It was usually associated with hemolysis which resulted in red or pink plasma. Most patients exhibited depression, lethargy, or weakness at the time of presentation (Figure 5).

The presence of any one of these clinical signs and the order in which it was exhibited in relation to others is related no doubt to a number of factors: the type and amount of heavy metal ingested; the size of the particle(s) ingested; the length of time the heavy metal was within the gut; the coexistence of grit within the ventriculus, which would hasten the mechanical breakdown of the metal; and the preexisting health status of the animal.

Giddings reported rapid onset of anorexia, depression, incoordination (inability to perch), loose droppings ("contained small amount of blood") in a mature double yellow-headed Amazon parrot (*A. ochrocephala oratrix*) suffering from plumbism.[30] Zook et al., in a retrospective study, reported on the clinical signs of 11 psittacines that perished from lead poisoning in a large zoological park collection over a 2½-year period.[28] Six of these parrots were found dead in their cages; two exhibited seizure activity; two were unable to fly and exhibited ataxia; and one exhibited only lethargy prior to death. Janssen et al., in a concise summary of lead poisoning in captive birds, indicated that the signs were often inconclusive, including nonspecific gastrointestinal and neurological signs (seizures, incoordination, alimentary stasis, and behavioral changes).[26] They also reported other commonly noted signs: anorexia, green diarrhea, weakness, and wing droop. The latter clinical sign was noted in one sandhill crane (*Grus canadensis*) suffering from lead poisoning secondary to the ingestion of lead-based paint.[27] The wings of this bird drooped from the carpal joint because of extensor muscle paralysis. This has also been noted in poultry[7] and waterfowl[12] and is considered analogous to wrist drop in humans suffering from plumbism. Droopy wings (Figure 5) were noted in a number of patients in this study, but this sign was attributed to the stressed and debilitated condition of the patients. This posture is typical of seriously ill birds, especially just prior to death.

Watery green or lime-green feces have been reported in birds of prey,[22,23] waterfowl,[12,15,18] and poultry[7] suffering from lead poisoning. Often, green, bile staining of the vent feathers is mentioned, especially in waterfowl prior to death or at necropsy. Diarrhea was not a consistent clinical sign in the authors' study. One cockatiel exhibited chartreuse vent feathers but the diarrhea produced by this bird was light brown.

Regurgitation was mentioned only once in the literature as a specific clinical sign of plumbism in caged birds.[29] Redig et al. noted vomiting in a female prairie falcon (*Falco mexicanus*) fed shotgun-killed ducks and pheasants.[22] In the authors' survey, this clinical sign was frequently but not consistently noted.

Polydipsia was another frequently but not consistently noted clinical sign of plumbism in the authors' study. Their literature search found polydipsia associated with plumbism mentioned only in regard to poultry.[7] It is possible, however, that the watery or loose droppings so often reported as diarrhea were really a reflection of polyuria, which would most likely be accompanied by an obligatory polydipsia.

Neurologic signs were noted in many of the avian species in which plumbism has been reported. Ataxia, amaurosis, and epileptiform seizures were noted in the aforementioned female prairie falcon.[21] Petrak included the same three signs in her report of lead poisoning in caged birds.[29] Jacobson et al. noted incoordination and a head tilt in an immature bald eagle (*Haliaeetus leucocephalus*) suffering from lead poisoning which resulted from the bird's ingestion of hunter-wounded prey.[23] Decker et al. reported ataxia and apparent incoordination in an adult male king vulture (*Sarcohampus papa*) that died of plumbism.[25] It is possible that the incoordination noted in these accounts was at least in part a manifestation of weakness in the patient. Nevertheless, the authors' study and that of Zook et al.[28] clearly indicate that neurologic signs (especially central nervous system signs) are common among psittacines suffering from lead poisoning.

Nowhere in the literature was hemoglobinuria mentioned as a clinical sign of lead poisoning. It was noted in only 4 of the authors' 13 cases; all of these involved Amazon parrots, and in most cases the hemoglobinuria was associated with hemolysis. Blackwell reported hemoglobinuria in a ewe suffering from chronic lead toxicosis but indicated that it is not a commonly observed sign in this disease of sheep.[8]

In summary, the avian practitioner should include lead poisoning in the differential diagnosis when the clinical signs of the patient include one or more of the following: vomiting, diarrhea, polyuria and polydipsia, hemoglobinuria, central nervous system signs, generalized depression, and weakness.

Radiographic Findings

Of the 13 typical clinical cases of heavy-metal intoxication, only six of the patients were presented with the owner's knowing that the bird had ingested heavy metal. In each of these cases, the existence of heavy-metal particles within the gastrointestinal tract of the patient was subsequently confirmed radiographically. Of the other cases, the presence of heavy metal within the gut was confirmed radiographically because the history suggested the possibility of plumbism (in three cases); other diagnostic tests performed previously had not elucidated the cause of the signs and x-rays were therefore undertaken (in two cases); radiography was included as part of the routine data base on the patient upon presentation (in one case); or heavy-metal intoxication was suspected after the patient's death (in one case).

In every case, radiography was done, and this revealed a variable number of heavy-metal–dense particles within the gut. It should be emphasized that the presence of such particles confirmed on x-ray does not confirm the diagnosis of lead poisoning; it only suggests the possibility of heavy-metal intoxication. A thorough history, a determination of the concentration of lead in the blood of the patient, and the retrieval and analysis of the radiopaque material are methods that can be used to confirm the diagnosis of plumbism (or other heavy-metal poisoning).

In Table III the dynamics of these particles in and as they pass through the gastrointestinal tract of the patient are detailed. In each case, subsequent radiographs revealed a definite decrease in the number or the size of the heavy-metal–dense particles within the gut, regardless of the amount of time that had elapsed between the radiographs. No correlation could be made between these dynamic changes and the existence of grit within the ventriculus. However, the presence of grit within the ventriculus along with the heavy metal would hasten the latter's mechanical degradation and subsequent passage out of the patient. Subsequent radiographs in some of the cases revealed heavy-metal–dense particles within the intestines when prior radiographs had indicated that the particles were within the ventriculus. This suggests that the particles are passed out of the patient prior to their complete degradation and dissolution by the action of the gizzard and intestinal fluids. In none of the cases could heavy-metal fragments be found within the droppings.

The cases involving the ingestion of a few relatively large, discrete heavy-metal particles (Amazon parrot 6) and the ingestion of a single lead pellet (green-winged macaw) reveal several interesting points. These larger particles do not tend to move out of the ventriculus, as do the smaller fragments, but they do undergo a visible reduction in size (no doubt resulting from mechanical degradation and absorption) with time. This information strongly suggests that surgical intervention (ventriculotomy)[23] may be more expedient in the management of certain heavy-metal toxicosis cases than a medical approach (to be discussed in Part II of this article).

Clinical Pathology

The important features in Table IV are the leukocytosis, hemolysis, regenerative anemia, absence of basophilic stippling of erythrocytes, evidence of renal compromise (elevations of both creatinine and uric acid), and serum aspartate aminotransferase (SAST, or SGOT) elevation, suggesting hepatic toxicity. The leukocytosis and the regenerative anemia were the most consistent hematologic findings.

No basophilic stippling of erythrocytes was noted by the laboratory, even in cases where lead ingestion by the patient was known when the blood sample was submitted and examination of the blood films for this morphologic peculiarity was requested. Basophilic stippling has been noted in the blood smears of puppies and cats suffering from plumbism.[2,3,5,38] Zook et al. found this to be a nearly consistent finding in their study of plumbism in 60 puppies.[2] They concluded that the appearance of large numbers of immature (especially nucleated) RBCs and basophilic stippling of erythrocytes with a normal or slightly lowered hematocrit is nearly pathognomonic of lead poisoning in the dog. In contrast, Knecht et al., in their more recent investigation of the same subject, did not find basophilic stippling of erythrocytes and circulating nucleated RBCs to be common.[3] Janssen et al. reported that a lowered hematocrit and basophilic stippling of RBCs are indicative of lead intoxication in birds.[26] However, the authors could find only one reference to this morphologic peculiarity, and it was regarding wild ducks afflicted with lead poisoning.[11] Therefore it seems that the practitioner should not depend on this finding to aid in the diagnosis of plumbism in caged birds.

Anticoagulants such as EDTA and potassium oxalate lessen the appearance of basophilic stippling in canine erythrocytes.[4,38] All blood smears taken from the avian patients in this study were made from blood as it flowed directly from a clipped toenail.[39]

The blood of at least two of the patients in this study exhibited hemolysis. More consistent findings included a mild to moderate decrease in the hematocrit and marked polychromasia. No abnormally shaped RBCs were noted, as has been reported elsewhere.[12]

The observed elevations in the SAST and the creatinine and uric acid values (although not consistent) probably reflect toxic damage to the liver and kidneys, respectively, of the affected caged birds. These elevated values are not diagnostic of plumbism by themselves but are contributory when the history, physical examination, radiographic evidence, and the other hematologic parameters of the patient are evaluated.

Toxicology

Determination of blood lead concentration and the toxicologic analysis of tissues for lead in a caged bird at necropsy are usually economically prohibitive in clinical practice. The former determination was once more difficult because of the relatively large volume of blood needed for the assay. However, this constraint is much less of a problem now because there are laboratories (human or otherwise) that can run this assay using as little as 20 μl of plasma.

Janssen et al. indicated that lead poisoning was most reliably diagnosed by determination of blood lead concentration and noted that values ranging from 146 mg/dl to 378 mg/dl have been reported.[26,27] Zook et al. reported a whole-blood lead concentration of 40 mg/dl in an ataxic kea parrot (*Nestor notabilis*) that was suspected to have ingested lead-based paint.[28] No other hematologic abnormalities in this patient were noted.

It is the authors' opinion that if heavy-metal densities are discovered on radiographs of a patient exhibiting signs consistent with heavy-metal toxicosis and the history provided does not reveal the source or identity of the metal, the initiation of chelation therapy should have precedence over the collection of blood for blood lead concentration determination. This clinical approach is justified in situations where economics dictates a conservative workup. The treatment program will not harm the patient and will usually render it asymptomatic by the time the toxicology results are reported.

If blood is to be collected for this toxicologic test, hematology, and blood chemistry, it must be done prior to the onset of chelation therapy. However, this may not be possible because of the stress imposed on the already debilitated patient during the blood collection procedure. The empirical treatment program should therefore take precedence.

REFERENCES

1. Smith HA, Jones TC, Hunt RD: *Veterinary Pathology*. Philadelphia, Lea & Febiger, 1972, pp 956-961.
2. Zook BC, Carpenter JL, Leeds EB: Lead poisoning in dogs. *JAVMA* 155:1329-1342, 1969.
3. Knecht CD, Crabtree J, Katherman A: Clinical, clinicopathologic, and electroencephalographic features of lead poisoning in dogs. *JAVMA* 175(2):196-201, 1979.
4. Kowalcyzk DF: Lead poisoning in dogs at the University of Pennsylvania Veterinary Hospital. *JAVMA* 168:428-432, 1976.
5. Jacobs G: Lead poisoning in a cat. *JAVMA* 179(12):1396-1397, 1981.
6. Blood DC, Henderson JA: *Veterinary Medicine*, ed 4. Baltimore, The Williams & Wilkins Co, 1974, pp 784-789.
7. Siegmund OH (ed): *The Merck Veterinary Manual*, ed 4. Rahway, NJ, Merck and Co, Inc, 1973, pp 935; 1087.
8. Blackwell JG: Chronic lead poisoning (chronic plumbism) in a ewe. *VM SAC* 72(12):1879-1882, 1977.
9. Martin DP: Primates, in Fowler ME (ed): *Zoo and Wild Animal Medicine*. Philadelphia, WB Saunders Co, 1978, p 547.
10. Beyers RK: Lead poisoning. *Pediatrics* 23:585-603, 1959.
11. Johns FM: A study of punctate stippling as found in the lead poisoning of wild ducks. *J Lab Clin Med* 19:514-517, 1934.
12. Coburn DR, Metzler DW, Treichler R: A study of absorption and retention of lead in wild waterfowl in relation to clinical evidence of lead poisoning. *J Wildl Mgmt* 15:186-192, 1951.
13. Bellrose F: Lead poisoning as a mortality factor in waterfowl populations. *Bull IL Nat Hist Surv* 27:235-288, 1959.
14. Rosen MN, Bankowski RA: A diagnostic technique and treatment for lead poisoning in swans. *Cal Fish Game* 46:81-90, 1960.
15. Trainer DO, Hunt RA: Lead poisoning of whistling swans in Wisconsin. *Avian Dis* 9:252-264, 1965.
16. Locke LN, Bagley GE, Irby HD: Acid-fast intranuclear inclusion bodies in the kidneys of mallards fed lead shot. *Bull Wildl Dis Assoc* 2:127-131, 1966.
17. Bagley GE, Locke LN: Lead poisoning in Canada geese in Delaware. *Avian Dis* 11:601-608, 1967.
18. Humphreys P: Noninfectious diseases, in Fowler ME: *Zoo and Wild Animal Medicine*. Philadelphia, WB Saunders Co, 1978, p 204.
19. Grandy JW, Locke LN, Bagley GE: Relative toxicity of lead and five proposed substitute shot types to pen-reared mallards. *J Wildl Mgmt* 32:483-488, 1968.
20. Locke LN, Bagley GE: Lead poisoning in a sample of Maryland mourning doves. *J Wildl Mgmt* 31:515-518, 1967.
21. Bagley GE, Locke LN: The occurrence of lead in tissues of wild birds. *Bull Environ Contam Toxicol* 2:297-305, 1967.
22. Redig PT, Stowe CM, Barnes DM, Arent TD: Lead toxicosis in raptors. *JAVMA* 177(9):941-943, 1980.
23. Jacobson E, Carpenter JW, Meliton N: Suspected lead toxicosis in a bald eagle. *JAVMA* 171:952-954, 1977.
24. Locke LN, Bagley GE, Frickie DN, Young LT: Lead poisoning and aspergillosis in an Andean condor. *JAVMA* 155:1052-1056, 1969.
25. Decker RA, McDermid AM, Prideaux JW: Lead poisoning in two captive king vultures. *JAVMA* 175(9):1009, 1979.
26. Janssen DL, Robinson PT, Ensley PK: Lead poisoning in birds. *JAVMA* 178(2):150, 1981.
27. Kennedy S, Crisler JP, Smith E, Bush M: Lead poisoning in sandhill cranes. *JAVMA* 171(9):955-958, 1977.
28. Zook BC, Sauer RM, Garner FM: Lead poisoning in captive wild animals. *J Wildl Dis* 8(3):264-272, 1972.
29. Petrak ML: Digestive system disturbances in cage birds (lead poisoning). *Vet Clin North Am* 3(2):196-197, 1973.
30. Giddings RF: Lead poisoning in a parrot. *VM SAC* 75(6):1015-1016, 1980.
31. Rosskopf WJ Jr, Woerpel RW: Lead poisoning in a cockatiel. *Mod Vet Pract* 63(1):46-48, 1982.
32. Rosskopf WJ Jr, Woerpel RW: Removal of a lead pellet by gizzard-otomy (ventriculotomy) in a green-winged macaw. *VM SAC* 77(6):969-974, 1982.
33. Fudge AM: Clinical findings in an Amazon parrot with suspected lead toxicosis. *Calif Vet* 36(5):23-25, 1982.
34. *Case Record #96564*. Downey, CA, Section of Comparative Pathology, Los Angeles County Dept of Health Services.
35. *Case Record #91075*. Downey, CA, Section of Comparative Pathology, Los Angeles County Dept of Health Services.
36. Petrak ML (ed): *Diseases of Cage and Aviary Birds*. Philadelphia, Lea and Febiger, 1969, p 500.
37. Burke TJ: Personal communication, University of Illinois, 1977.
38. Zook BC, McConnell G, Gilmore CE: Basophilic stippling of erythrocytes in dogs with special reference to lead poisoning. *JAVMA* 157:2092-2099, 1970.
39. Woerpel RW, Rosskopf WJ Jr: Avian handling techniques: Part II. *Anim Health Tech* 3(2):81-86, 1982.
40. Rosskopf WJ Jr, Woerpel RW, Van De Water D, Rosskopf G: Normal hematologic and blood chemistry values for commonly kept pet avian species. *VM SAC*, in press.

Heavy-Metal Intoxication in Caged Birds—Part II

Richard W. Woerpel, MS, DVM
Walter J. Rosskopf, Jr., BS, DVM

Animal Medical Centre of Lawndale
Hawthorne, California

Heavy-metal intoxication is common among caged birds, but it is frequently not diagnosed. Part I of this article summarized the existing literature on the subject and presented an in-depth discussion of lead toxicosis in caged birds, focusing on the sources, clinical signs, radiographic findings, clinical pathology, and toxicology of lead poisoning. In Part II, treatment and pathology are discussed, and three case reports are presented.

Treatment

Petrak has described the use of calcium ethylenediaminetetraacetic acid (Ca EDTA) for treating plumbism in caged birds.[1] Intramuscular injections of 20 to 45 mg/kg were given two to three times daily. The drug was mixed in normal saline or 5% dextrose solution prior to administration. Giddings reported using calcium disodium edetate[a] to treat an Amazon parrot for lead poisoning at a dose of 110 mg/kg in two and later three divided doses daily for four days.[2] The drug was initially given intravenously (diluted 1:2 with 5% dextrose solution) and later intramuscularly (diluted 1:4 with 5% dextrose solution). Janssen et al. used a dose of 35 mg/kg of Ca EDTA, given intramuscularly twice daily for five days for treatment of plumbism in birds.[3] This same dosage was used by Kennedy et al. in treating sandhill cranes suffering from lead poisoning.[4]

In treating caged birds suffering from plumbism, the authors have used calcium disodium edetate[b] dosages between 35 and 50 mg/kg given by intramuscular injection three times daily for five to seven days.[5-7] They do not dilute the drug before administering it intramuscularly and have had no problems. They have found, as did the authors mentioned above, the therapeutic response to be dramatic. Often the prominent clinical signs disappear within the first 24 to 48 hours of treatment. No side effects have been seen from using this drug as often as three times daily by intramuscular injection. The authors have also sent home patients on double their injectable dose of Ca EDTA to be given directly per os three times daily (in lieu of injections). This latter therapeutic method has kept patients asymptomatic during the time that heavy metal is being cleared from their gastrointestinal tracts. In addition to

[a]Havidote®, Haver-Lockhart, Shawnee, KS 66201.
[b]Calcium Disodium Versenate®, Riker Laboratories, Inc., Northridge, CA 91324.

Ca EDTA, the authors also routinely use parenteral ampicillin[c] prophylactically twice daily and injections every other day of stanozolol[d] to stimulate erythropoiesis, in addition to routine supportive care (e.g., force-feeding and fluids).

Some authors have used a noninvasive suction technique to aspirate heavy-metal particles from the stomach or gizzard of an afflicted bird in lieu of gastrotomy or ventriculotomy.[8,9] The authors have performed both cropotomy[10] and ventriculotomy[6] procedures in the treatment of lead-poisoned caged birds, in addition to medical therapy with Ca EDTA.

When radiography reveals heavy-metal particles within the crop of the patient, a cropotomy must be performed to prevent their inevitable movement into the ventriculus. However, the authors recommend that general anesthesia *not* be used for this procedure because of the potential risks to the patient. With the use of only physical restraint, the procedure is simple, quick, and not dependent on the total relaxation of general anesthesia for its success.[10]

One of the authors' cases involved an African grey parrot. The client knew the bird had recently ingested lead from a leaded window. Survey radiographs revealed numerous heavy-metal–dense particles within the crop and gizzard (Figure 1). Because of the large number of particles within the crop destined to become sequestered within the gizzard and result in systemic absorption of lead, and because the bird was exhibiting signs of plumbism, a cropotomy was elected. The patient was given 15 mg of intramuscular ketamine, and the surgery (Figure 2) resulted in successful removal of all the lead fragments. Unfortunately, the parrot never recovered from the anesthetic. Retrospectively, if faced with the same clinical circumstances, the authors would definitely elect to perform a cropotomy. They would, however, use only physical restraint and not take the risks of general anesthesia.

[c]Polyflex™, Bristol Laboratories, Syracuse, NY 13201.
[d]Winstrol®-V, Winthrop Laboratories, New York, NY 10016.

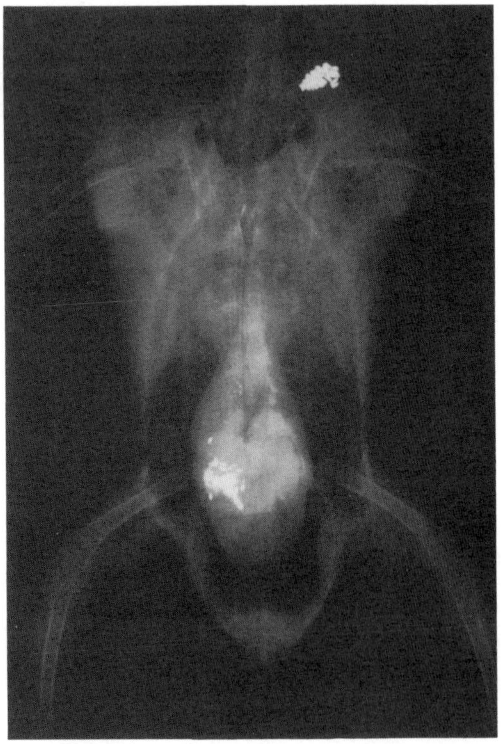

Figure 1—Radiograph of an African grey parrot suffering from clinical plumbism. Note heavy-metal–dense particles within the crop and gizzard.

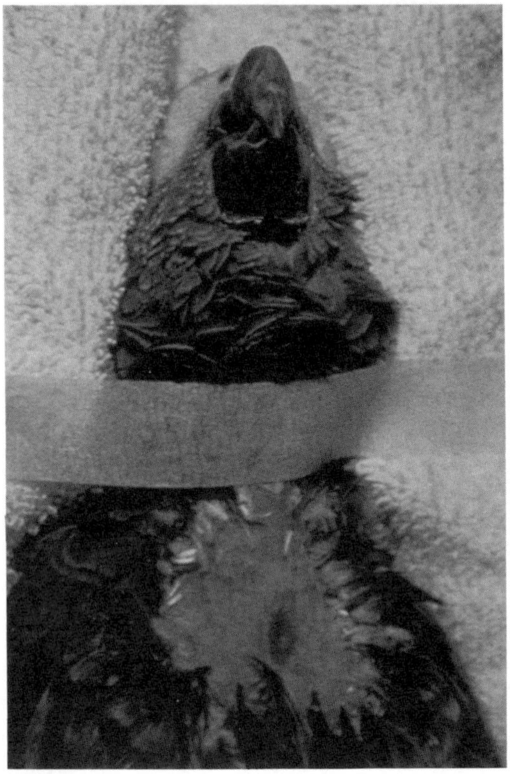

Figure 2—African grey parrot (shown in Figure 1) under ketamine anesthesia during cropotomy to retrieve lead particles.

The decision to perform a cropotomy should be made as soon as possible after radiography has confirmed the presence of heavy-metal particles within the crop of a patient showing signs of intoxication. Chelation therapy may be initiated prior to the surgery, but surgery cannot be delayed to await a clinical response. The decision to perform a ventriculotomy for retrieval of one or more heavy-metal particles (Figure 3), on the other hand, need not be as hasty. The patient probably should be receiving chelation therapy and should be asymptomatic before this procedure is attempted. The authors have performed only one ventriculotomy for this purpose, and it was successful.[6] They attribute their success to the stability of the patient, achieved by prior treatment with Ca EDTA.

Pathology

Zook et al. estimated the incidence of plumbism in psittacines necropsied at the National Zoological Park from January 1969 to May 1971 to be 50%.[11] This figure was based on the presence of multiple acid-fast, intra-

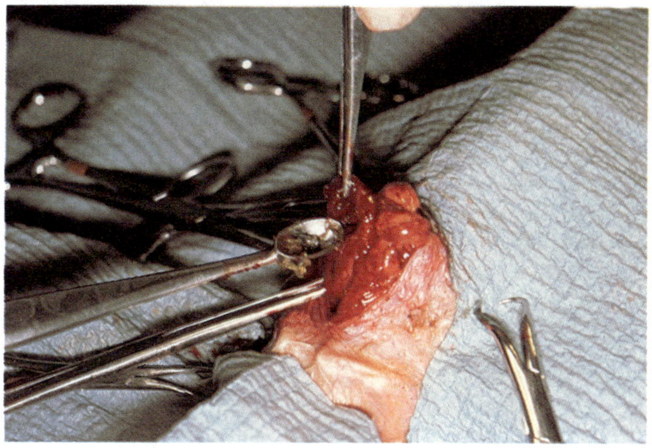

Figure 3—Ventriculotomy performed on a green-winged macaw. Note the lead pellet (from 177-caliber airgun) in the surgical spoon.

nuclear inclusion bodies within proximal tubular epithelial cells of the kidney or within hepatocytes. These inclusion bodies within the kidney and/or the liver are specific for lead-poisoned mammals and are thought to function in the storage of lead.[12] Many other authors have reported their presence within the kidney in relation to lead-poisoned avian species.[13-19] It should be noted, however, that nearly an equal number of investigators (including the authors) have not found these inclusion bodies upon histopathologic examination of the kidney and/or liver using acid-fast stains.[4,9,20-22] Locke et al. reported that the amount of lead absorbed, the period of exposure, and the diet of the individual affected the occurrence of intranuclear inclusion bodies;[14] other unknown factors also probably influence the presence or absence of intranuclear inclusion bodies within the tissues.

Few other authors have reported the existence of hemoglobin casts within the renal tubules,[19] but a number have noted evidence within the liver of hemolysis (e.g., hemosiderin).[4,18,21,22] These same authors also noted definite evidence of hepatocellular degeneration and/or necrosis. None mentioned the existence of any pathology involving the tissues of the central nervous system.

Very little has been written regarding the pathological changes (both gross and microscopic) that accompany plumbism in psittacines. This is in part because the disease, when properly diagnosed, is treatable, and when it is not diagnosed antemortem, there are few lesions (without the use of special stains) that suggest plumbism to the pathologist.

The discovery within the gizzard or elsewhere in the gastrointestinal tract of one or more heavy-metal fragments that could be analyzed for lead content would be the most rewarding finding at necropsy on a lead-poisoned psittacine. No other gross findings should be expected. Interestingly, many investigators have noted in the tissues of lead-poisoned poultry, waterfowl, or raptors one or more of the following gross findings: gross distention of the gallbladder;[18-23] emaciation;[18-20,23] eroded mucosa of gizzard (stomach)[8,21] with bright green staining of its contents;[8,21,23] atrophy of liver and/or heart;[19,20,23] increased amount of pericardial fluid;[18,21,23] and impaction of the proventriculus.[8,21] It should be noted that a gallbladder is lacking in the budgerigar and in some species of parrots,[24] and therefore, gross distention of the gallbladder is rarely seen in caged birds. It should also be noted that in all cases the gross lesions mentioned were the result of chronic plumbism. Psittacine species, in contrast, seem to manifest clinical signs within a relatively short time following the ingestion of a critical amount of heavy metal. Therefore, these lesions would be rarely encountered during the necropsy of a parrot that succumbed to lead poisoning.

Case Report 1

A red-lored Amazon parrot (*Amazona autumnalis autumnalis*) of unknown age and sex was presented to the authors' clinic on 4/7/79 with a history of lead ingestion. The bird had apparently broken the plastic covering of a toy penguin and eaten some of its lead core. The client did not know how long the bird had been ingesting the lead.

Physical examination revealed a well-muscled bird with pronounced central nervous system signs (head tilt, torticollis, and incoordination) that was unable to perch. A blood sample was collected for hematology and chemical evaluation, and survey radiographs were obtained (Amazon 4 of Table III in Part I of this article). The latter revealed more than 50 heavy-metal–dense particles within the gizzard. The patient was immediately given 10 mg intramuscular Ca EDTA, 25 mg intramuscular ampicillin, and 0.5 mg intramuscular dexamethasone. The patient was hospitalized for the next four days, during which time it received 10 mg Ca EDTA three times daily, 30 mg ampicillin once daily, and parenteral B vitamins.

The blood test results revealed only an elevated creatinine value. All other parameters were within normal limits. Throughout its stay in the hospital, the patient exhibited only slight improvement. The central nervous system signs and weakness continued. Hospitalization was terminated for financial reasons. The parrot was released on Ca EDTA to be given orally at 20 mg three times daily. On 4/13 the client indicated that the bird's general condition was not improved and that it was manifesting definite signs of blindness. The owner was instructed to continue the medication as previously directed. The patient was reexamined on 4/16. At that time the parrot was clinically normal. Radiography of the patient revealed approximately 20 particles of lead within the gizzard and gut. The owner was instructed to continue the oral Ca EDTA. The bird remained clinically normal and was reradiographed on 4/19. The x-rays revealed only three lead particles within the gut. The owner was told to stop the chelation therapy and present the parrot for final radiography on 4/21. On this date the radiographs revealed no heavy metal. The bird made a complete recovery.

This case is reported because it is typical of those seen in private practice and because it demonstrates the relative severity of the central nervous system signs sometimes seen with plumbism and the response of the patient to specific chelation therapy (even when it is administered orally).

Case Report 2

On 5/30/81, an 11-year-old blue-fronted Amazon parrot (*A. aestiva aestiva*) of unknown sex was presented with acute onset of signs that were suggestive of plumbism. The owner had noted chocolate-milk–colored droppings that morning. She indicated that the bird had suffered lead intoxication approximately 10 years previous to this visit. When questioned about the current possibility of plumbism and the availability of lead within the parrot's environment (the owner admitted that the bird was allowed substantial freedom from its cage), the owner stated that her husband frequently prepared and loaded ammunition within the house.

Physical examination of the patient revealed obvious hemoglobinuria (see Figure 3 in Part I) and a weak, stressed parrot of 375 g body weight. Survey radiographs and blood for hematology and chemical evaluation were obtained. The radiographs revealed no heavy-metal–dense fragments of any kind within the bird. Whole blood was collected in heparinized microhematocrit tubes and centrifuged, and the packed-cell volume (PCV) (23%) was recorded. It was noted that the plasma was clear and red (hemolysis). The anemia and hemolysis and presenting signs continued to suggest lead toxicosis as the likely diagnosis. The owner was again questioned regarding the possibility of the parrot's past or present exposure to heavy metal. She then mentioned that her husband had melted lead #2 alloy on the stove in the kitchen of the home on each of two days prior to 5/30 and had done so many times before. The bird had been in the living room, and her husband usually carried out this procedure with the kitchen ventilation fan on and the windows open. She was vague as to whether these two precautions had been taken this last time and mentioned the presence of smoke in the house. The tentative diagnosis was plumbism secondary to inhalation of the heavy metal.

Upon hospitalization the patient was given intramuscular injections of 30 mg ampicillin, 10 mg Ca EDTA, 12.5 mg stanozolol, 0.4 mg dexamethasone, and 1.0 mg vitamin K.[e] During its four-day stay, the parrot received 25 mg ampicillin twice daily, 20 mg Ca EDTA twice or three times daily, and every-other-day injections of 1.0 mg vitamin K and 12.5 mg stanozolol.

On the day following hospitalization, the droppings were nearly normal (Figure 4) and the bird seemed a little stronger. The blood test results were obtained on the following day and revealed no basophilic stippling, a mild leukocytosis with a heterophilia and basophilia, slight thrombocytopenia (qualitative assessment), elevated total protein, and normal values for serum aspartate aminotransferase (SAST, or SGOT) and creatinine. On each successive day of hospitalization the patient grew stronger and more aggressive. There was no hemoglobinuria noted after the day of presentation. A PCV performed on 6/2/81 (three days postpresentation) was 21% with no evidence of hemolysis. This was not considered a decrease in red cell mass because the first PCV and total protein value obtained on 5/31 were probably falsely elevated as a result of dehydration of the patient.

The patient was released on 6/3/81 and was not returned one week later as requested for a recheck. One year later it was alive and well with no repeat of similar signs. The husband continues to melt lead tape in the home, but the parrot is placed outdoors during this procedure.

This case is of particular interest because the history, physical examination, and clinical pathology results strongly suggested plumbism, but radiography could not confirm the expected presence of heavy metal within the gut of the patient. The tentative diagnosis of inhalation plumbism was never confirmed but remains the most plausible explanation for the clinical signs and dramatic response to treatment. Plumbism has been reported in horses as a result of their frequent exposure to fumes from lead smelters, and in other domestic animals as a result of exposure to fumes from burning storage batteries or from cutaneous absorption of gasoline containing tetra-ethyl lead.[12,23] Cotter reported on an inhalation lead intoxication syndrome in humans which resulted from chronic exposure of welders to fumes from the burning of lead-painted surfaces.[25]

Case Report 3

This case report involves zinc toxicosis in a seven-year-old green-winged macaw (sex unknown). This disorder resulted from the bird's ingestion of a zinc-aluminum alloy, the source of which was later determined to be a toy.

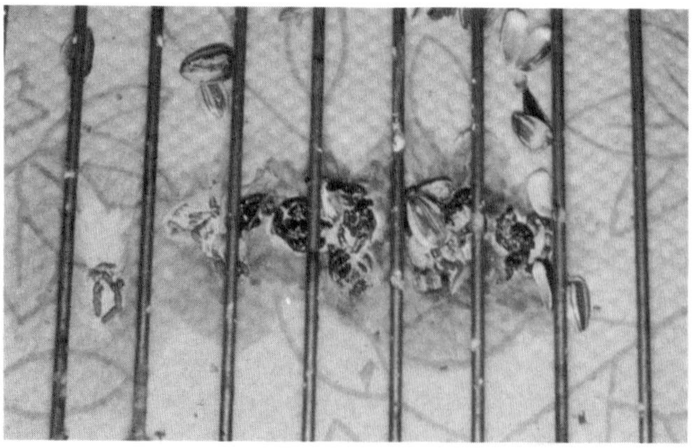

Figure 4—Droppings from a blue-fronted Amazon parrot with probable inhalation plumbism one day after presentation. The droppings from this bird on the day of presentation are shown in Figure 3 of Part I of this article.

[e] AquaMEPHYTON®, Merck Sharp & Dohme, West Point, PA 19486.

The macaw was first presented on 1/5/81 because of a relatively sudden onset of lethargy, vomiting, and diarrhea. The physical exam was unremarkable (weight—1245 g). Blood was collected for clinical pathology (hematology and chemical evaluation), and the bird was sent home on 50 mg ampicillin to be given intramuscularly once a day for seven days. The blood examination revealed only leukocytosis with heterophilia and eosinophilia. The patient was returned for a progress check on 1/12/81, at which time the owner indicated that the bird was nearly 100% normal. A blood sample collected at this time revealed that the white blood cell (WBC) count had fallen into the high normal range, with complete disappearance of monocytes and eosinophils from the differential count.

The bird was normal until 6/3/81 at which time it was presented to the authors' clinic because of anorexia, diarrhea, and a change in color of the feces. Physical examination was unremarkable (weight—1245 g). A blood sample (hematology only) was taken and the bird was sent home on parenteral ampicillin, as before, for one week. The WBC and differential counts were essentially normal. On 6/5 the bird was not doing well and had started to vomit. The macaw was reexamined on 6/10. Its weight had fallen to 1103 g and its droppings revealed green feces without form and yellow urine and urates. Another blood sample (hematology and chemical evaluation) was collected. All values were within normal limits.

The macaw continued to do poorly at home and the owner agreed to hospitalize the bird on 6/12. During its 10-day period of hospitalization the patient received parenteral antibiotics, antiemetic medication,[f] vitamins (B complex and A, D, and E[g]), and anabolic steroids (stanozolol), in addition to aggressive force-feeding. Blood examination (hematology and chemical evaluation) done on 6/16 indicated severe leukocytosis (WBC = 35,000 to 40,000/mm^3) with many toxic heterophils, with extreme elevations in both SAST (1426 IU/L) and lactate dehydrogenase (LDH) (2498 IU/L) values, suggesting severe hepatitis (probable toxic cause).

The patient continued to lose weight (on 6/19 it weighed 996 g) and exhibit intermittent vomiting and continuous diarrhea. On 6/19 the macaw was x-rayed. The radiographs revealed approximately 25 particles of heavy-metal–dense material of varying sizes, all of which appeared to be within the gizzard. The bird was started on parenteral Ca EDTA at 25 mg three times daily. A blood lead concentration determination was not done. The patient's weight and overall condition continued to decline in spite of chelation therapy and the aggressive supportive care outlined above. A blood sample (hematology and chemical evaluation) taken on 6/22 revealed a high normal WBC count with heterophilia and monocytosis and a rising SAST value (2218 IU/L).

[f]Centrine®, Bristol Laboratories, Syracuse, NY 13201.
[g]Injacom®, Roche Chemical Div., Nutley, NJ 07110.

The bird was allowed to go home on 6/22 for a short stay; the authors hoped that a more familiar environment would stimulate its appetite. No medications were sent home with the patient. On 6/24, the macaw was returned in an extremely weakened condition. Its weight had dropped to 827 g and its droppings still reflected yellow brown urates and diarrhea. Radiographs taken on this day revealed a slight decrease in the total number of particles and not all were located within the gizzard. Chelation therapy and supportive care (including force-feedings three times daily) were reinstituted and 1 mg parenteral dexamethasone was given additionally for the next three days.

On 6/26 the bird began to show mild improvement and began to gain weight. The patient was released on 6/27. No medication was sent home with the bird. It continued to exhibit gradual and steady improvement each day. The client returned the bird on 7/3, at which time it weighed 999 g. Radiography revealed no more heavy metal within the gut. Blood examination (hematology and chemical evaluation) revealed a normal WBC and differential and a nearly normal SAST (422 IU/L) value.

This green-winged macaw made a complete recovery and regained its original weight (1210 g) by 7/11/82. The owner had the toy analyzed by a private laboratory (98.8% zinc; 1.2% aluminum).

This case is noteworthy because it involves an atypical heavy-metal intoxication, where the source of the metal was zinc rather than lead. The course of the illness was chronic, which is unlike plumbism cases treated by the authors. It is impossible to ascertain just how long the zinc-aluminum particles had been in the gut. The history and clinical signs suggest that they may have been present in the bird prior to the first complaint of gastrointestinal signs on 1/5/81. They remained within the gut for a substantial period of time, probably because of their relatively large size.

The major clinical signs in this case were those of gastroenteritis. It is not known whether these signs were primary or secondary to the hepatic involvement. The salient clinical pathologic findings were leukocytosis with heterophilia and evidence of hepatic involvement (grossly elevated SAST and LDH values). The cause of the hepatitis was undoubtedly toxic.

It is interesting that this case was comparatively refractory to Ca EDTA treatment. The patient did not exhibit the rapid, dramatic improvement characteristic of lead-poisoned patients receiving chelation therapy and did not seem to benefit from it. The authors are still unsure of what caused the course of the bird's illness to reverse itself on 6/26. The mass of heavy metal within the bird had been gradually decreasing and it is possible that the amount remaining dropped below the critical level necessary to cause clinical illness.

Nevertheless, this case clearly demonstrates how aggressive supportive care and frequent monitoring of the patient (e.g., weight and hematologic parameters) can result in the successful resolution of very serious disease problems in caged birds. This bird would surely have perished without this attentive nursing care.

REFERENCES

1. Petrak ML: Digestive system disturbances in cage birds (lead poisoning). *Vet Clin North Am* 3(2):196-197, 1973.
2. Giddings RF: Lead poisoning in a parrot. *VM SAC* 75(6):1015-1016, 1980.
3. Janssen DL, Robinson PT, Ensley PK: Lead poisoning in birds. *JAVMA* 178(2):150, 1981.
4. Kennedy S, Crisler JP, Smith E, Bush M: Lead poisoning in sandhill cranes. *JAVMA* 171(9):955-958, 1977.
5. Rosskopf WJ Jr, Woerpel RW: Lead poisoning in a cockatiel. *Mod Vet Pract* 63(1):46-48, 1982.
6. Rosskopf WJ Jr, Woerpel RW: Removal of a lead pellet by gizzardotomy (ventriculotomy) in a green-winged macaw. *VM SAC* 77(6):969-974, 1982.
7. Woerpel RW, Kosskopf WJ Jr: Avian therapeutics. *Mod Vet Pract* 62(12):947-949, 1981.
8. Humphreys P: Noninfectious diseases, in Fowler ME: *Zoo and Wild Animal Medicine*. Philadelphia, WB Saunders Co, 1978, p 204.
9. Redig PT, Stowe CM, Barnes DM, Arent TD: Lead toxicosis in raptors. *JAVMA* 177(9):941-943, 1980.
10. Rosskopf WJ Jr, Woerpel RW, Pitts BJ: Cropotomy in a parrot. *Mod Vet Pract* 63(3):219-222, 1982.
11. Zook BC, Sauer RM, Garner FM: Lead poisoning in captive wild animals. *J Wildl Dis* 8(3):264-272, 1972.
12. Smith HA, Jones TC, Hunt RD: *Veterinary Pathology*. Philadelphia, Lea & Febiger, 1972, pp 956-961.
13. Bellrose F: Lead poisoning as a mortality factor in waterfowl populations. *Bull IL Nat Hist Surv* 27:235-288, 1959.
14. Locke LN, Bagley GE, Irby HD: Acid-fast intranuclear inclusion bodies in the kidneys of mallards fed lead shot. *Bull Wildl Dis Assoc* 2:127-131, 1966.
15. Bagley GE, Locke LN: Lead poisoning in Canada geese in Delaware. *Avian Dis* 11:601-608, 1967.
16. Grandy JW, Locke LN, Bagley GE: Relative toxicity of lead and five proposed substitute shot types to pen-reared mallards. *J Wildl Mgmt* 32:483-488, 1968.
17. Locke LN, Bagley GE: Lead poisoning in a sample of Maryland mourning doves. *J Wildl Mgmt* 31:515-518, 1967.
18. Locke LN, Bagley GE, Frickie DN, Young LT: Lead poisoning and aspergillosis in an Andean condor. *JAVMA* 155:1052-1056, 1969.
19. Decker RA, McDermid AM, Prideaux JW: Lead poisoning in two captive king vultures. *JAVMA* 175(9):1009, 1979.
20. Coburn DR, Metzler DW, Treichler R: A study of absorption and retention of lead in wild waterfowl in relation to clinical evidence of lead poisoning. *J Wildl Mgmt* 15:186-192, 1951.
21. Trainer DO, Hunt RA: Lead poisoning of whistling swans in Wisconsin. *Avian Dis* 9:252-264, 1965.
22. Jacobson E, Carpenter JW, Meliton N: Suspected lead toxicosis in a bald eagle. *JAVMA* 171:952-954, 1977.
23. Siegmund OH (ed): *The Merck Veterinary Manual*, ed 4. Rahway, NJ, Merck and Co, Inc, 1973, pp 935; 1087.
24. Petrak ML (ed): *Diseases of Cage and Aviary Birds*. Philadelphia, Lea & Febiger, 1969, pp 82; 115.
25. Cotter LH: Lead intoxication by inhalation. *J Ind Hyg Toxicol* 28:44-46, 1946.

Disorders of the Avian Crop

Terry W. Campbell, DVM
Department of Laboratory Medicine
College of Veterinary Medicine
Kansas State University
Manhattan, Kansas

The crop (ingluvies) is a dilatation or diverticulum of the esophagus in birds. It is subject to several medical disorders, and the knowledge of these conditions is important to the avian practitioner. Common noninfectious surgical disorders include fistulas, lacerations, and obstructions. Common infectious crop disorders are candidiasis, trichomoniasis, and sour crop. This article provides a basic understanding of crop anatomy and physiology and describes the various crop disorders and current treatments.

Anatomy

The crop is a specialized, permanent diverticulum or expansion of the esophagus. The esophagus is divided into two sections in relation to the crop, the pars cervicalis (the area between the pharynx and crop) and the pars thoracica (the area between the crop and proventriculus). The esophagus and crop generally lie to the right of the midline and in the subcutaneous space bound by delicate fascia and adipose tissue. Gallinaceous, psittacine, and columbiform birds have a muscular sling that surrounds the crop and inserts into the skin.[1,2] This sling aids in emptying of the crop. Depending upon age, species, and size of the bird, the crop usually lies near the thoracic inlet. A full crop in hawks extends ventrally. It also extends ventrally in parrots, whereas in some psittacines it protrudes laterally and dorsally. Not all crops are identical, nor do all birds have crops. The crop may be a spindle-shaped enlargement of the esophagus, a unilateral enlargement or evagination, a unilateral sac, or a bilateral double sac.[3] The parakeet crop is a fusiform widening of the esophagus that narrows at the pectoral end.[4] Some birds (e.g., canaries, owls, and gulls) do not have crops but can store food by temporary expansion of the esophagus.[3,5]

Avian esophageal and crop tissues have the same general organization as the mammalian esophagus. The musculature of the crop, the tunica muscularis, is in three layers in the chicken and two layers in psittacines and birds of prey.[2] The external longitudinal muscle is usually thin, while the circular and interlongitudinal muscle layers are well developed.[3] The epithelium (lamina epithelialis mucosae) varies in thickness with species, and the outer layer may be cornified into a stratum corneum. In some passerines the epithelium is thickest in the crop with the greatest cornification in the pars cervicalis. The tunica mucosa of the crop contains mucous glands, which vary in location among species.[2] The glands are tubular to alveolar and have merocrine secretion.

The crop is innervated by esophageal branches of the glossopharyngeal nerve anastomosing with recurrent branches of the vagus.[6] Normal peristalsis is maintained by the vagal efferent input and the myenteric nervous system. The vagus also controls the crop sphincter.[3] The crop of pigeons and chickens has stronger rhythmic contractions when empty than when full. Feeding or cerebral inhibition causes a temporary cessation of these movements. Birds that swallow large food particles (i.e., raptors) temporarily store the food in the crop before peristaltic contractions move it into the proventriculus.

The crop is supplied by the left ascending esophageal artery, which is a branch from the common carotid artery. The venous return is through the esophageal veins draining into the left and right caudal veins of the crop. These veins enter the jugular directly.

Crop Function

The crop functions as a food storage chamber where ingesta undergoes softening, moistening, and swelling.[7] The crop supplies ingesta to the proventriculus at an appropriate rate for digestion. Food initially consumed may be delivered directly to the proventriculus without entering the crop. Later, the crop sphincter relaxes allowing food to enter the crop. Ingesta leaves the crop at irregular intervals reflexively controlled by the degree of fullness of the gastrointestinal tract.[3] The crop allows the bird to consume large quantities of small food rapidly, thus minimizing exposure time to predation.[7] Food to feed the young is stored in the crop from which it is regurgitated by reverse peristalsis in such birds as hawks, parrots, and pigeons. Maximum storage capacity is obtained by the saclike diverticula-style crops.

The role of the crop in chemical digestion is controversial. Some authors feel that starch digestion within the crop is due to amylase activity derived from saliva and crop secretions.[8] Others believe carbohydrate digestion is primarily microbial in origin.[9] Lactic acid can be found in significant concentration within the crop lumen, indicating carbohydrate hydrolysis. Protein digestion probably occurs from proventricular proteinases regurgitated into the crop. Any chemical digestion within the crop is of minor importance since it precedes the physical digestion by the gizzard.

Some birds produce a milklike secretion (crop milk) that is formed in the crop and regurgitated to feed nestlings. In pigeons and doves, this fluid is produced by the desquamation of fat-laden cells of the crop. In both sexes prior to hatching, this superficial nutritive cell layer begins to proliferate under the stimulation of oxytocin and prolactin.[7,10,11] The liquid produced is rich in fat and protein but low in carbohydrates and is fed to the young during the first two weeks of life.[3] Crop milk production allows parents to feed at irregular intervals while providing nestlings with a stable and constant food supply.[12]

The crop functions in courtship behavior in some birds. Males of certain species (i.e., grouse and pigeons) have inflatable esophageal diverticula, which act as resonating chambers or display devices.[3]

Examination of the Crop

Examination of the crop should be included in the physical examination of the avian patient. The crop is palpated to determine the degree of fill and consistency of its contents. Presence (or absence) of contents, dilatation, loss of tone, and masses inside the crop wall should be noted. An impacted crop may be enlarged, doughy, or firm upon palpation. An extremely dilated, atonic, fluid-filled crop can result from obstruction distal to the crop (i.e., in the proventriculus or gizzard). Crop atony can result from bacterial, protozoal, or mycotic infections. Parrots with access to food should have food in the crop;[13] thus, an empty crop is abnormal. In some birds the crop can be visualized through the skin by wetting the feathers. Better visualization is achieved by transillumination of the skin and crop wall with a bright light, such as that of an otoscope.

Contrast radiology is useful in the diagnosis of certain crop disorders. A 10 to 25% solution of barium sulfate is introduced into the crop using an infant feeding tube. The barium dosage for birds the size of a parakeet (30 gm) is 0.5 to 2.0 ml and for parrots is 5.0 to 10.0 ml.[14,15] Survey radiographs are taken before the barium is given. Second radiographs are taken immediately after barium administration. Subsequent radiographs are taken at 10- to 30-minute intervals. Barium should be in the proventriculus within 15 minutes and the small intestine within 30 minutes. The usual transit time of barium through the gastrointestinal tract is less than three hours.[14] Air can be used as the contrast medium for contrast radiology of the crop.[16,17]

Aspiration and evaluation of the crop contents is valuable in the diagnosis of crop disease. Whenever a crop disorder is suspected, aspiration of the crop contents should be considered. Sterile disposable feeding tubes are used (Figure 1). Tube sizes include No. 5 French for birds the size of a parakeet or smaller, No. 8 to No. 10 French for birds the size of cockatiels and medium-sized parrots (i.e., conures), and No. 14 to No. 18 French for larger birds (i.e., Amazon parrots, macaws, and raptors). A speculum will aid passage of the tube through the mouth. In parakeets or smaller birds, a small paper clip or thumb forceps can be used for this purpose; a larger paper clip or laboratory animal speculum can be used in a cockatiel or medium-sized parrot. An open-handle–style hoof pick or laboratory animal speculum can be used for aid in passing a feeding tube into the mouth of large parrots.

The head and neck should be extended to straighten the esophagus when inserting a tube into the crop. The tube is inserted into the mouth and passed over the tongue into the esophagus. The tube should pass easily into the crop and can be palpated through the skin. If

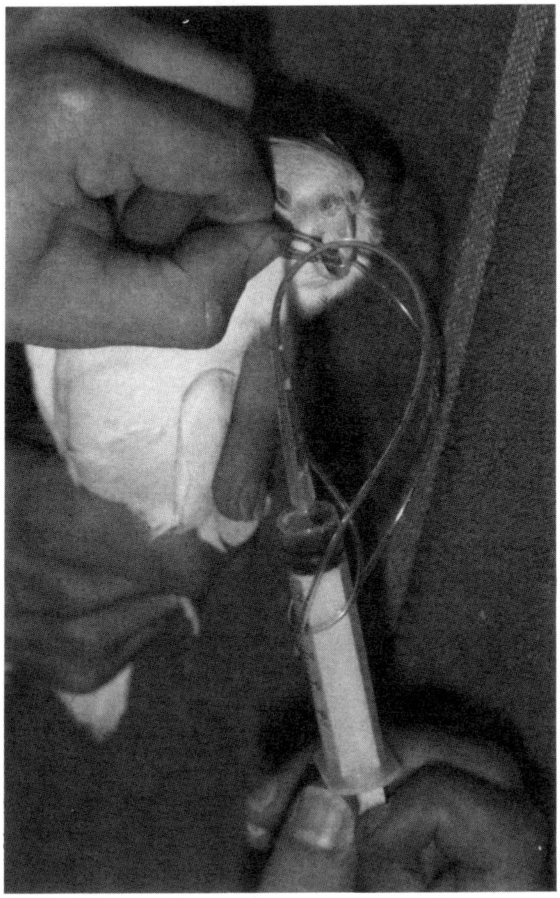

Figure 1—Crop aspiration technique using a sterile feeding tube.

any resistance occurs during the passage of the tube, the process should be stopped and repeated. The wall of the esophagus and crop is easily punctured, and excessive force should be avoided. In larger birds the mouth can be examined to insure the tube is in the esophagus and not in the trachea. When the end of the tube is within the crop, contents of the crop can be aspirated with a sterile syringe attached to the external end of the tube. Aspirated crop material should be submitted for mycotic and bacterial culture, antibiotic sensitivity, and cytologic examination. A wet mount is examined for trichomonads or other protozoa. An air-dried smear can be stained with Diff Quik®,[a] Wright's stain, or other suitable cytologic stain. The stained smear is examined for the presence of inflammatory cells, *Candida*, or any other abnormal content.

Ingluvotomy

Crop disorders that require surgery include lacerations, foreign bodies, calculi, fistulas, punctures, impactions, obstructions, and chronic dilatation. An ingluvotomy is indicated for removal of foreign bodies or obstructing material and repair of chronic dilatation. General anesthesia is usually required, although the procedure may be done without anesthesia in young birds.[17] Since the crop is relatively avascular and subcutaneous in location, surgery is relatively easy. However, the crop wall is thin and easily torn and care should be taken when handling the tissue. The crop should be emptied of excess gas and liquid prior to surgery using the crop aspiration technique described above. Patency of the esophagus and crop is maintained before and after surgery with a soft feeding tube or catheter placed in the esophagus and crop. The bird is placed in dorsal recumbency with proper consideration for preservation of body temperature. Feathers are removed from the incision site. The skin is prepared with a gentle surgical scrub and swabbed with tincture of iodine. A skin incision is made using a scalpel blade. The crop is bluntly dissected from surrounding tissue, and an incision is made into the crop for the removal of foreign bodies or obstructing material. The skin and crop should be sutured separately when closing.[10,18-20] The crop wall is closed using an inverting pattern (i.e., continuous Lembert suture) using 3-0 to 5-0 surgical gut or 4-0 absorbable suture on an atraumatic needle. The skin is closed with a simple interrupted or continuous pattern using 2-0 to 4-0 surgical gut. Optimum healing is obtained if suture lines of the crop and skin are offset.

Food and water should be withheld as long as possible following surgery, but no longer than 18 hours depending upon the size and condition of the bird.[21] Generally, food and water are withheld for three to four hours postoperatively and small amounts of soft foods are offered for 12 to 24 hours. Normal feeding is resumed after 24 hours. A common complication of ingluvotomy is a fistula, which requires resuturing. An Elizabethan collar may be required to prevent the bird from removing the sutures.

Crop Fistula

Crop fistulas result from postoperative ingluvotomy complications, lacerations, penetration of foreign bodies, and trauma or necrosis of the crop lining. A puncture of the crop occurs frequently in birds being force-fed using feeding tubes. Baby birds often develop marked edema and bruising in the area where the crop was punctured by a feeding tube and die quickly. Necrosis of the crop mucosa also may result from trauma induced by a tube or hot foods. The subcutaneous location of the crop predisposes it to punctures and lacerations (a common occurrence from encounters with cats). Raptors may suffer from punctures of the esophagus or crop as a result of bones ingested with their prey.[22,23] Crop fistulas can be difficult to treat and require immediate attention. Examination of the bird may reveal only a small opening and a few feathers matted with crop content. In acute cases the bird appears healthy, but a ravenous appetite and marked weight loss may be associated with a more chronic disorder. After feeding, the food may be deposited externally or subcutaneously; the latter is usually fatal.[24]

Repair of a fistulated crop requires debridement and separation of the crop wall from the skin. The freshened

---

[a]Harleco, Gibbstown, NJ 08027.

edges of the opened crop and skin are closed independently as in an ingluvotomy. Altman[25] suggests using 4-0 nylon to repair the crop because of the rapid absorption of 4-0 surgical gut. If more than eight hours have elapsed, the crop tissue becomes difficult to dissect from the surrounding tissue.[25] If the fistula repair is delayed longer than 24 hours, the prognosis is guarded.[10] A soft, seedless diet should be fed for the first 24 to 48 hours following fistula repair. Soaked and softened seed and soft foods should be continued for one week postoperatively.[11] A broad-spectrum oral antibiotic for one week is recommended.

Crop Impaction

Impaction of the crop is uncommon in caged birds. When it occurs, the impaction usually is due to a dry food mass resulting from obstructive foreign bodies, greedy feeding, inflammation lower in the gastrointestinal tract, or neuromuscular stasis of the crop.[26] Chickens, quail, and pheasants deprived of greens often gorge themselves when given access to long grass and this may result in crop impactions.[11,27] Ingestion of certain types of foods (e.g., oatmeal) or seeds (e.g., soybeans) frequently results in crop impactions.[11,28,29] If a large amount of these foods is ingested, crop impaction can result when the food rapidly swells within the crop. Grit impactions frequently occur when a bird denied access to grit suddenly is given grit free choice.

Raptors ingest large chunks of food or the entire carcass of small prey. The undigested parts are regurgitated as a pellet or casting, which involves gastric and esophageal antiperistalsis. Crop impactions in captive birds of prey often occur when a diet containing no castings (or roughage) is suddenly changed to one with castings.[30] Calculi causing crop impaction (crop lithiasis) are rare but have been reported.[11,31]

Clinical signs of crop impaction include repeated nonproductive regurgitation attempts, an interest in food but reluctance to eat, and picking at the base of the neck in the area of the crop. The crop is usually enlarged, has a doughlike consistency, and fails to empty. Acute impactions lead to crop rupture, toxicity due to absorbed toxins, or compression of the trachea. Chronic impactions result in emaciation and death due to starvation.[11]

Nonsurgical attempts to relieve the impaction should be attempted. In small birds a few drops of mineral or vegetable oil are given by crop gavage followed by gentle manual massage to break up the mass.[26] In raptors and gallinaceous birds 20 to 30 ml of vegetable oil can be given to soften the mass. Flushing or purging of the mass with warm isotonic saline may be attempted, but care must be taken to prevent respiratory aspiration of the fluid. If nonsurgical attempts fail, then an ingluvotomy to remove the impacted material is indicated.

Young hand-fed psittacines frequently develop crop impactions. Predisposing conditions include feeding foods that are cold, low in fiber, or spoiled; introducing air into the crop during feeding; and overfeeding the bird.[32] These conditions result in delayed emptying or impaction of the crop. Treatment should be prompt and requires evacuation of the crop by turning the chick upside down and milking out the contents. The bird is then fed small amounts of food at frequent intervals. If the retained food has fermented, then treatment may require administering a sodium bicarbonate solution (1 tsp/pt of water).

Chronic Dilatation of the Crop (Pendulous Crop)

The crop may become extremely dilated as a result of chronic obstruction distal to the crop, excessive food intake, atony from crop infections (bacterial, protozoal, or fungal), or unknown causes. This disorder frequently leads to ingluvitis, frequent regurgitation, and malnutrition. Birds with chronic dilatation of the crop lose body weight, as most of the ingested food is unable to pass out of the enlarged crop. Physical examination reveals an extremely enlarged and flaccid, fluid-filled crop that lies over the cranial aspect of the thorax. This condition is seen in older parakeets with a history of excessive food intake or hand-fed young psittacines that have been overfed. It can also be secondary to gastrointestinal tract obstruction (i.e., impaction of the proventriculus or gizzard) or pressure due to lesions at the thoracic inlet (i.e., abscess, neoplasia, fat deposits, or thyroid dysplasia). (See Figure 2.) Once the crop has been distended, it rarely corrects itself.

Diagnosis of the primary lesion may require crop aspiration for cytologic evaluation, culture of the crop contents, and contrast radiology to reveal obstructive lesions distal to the crop. Treatment of the primary lesion should be the first consideration. Excess crop fluid can be removed by turning the bird upside down and quickly milking the fluid out. The crop may require emptying two to three times a day. Force-feeding small amounts of a liquid diet at frequent intervals may be required, especially in obstructive cases. Oral antibiotics, as indicated from bacterial culture and sensitivity tests, should be given. Chloramphenicol palmitate[b] (0.05 to 0.01 ml/50 gm body weight) is a good broad-spectrum antibiotic to use while waiting for antibiotic sensitivity test results. Nystatin[c] (given at 0.05 to 0.01 ml/50 gm body weight) is indicated for candidiasis. Obese birds with fat deposits at the thoracic inlet should be fed reducing diets. Thyroid dysplasia should be treated by adding 10% sodium iodide to the drinking water (1 drop/30 ml). The distended crop is often refractory to medical treatment and usually requires a partial ingluvectomy. Using the technique described for an ingluvotomy, 40 to 60% of the distended crop wall can be removed with a fair to good prognosis.[21] Distention may recur, especially if the primary lesion is uncorrected.[20]

[b]Chloromycetin® Palmitate, Parke-Davis, Morris Plains, NJ 07950.
[c]Mycostatin®, E.R. Squibb & Sons, Inc., Princeton, NJ 08540.

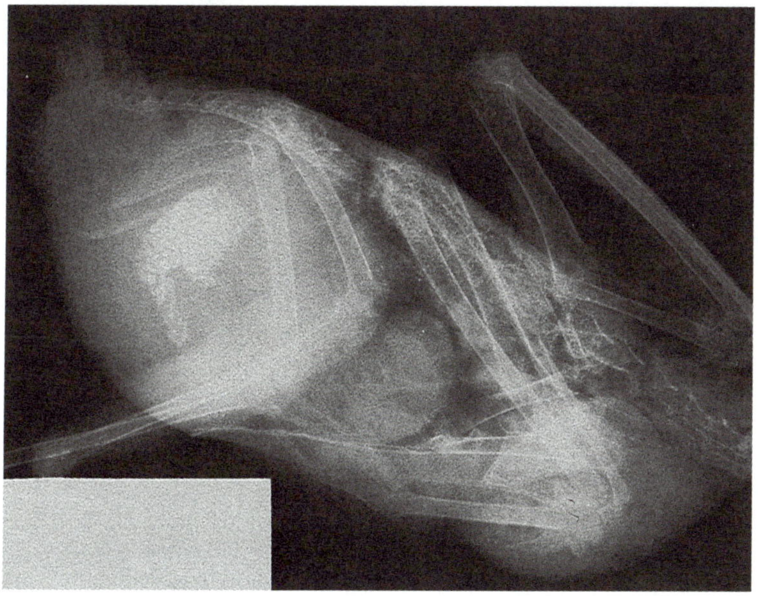

Figure 2—Lateral radiograph showing dilatation of the crop resulting from an obstruction of the proventriculus.

Ingluvitis (Inflammation of the Crop)

Ingluvitis can be caused by infectious agents such as bacteria, protozoa, and fungi; by chemical irritants, including such toxic plants as ivies, lilies, and oleander; by nutritional imbalances or deficiencies; and by unknown etiologies. Regurgitation is a common clinical sign. The crop becomes flaccid and filled with mucoid fluid, which is frequently regurgitated and flipped on the bird's head and objects in its cage. This material will paste head feathers together. Polydipsia is common.[33] The diagnosis is based upon clinical signs of regurgitation, the presence of an enlarged atonic crop, and cytologic evidence of inflammation on examination of the crop contents.

Cytologically, a normal crop aspirate from seed-eating birds has moderate numbers of cornified squamous epithelial cells and extracellular bacteria with a variety of morphologic types (Figure 3). An occasional *Candida*-like yeast can be seen, and there is a moderate amount of debris and plant fibers depending upon the sample. A Gram's stain reveals primarily gram-positive cocci and small to medium rods. Presence of many inflammatory cells (i.e., heterophils and macrophages) and an increased number of bacteria (especially intracellular), protozoa, or yeasts is indicative of ingluvitis (Figure 4). A smear with a large number of bacteria predominantly of one morphologic type or many gram-negative bacteria (in seed-eating birds) is abnormal.

Treatment requires emptying the crop two to three times a day and using oral antibiotics based upon the culture and sensitivity tests. Liquid vitamins are recommended. Supplemental digestive enzymes, lactobacillus, and nutritional yeasts may aid in restoration of normal crop flora. Ingluvitis has an inconsistent prognosis and can become a chronic or recurrent condition.

Sour Crop

Sour crop is an inflammation or ulceration of the crop associated with a foul-smelling, fermenting crop

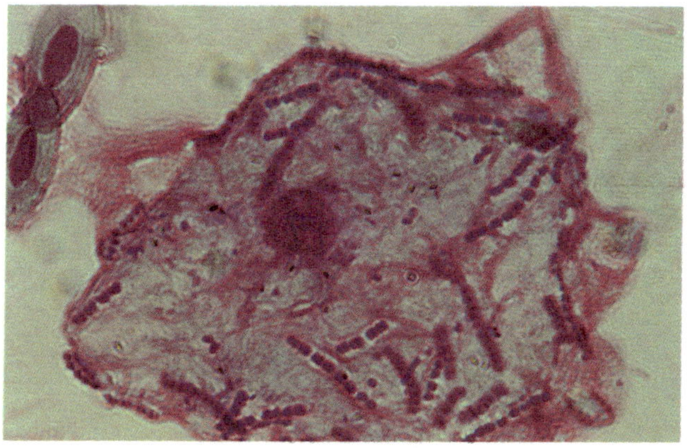

Figure 3—Crop aspirate from a scarlet macaw showing *Alysiella filiformis*, a normal bacterial inhabitant of the avian crop frequently seen on the surface of squamous epithelial cells. (Diff Quik, 100×)

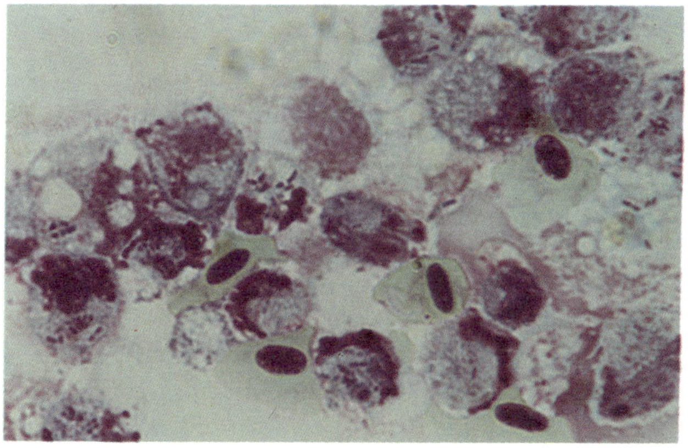

Figure 4—Septic ingluvitis in a cockatiel. Cytology of the crop aspirate shows a marked number of heterophils and macrophages with phagocytosis of bacteria. (Diff Quik, 100×)

fluid. Crop content is often acidic, which is presumably due to excessive lactate production (normal crop pH of seed-eating birds is between 4.5 and 6.7).[3] Predisposing factors include ingestion of spoiled food, irregular feeding, chilling, lower digestive tract disorders, vitamin deficiencies, protein deficiencies, regurgitation of the proventriculus content into the crop, and such infectious agents as *Candida* and *Trichomonas*.[11] Disorders causing delayed emptying of the crop predispose to this condition. Death results from malnutrition and dehydration due to vomiting and diarrhea.[11] Treatment requires emptying the crop several times a day. A broad-spectrum antibiotic (e.g., chloramphenicol palmitate), an antacid (e.g., sodium bicarbonate), and a digestive tract protectant (i.e., Kaopectate®[d]) should be given. A liquid diet given every two hours for one to three days is followed by a semisolid diet and finally a normal diet after three to five days.[11] Specific treatment for any infectious agent should be provided.

Candidiasis of the Crop

Candidiasis is caused by a fungus in the genus *Candida. Candida albicans* is the most common species isolated. The organism is part of the normal intestinal flora and is frequently isolated from droppings of healthy birds.[34-36] *Candida* is usually found in low numbers but will cause disease if allowed to overgrow. Predisposing factors to candidiasis include prolonged antibiotic treatment, avitaminosis (especially in avitaminosis A), nutritional disorders, bacterial or viral infections, feeding damp spoiled foods, and poor sanitation.[36,37] Jungerman and Schwartzman[36] list possible reasons for antibiotic enhancement of candidiasis: (1) direct stimulation of mycotic growth, (2) removal of bacteria competing for nutrients, (3) removal of organisms producing antifungal substances, (4) direct tissue damage allowing local invasion by *Candida*, (5) conversion of *Candida* to a more invasive form, (6) toxic products produced by *Candida*, (7) depression of the host immune response, (8) destruction of the normal flora resulting in avitaminosis that leads to lower tissue resistance to *Candida* invasion, and (9) use of certain antibiotics (especially tetracyclines) by *Candida* as a nitrogen source.

Young birds are more susceptible to candidiasis. *Candida* and bacterial infections of the crop are common causes of crop impaction and death in baby psittacines.[37] The organism is usually confined to the crop, causing delayed emptying of the crop and malnutrition. Cytologic evaluation of the crop contents shows an absence of inflammation (i.e., no heterophil or macrophage infiltration). The organism can invade the mouth, infraorbital sinuses, esophagus, proventriculus, gizzard, and intestinal tract.[36,38] Systemic infections can occur, especially in young birds. Venereal candidiasis has been reported in geese.[39]

A normal healthy crop has a white to pale pink mucosal lining with many smooth convoluted folds. Candidiasis causes crop mucosa to become rough and thickened. The crop surface may be coated with a catarrhal to mucoid tenacious exudate.[36] Infected crops show mild white streaking, erosions, pseudomembranous white areas, or diphtheritic membrane formation.[40] Oral lesions are not always present with crop lesions.

Clinical signs are variable. They include general malaise, loss of body weight (often with an increased appetite), delayed emptying of the crop, frequent regurgitation, and a thickened or dilated crop. Crop candidiasis in raptors is characterized by pseudomembranous patches of epithelium, foul-smelling crop contents, and impairment of ingestion.[30] Frequently, the only sign is of general malaise.

Suspicion of candidiasis of the crop is based on clinical signs, a history with predisposing factors, and demonstration of crop lesions. A presumptive diagnosis is based on the identification of the organism either by microscopic examination or mycotic culture of the crop contents. If blastospores and pseudohyphae (or true mycelia) are present, a presumptive diagnosis of candidiasis can be made, since these forms indicate tissue invasion (Figure 5).[36] Aspiration of the crop contents will usually reveal oval, thin-walled budding yeasts measuring 3 to 6 μ in diameter. Dry smears stained with Diff Quik®,[a] Gram's stain, or new methylene blue or a wet mount stained with lactophenol cotton blue will aid in identifying the yeasts (Figure 6). Selective media are required to culture *Candida*. The organism grows on blood or Sabouraud's agar producing soft, white, smooth colonies with a characteristic yeast odor. Older colonies will show feathery margins due to mycelial growth. Cornmeal agar is used to identify *Candida albicans*, which produces characteristic chlamydospores.[36,41] Differential diagnosis for avian candidiasis includes pox, trichomoniasis, histomoniasis, and avitaminosis A lesions.

Treatment of crop candidiasis involves correcting the predisposing factors. Specific medications include nystatin,[c] chlorhexidine,[e] ketaconizol,[f] amphotericin B,[g] and iodine.[37] Supplemental A and B-complex vitamins are indicated. Nystatin[c] is commonly used to treat *Candida* at a dose of 100,000 units/300 gm body weight once or twice a day for seven days.[37,42] Other antifungal drugs, amphotericin B[g] and flucytosine,[h] are used in cases refractory to nystatin.[37] A 2% chlorhexidine solution[e] in the water or 15% formic acid solution sprayed on the food can be used to treat flocks.[37,43]

Trichomoniasis

Trichomoniasis is a common disease affecting the crop in pigeons, doves, and raptors. It has been reported

[d]The Upjohn Co., Kalamazoo, MI 49001.

[e]Nolvasan®, Fort Dodge Laboratories, Fort Dodge, IA 50501.
[f]Nizoral®, Janssen Pharmaceutica, Inc., New Brunswick, NJ 08903.
[g]Fungizone®, E.R. Squibb & Sons, Inc., Princeton, NJ 08540.
[h]Ancobon®, Roche Products, Inc., Manati, PR 00701.

in chickens, turkeys, finches, canaries, and rarely in psittacines.[44-46] Trichomoniasis is called "canker" by pigeon fanciers and "frounce" by falconers. The disease is caused by *Trichomonas gallinae*, an ellipsoid or piriform flagellate protozoan. The organism measures 5 to 19 μ by 2 to 9 μ and has four anterior flagella, a narrow axostyle that protrudes 2 to 8 μ from the body, an undulating membrane, and no posterior flagellum.[45,47,48] The disease primarily affects young birds. Adult pigeons and doves may be healthy carriers and transmit the organism through the crop milk to their young. Trichomonads are sensitive to drying and do not form cysts, therefore direct transmission or contamination of food and water by material from the mouth (but not the feces) is necessary.[15,49] Raptors become infected by eating feral pigeons and doves. The susceptibility of pigeons and doves varies among breeds and the pathogenicity varies among strains of *T. gallinae*. Stress due to concurrent illness or environmental changes may predispose the bird to infection. Young pigeons appear to be most susceptible during weaning or molting.[45] Chemical irritants affecting the mucosa of the upper digestive tract will allow the normal protozoan population to become pathogenic.[50]

Trichomonas infections have an affinity for the esophagus and crop. Early lesions are small, white or yellow caseous nodules on the mucosa that may develop into large necrotic masses, which can occlude the lumen.[45] These firm masses may extend between folds in the mucosa and are often palpated as hard masses in the esophagus and crop. Soft, moist lesions occur with acute forms whereas dry, firm, cheesy lesions are seen in chronic forms.[11] Lesions may involve the oral cavity and upper respiratory tract. Highly pathogenic strains are invasive with lesions extending into the head and neck musculature or causing systemic infection.[51,52]

Clinical signs of trichomoniasis are more severe in young birds. Initially, regurgitation may occur due to invasion of the esophagus or crop mucosa. Sudden death without signs of illness occurs in some acute cases. Clinical signs of the chronic forms depend upon the severity and location of the lesions. Common signs include anorexia, weight loss, dyspnea, general malaise, and depression. The bird with occlusion of the esophagus or crop may die from starvation. A large amount of foul-smelling fluid may accumulate in the crop and may exude from the mouth.

The lesions caused by trichomoniasis must be differentiated from those of candidiasis, avitaminosis A, pox, and bacterial abscess. The diagnosis is based on history, clinical signs, and demonstration of the organisms from lesions or crop contents. A sample is collected by swabbing the crop with a moist cotton swab or aspirating the contents. A wet mount is prepared and the organisms can be seen microscopically. Trichomonads move through the fluid, and a wavy motion of the flagella and undulating membrane can be seen. The organisms can also be cultured in the laboratory (Figure 7).

Treatment for trichomoniasis involves use of antiprotozoal drugs. Dimetridazole[i] has been used successfully at a dose of 50 mg/kg body weight orally for two to seven days or 0.6 mg/L drinking water (2.27 g/gal) for six to seven days.[27,37,44,48,52] A single oral dose of 500 mg dimetridazole[i]/kg body weight has also been recommended.[42] Metronidazole[j] can be used orally at a dose of 50 to 60 mg/kg body weight or 66 mg/L (250 mg/gal) of drinking water for five to seven days.[42,52] The drug, 2-amino-5-nitrothiazole[k] can be used orally at a dose of 30 to 45 mg/kg body weight or 1 to 2 g/L of drinking water for seven days.[27,42,45,48] Ipronidazole[l] at a dose of 132 mg/L (500 mg/gal) of drinking water for seven days has also been used.[37] Broad-spectrum antibiotics and vitamin supplementation by crop gavage may aid in preventing secondary bacterial infections and vitamin deficiencies.

Recovery from infection or previous exposure to trichomonads will lead to immunity. Infection with an avirulent strain produces immunity against virulent strains, and passive immunity using serum from an infected bird provides protective immunity.[45] Trichomoniasis is controlled by eliminating carrier birds with treatment, preventing feral birds from contaminating food and water, and regular cleaning of food and water containers.

Neoplasia of the Crop

Neoplasms affecting the crop are rare. Petrak[53] describes a leiomyosarcoma of the crop in a budgerigar. The tumor measured 5 cm in diameter and was attached to the crop wall. A green-wing macaw with multiple papillomas affecting the esophagus, crop, and cranial proventriculus was referred to the author's clinic.[54] The bird was extremely emaciated, weak, and had inspiratory wheezing. Physical examination revealed marked weight loss, marked stress barring of the feathers, and a small papilloma in the glottis. Radiographs, hemogram, and blood chemistry results were within normal limits except for a slight elevation of aspartate aminotransferase. The bird continued to eat but was supplemented by tube feeding. Necropsy revealed multiple papillomatous growths partially occluding the lumen of the esophagus, crop, and proventriculus (Figure 8).

---

[i] Emtryl®, Salsbury Labs, Charles City, IA 50616.
[j] Flagyl®, Searle & Co., San Juan, PR 00936.
[k] Enheptin®, American Cyanamid Co., Princeton, NJ 08540.
[l] Ipropran®, Roche Chemical Div., Nutley, NJ 07110.

REFERENCES

1. Vanden Berge JC: Aves myology, in Getty R (ed): *Sisson and Grossman's The Anatomy of the Domestic Animals*. Philadelphia, WB Saunders Co, 1975, p 1803.
2. Koch T: *Anatomy of the Chicken and Domestic Birds*. Ames, IA, The Iowa State University Press, 1973, pp 70-71.
3. Ziswiler V, Farner DS: Digestion and the digestive system, in Farner DS, King JR (eds): *Avian Biology*, vol 2. New York, Academic Press, 1972, pp 343-430.
4. Stone RM: Clinical examination and methods of treatment, in

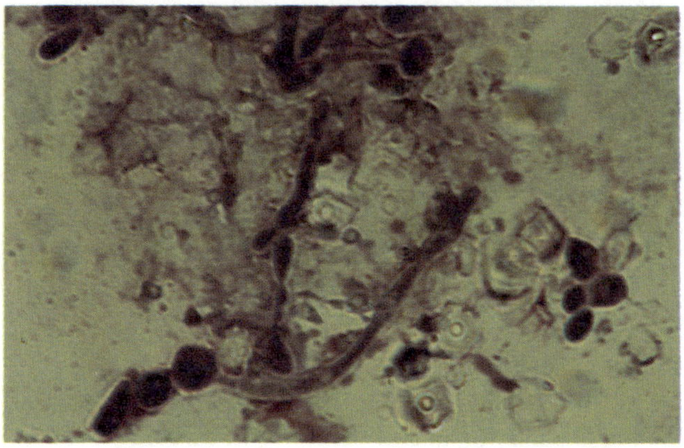

Figure 5—Candidiasis in a young cockatiel. The crop aspirate shows budding yeasts, pseudohyphae, and chlamydospores of *C. albicans*. (Diff Quik, 100×)

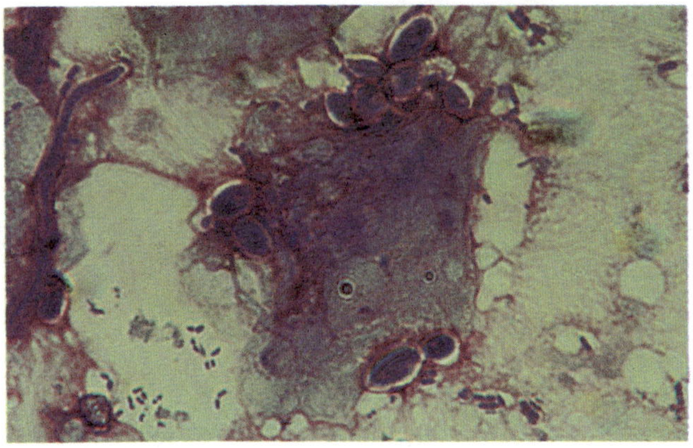

Figure 6—Candidiasis in a yellow-naped Amazon parrot. Note the thin-walled budding yeasts. (Diff Quik, 100×)

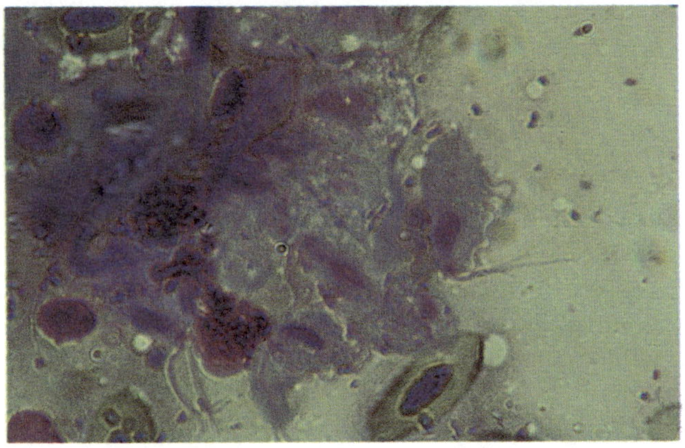

Figure 7—Crop aspirate from a pigeon with trichomoniasis. Note the piriform flagellate protozoa with anterior flagella and the undulating membrane. (Diff Quik, 100×)

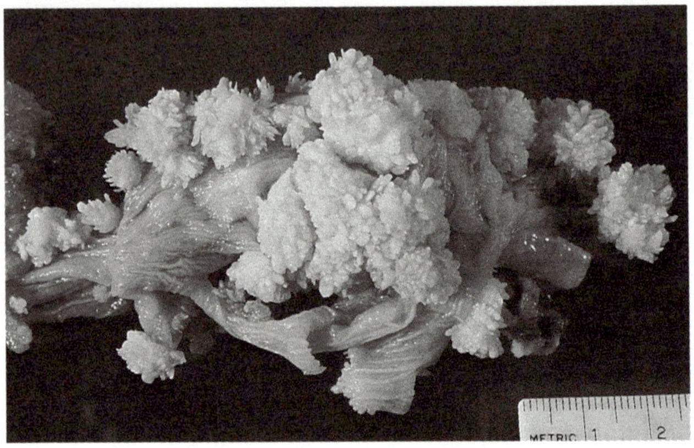

Figure 8—Multiple papillomatous growths partially occluding the esophagus and crop in a green-wing macaw.

Petrak ML (ed): *Diseases of Cage and Aviary Birds*. Philadelphia, Lea & Febiger, 1982, p 261.

5. Duke GE: Raptor physiology, in Fowler ME (ed): *Zoo and Wild Animal Medicine*. Philadelphia, WB Saunders Co, 1978, p 225.
6. McLelland J: Aves digestive system, in Getty R (ed): *Sisson and Grossman's The Anatomy of the Domestic Animals*. Philadelphia, WB Saunders Co, 1975, p 1867.
7. McCauley WJ: *Vertebrate Physiology*. Philadelphia, WB Saunders Co, 1971, p 200.
8. Prosser CL: Nutrition, in Prosser CL (ed): *Comparative Animal Physiology*. Philadelphia, WB Saunders Co, 1973, p 134.
9. Ivorec-Szylit O, Mercier C, Raibaud P, Calet C: Contribution a l'e'tude de la de'gradation des glucides dans le jabot du Coq. Influence du taux de glucose du re'gime sur l'utilisation de l'amidon. C.R. *Acad Sci* 261:3201-3203, 1965.
10. Stunkard JA: *A Guide to Diagnosis, Treatment and Husbandry of Caged Birds*. Bonner Springs, KS, Veterinary Medicine Publishing Co, 1980.
11. Arnall L, Keymer IF: *Bird Diseases*. Neptune City, NJ, TFH Publications, Inc, 1975.
12. Schmidt-Nielsen K: *Animal Physiology*. Cambridge, Cambridge University Press, 1979, p 128.
13. Spira A: Practice tips from an avian practice. *Proc AAHA 47th Annual Meeting*:56, 1980.
14. Galvin C: Laboratory diagnostic aids in pet bird practice. *Proc AAHA 47th Annual Meeting*:50, 1980.
15. Altman R: Radiology, in Fowler ME (ed): *Zoo and Wild Animal Medicine*. Philadelphia, WB Saunders Co, 1978, pp 364-367.
16. Evans SM: Avian radiographic diagnosis. *Compend Contin Educ Pract Vet* 3(7):660-666, 1981.
17. Rosskopf WJ, Woerpel RW, Pitts BJ: Cropotomy in a parrot. *Mod Vet Pract* 63(3):219-222, 1982.
18. Redig P: Orthopedic and soft tissue surgery in raptorial birds, in Fowler ME (ed): *Zoo and Wild Animal Medicine*. Philadelphia, WB Saunders Co, 1978, pp 246-253.
19. Madill DN: Avian Surgery, in Hungerford TG (ed): *Proceedings No. 55 Refresher Course on Aviary and Caged Birds*. Sydney, Australia, The Post-graduate Committee in Veterinary Science, 1981, pp 208-209.
20. Amand WB: General techniques for avian surgery, in Kirk RW (ed): *Current Veterinary Therapy VI*. Philadelphia, WB Saunders Co, 1977, p 713.
21. Gandal CP: Anesthetic and surgical techniques, in Petrak ML (ed): *Diseases of Cage and Aviary Birds*. Philadelphia, Lea & Febiger, 1982, p 316.
22. Brooks NG: Crop wall necrosis in a sparrowhawk. *Vet Rec* 111(22):513, 1982.
23. Pepper WJ: Crop wall necrosis. *Vet Rec* 111(25/26):591, 1982.
24. Lafeber TJ: Respiratory diseases. *Vet Clin North Am* 3(2):218, 1973.
25. Altman RB: Conditions involving the integumentary system, in Petrak ML (ed): *Diseases of Cage and Aviary Birds*. Philadelphia, Lea & Febiger, 1982, pp 368-381.
26. Minsky L, Petrak ML: Diseases of the digestive system, in Petrak ML (ed): *Diseases of Cage and Aviary Birds*. Philadelphia, Lea & Febiger, 1982, pp 432-448.
27. Schultz DJ: Alimentary tract disease, in Hungerford TG (ed):

Proceedings No. 55 Refresher Course on Aviary and Caged Birds. Sydney, Australia, The Post-graduate Committee in Veterinary Science, 1981, pp 535-562.

28. Hurst GA: Crop impactions in bobwhite quail in Louisiana. *J Wildl Dis* 14:355-357, 1978.
29. Jarvis RL: Soybean impaction of waterfowl, in Hoff GL, Davis JW (eds): *Noninfectious Diseases of Wildlife.* Ames, IA, The Iowa State University Prèss, 1982, pp 109-112.
30. Halliwell WH: Diseases of birds of prey. *Vet Clin North Am* 9(3):541-568, 1979.
31. Batwell R: Crop lithiasis in a budgerigar. *Aust Vet J* 54:452-453, 1978.
32. Eamens GJ: Zoonoses and other human diseases associated with aviary and cage birds, in Hungerford TG (ed): *Proceedings No. 55 Refresher Course on Aviary and Caged Birds.* Sydney, Australia, The Post-graduate Committee in Veterinary Science, 1981, p 546.
33. Perry RA: Aspects of examination, diseases and therapy of caged birds, in Hungerford TG (ed): *Proceedings No. 55 Refresher Course on Aviary and Caged Birds.* Sydney, Australia, The Post-graduate Committee in Veterinary Science, 1981, p 118.
34. Kocan RM, Hasenclever HF: Normal yeast flora of the upper digestive tract of some wild columbids. *J Wildl Dis* 8:365-368, 1972.
35. Kocan RM, Hasenclever HF: Seasonal variation of the upper digestive tract yeast flora of feral pigeons. *J Wildl Dis* 10:263-266, 1974.
36. Jungerman PF, Schwartzman RM: *Veterinary Medical Mycology.* Philadelphia, Lea & Febiger, 1972.
37. Clubb SL: Infectious diseases. *Proc 1982 Annual Meeting of the AAV*:91-119, 1982.
38. Humphreys PN: Debilitating syndrome in budgerigars. *Vet Rec* 101:248-249, 1977.
39. Beemer AM, Kuttin ES, Katz Z: Epidemic venereal disease due to *Candida albicans* in geese in Israel. *Avian Dis* 17:639-649, 1973.
40. Chute HL: Fungal infections, in Hofstad MS (ed): *Diseases of Poultry.* Ames, IA, The Iowa State University Press, 1972, pp 458-463.
41. Carter GR: *Essentials of Veterinary Bacteriology and Mycology.* East Lansing, MI, Michigan State University Press, 1976.
42. Woerpel RW, Rosskopf WJ: Avian therapeutics. *Mod Vet Pract* 62:947-949, 1981.
43. Wood NA: Treatment of established infections of candidiasis in partridges with formic acid. *Vet Rec* 87:656-658, 1970.
44. Keymer IF: Parasitic diseases, in Petrak ML (ed): *Diseases of Cage and Aviary Birds,* Philadelphia, Lea & Febiger, 1982, pp 538-539.
45. Levine ND: *Protozoan Parasites of Domestic Animals and of Man.* Minneapolis, Burgess Publishing Co, 1973, pp 102-104.
46. Ahmed A, Pandurang A, Acharya RS, Ali G: Some observations on trichomoniasis of the upper digestive tract of love birds (budgerigars) in Hyderabad, Andhra Pradesh. *Indian Vet J* 47:210-212, 1970.
47. Griffiths HJ: *A Handbook of Veterinary Parasitology.* Minneapolis, University of Minnesota Press, 1978.
48. Soulsby EJL: *Helminths, Arthropods and Protozoa of Domesticated Animals.* Philadelphia, Lea & Febiger, 1982, pp 562-564.
49. Greve JH: Parasitic diseases, in Fowler ME (ed): *Zoo and Wild Animal Medicine.* Philadelphia, WB Saunders Co, 1978, p 380.
50. Conrad R: Pigeons-hygromycin-trichomoniasis. *Proc 19th Western Poultry Disease Conference, 4th Poultry Health Symposia*:15, 1970.
51. Kocan RM, Banko W: Trichomoniasis in the Hawaiian barred dove. *J Wildl Dis* 10:359-360, 1974.
52. Fowler ME: Doves, hornbills, toucans, and tinamous, in Fowler ME (ed): *Zoo and Wild Animal Medicine.* Philadelphia, WB Saunders Co, 1978, p 330.
53. Petrak ML, Gilmore CE: Neoplasms, in Petrak ML (ed): *Diseases of Cage and Aviary Birds.* Philadelphia, Lea & Febiger, 1982, pp 623-624.
54. Campbell TW: Unpublished case report, Kansas State University, 1981.

Update

Capillariasis can occasionally affect the oral cavity, esophagus, and crop of birds. *Capillaria* spp. cause thickening of the crop mucosa and can be identified by the presence of the characteristic double operculated oval ova in crop aspirate or swab samples. Anthelmintics such as fenbendazole (Panacur®—American Hoechst Corporation), 10 to 50 mg/kg body weight given orally once a day for five days, or mebendazole (Telmintic™—Pitman-Moore), 25 mg/kg body weight given orally twice a day for five days, can be used for the treatment of capillariasis.

During the physical examination, the esophageal and crop mucosa can be inspected by direct endoscopy.

DOSAGES FOR ANTIBIOTICS AND PARASITICIDES USED IN EXOTIC ANIMALS

Elliott Jacobson, DVM, PhD
George V. Kollias, Jr., DVM
Larry J. Peters, DVM

University of Florida
Gainesville, Florida

This series of tables is for veterinarians who need quick reference to a treatment regimen after they diagnose a disease in an exotic animal. Dosages for antibiotics and parasiticides are given for common amphibians, reptiles, rodents, and rabbits.

There are relatively few antibiotics/parasiticides for which detailed pharmacokinetic studies have been performed in laboratory and exotic animal species. Many of the dosages have been extrapolated from human and domestic animal species with efficacy based upon clinical impressions. Pharmacokinetic studies of gentamicin have shown that the half-life of this antibiotic (given the same dosage) is considerably longer in reptiles than in birds and mammals. Thus strict extrapolation from species to species and group to group, where scientific information is lacking, should be cautiously considered. The following tables cover dosages of antibiotics/parasiticides for a wide range of vertebrate species, combining information gathered from the literature and information gathered from the authors' clinical experience. Species-related idiosyncratic reactions are yet to be documented. The dosages given in these tables are only to be used as guidelines until further investigations document the most efficacious dosing regimen.

TABLE 1. COMMON ANTIMICROBIAL AND PARASITICIDE DOSAGES FOR SALAMANDERS, FROGS, AND TOADS

Primary Diagnosis	Location	Pathogen	Drug	Treatment
Redleg	Multiple: Septicemia with cutaneous hemorrhage	*Aeromonas hydrophila*	Tetracycline	5 mg/30 g PO bid for 7 days
			Gentamicin	2–4 mg/kg IM every 3 days for 4 treatments & 50 mg/38 L of water as a dip for 1 hr/day
			Furanace (Nifurpirinol)	250 mg/38 L of water as a dip for 1 hr/day
Cutaneous mycoses	Integument: Cutaneous ulcerations	*Saprolegnia, Phialophora*	Malachite green	0.15 mg/L of water as a dip 1 hr/day
			Potassium permanganate	0.2 mg/L of water as a dip 5 min per day
			Tinactin® (Tolnaftate)	Topical application
Cestodiasis	GI tract	*Ophiotaenia, Nemataenia, Diphyllobothrium*	Niclosamide	150 mg/kg PO as a single dose repeated in 2 wk
			Bunamidine	50 mg/kg PO as a single dose repeated in 2 wk
Nematodiasis	Lungs	*Rhabdias*	Levamisole	10 mg/kg IP as a single dose repeated in 2 wk
	GI tract	*Ophidascaris*	Thiabendazole	50 mg/kg PO as a single dose repeated in 2 wk
		Cosmocercoides	Mebendazole	20 mg/kg PO as a single dose repeated in 2 wk
		Oxsomatium	Piperazine salts	50 mg/kg PO as a single dose repeated in 2 wk

TABLE 2. COMMON ANTIMICROBIAL/PARASITICIDE DOSAGES FOR TURTLES AND TORTOISES

Primary Diagnosis	Location	Pathogen	Drug	Treatment
Septicemic cutaneous ulcerative disease (SCUD)	Multiple: Septicemia with cutaneous necrosis	*Citrobacter freundii, Serratia marcescens*	Chloramphenicol	20 mg/kg IM bid for 9 days
Ulcerative shell disease	Carapace, plastron, skin	*Beneckea chitinovora*	Chloramphenicol	20 mg/kg IM bid for 9 days
			Ampicillin trihydrate	6 mg/kg bid for 2 wk
Ulcerative stomatitis	Oral cavity	*Aeromonas, Pseudomonas*	Chloramphenicol	Same as above
			Gentamicin	For aquatic turtles, 10 mg/kg q48hr for 4–5 treatments. For tortoises, 2–4 mg q72hr for 4–5 treatments
		Vibrio	Oxytetracycline	10 mg/kg PO sid for 1 wk
Mycotic pneumonia	Lungs	*Paecilomyces, Beauvaria*	Ketoconazole	25 mg/kg PO sid for 2 wk
			Thiabendazole	50 mg/kg PO sid for 2 wk
Mycotic dermatitis	Carapace, plastron	*Penicillium*	Ketoconazole	Same as above
			Thiabendazole	Same as above
		Mucor	Malachite green	0.15 mg/L of water as a dip 1 hr per day for 2 wk
Otitis media	Middle ear below postocular tympanic scale	*Escherichia coli, Proteus*	Chloramphenicol	Same as above
			Gentamicin	Same as above

TABLE 3. COMMON ANTIMICROBIAL DOSAGES FOR ALLIGATORS, CAIMANS, AND CROCODILES

Primary Diagnosis	Location	Pathogen	Drug	Treatment
Bacterial pneumonia	Lungs	*Pasteurella multocida, Staphylococcus*	Chloramphenicol	20 mg/kg IM sid or bid (depending on size) for 9 days
Septicemia	Multiple	*Aeromonas*	Chloramphenicol	20 mg/kg IM sid or bid (depending on size) for 9 days
			Gentamicin	2 mg/kg every 72 hr for 5 treatments
			Tetracycline	10 mg/kg PO sid for 9 days
Mycotic dermatitis	Footpads, toes	*Trichophyton, Mucor*	Ketoconazole	50 mg/kg PO sid for 2 wk, topical use of organic iodine ointments
Nematodiasis	GI tract	*Dujardinascaris multicaecum*	Thiabendazole	50 mg/kg PO as a single dose repeated in 2 wk
			Mebendazole	20 mg/kg PO as a single dose repeated in 2 wk
			Piperazine	50 mg/kg PO as a single dose repeated in 2 wk

TABLE 4. COMMON ANTIMICROBIAL DOSAGES FOR LIZARDS AND SNAKES

Primary Diagnosis	Location	Pathogen	Drug	Treatment
Ulcerative stomatitis	Oral cavity	*Pseudomonas, Aeromonas*	Chloramphenicol	20 mg/kg IM bid for 9 days.
			Gentamicin	2–4 mg/kg IM q72hr for 5 treatments.
			Amikacin	2 mg/kg IM q72hr for 5 treatments.
			Carbenicillin	100 mg/kg IM or PO sid for 2 wk. Often aminoglycosides & carbenicillin are used in combination; with aminoglycoside therapy, make sure animal is hydrated.
Subcutaneous bacterial granulomas	Integument	*Proteus, Escherichia coli, Pseudomonas, Salmonella*	Chloramphenicol, gentamicin, amikacin, carbenicillin	Dose regimens same as above.
Pneumonia	Lungs/air sacs	*Pseudomonas, Aeromonas, Arizona, Proteus*	Chloramphenicol, gentamicin, amikacin, carbenicillin	Dose regimens same as above. Reptiles may also be nebulized with gentamicin or amikacin at 2 mg/10 ml saline.
			Tylosin	5 mg/kg IM sid for 10 days.
Systemic bacterial infections	All internal organ systems	*Pseudomonas, Aeromonas, Arizona, Salmonella*	Chloramphenicol, gentamicin, amikacin, carbenicillin	Dose regimens same as above.
Enteritis	Small intestine, colon	*Arizona, Salmonella, Proteus*	Chloramphenicol, gentamicin, amikacin, carbenicillin	Dose regimens same as above. Additional oral administration via stomach tube may be indicated. In snakes, many cases of enteritis are associated with parasitisms, & appropriate parasiticides should be used.
Osteomyelitis	Skeleton, palpebra, cornea	*Pseudomonas, Aeromonas, Citrobacter, Edwardsiella*	Trimethoprim-sulfadiazine	15 mg/kg PO sid for 2 wk.
			Tetracycline, gentamicin, amikacin	10 mg/kg PO sid for 2 wk.
Wound infections	Integumentary system	*Staphylococcus, Pseudomonas*	Gentamicin, amikacin	Dose regimen same as above.
		Peptostreptococcus	Lincomycin	10 mg/kg PO bid for 2 wk.
Pyodermas	Integumentary system	*Staphylococcus, Pseudomonas, Citrobacter*	Carbenicillin, gentamicin, amikacin	Dose regimen same as above.
Superficial ocular infections	Conjunctiva	*Pseudomonas, Aeromonas*	Chloramphenicol, gentamicin	Topical application of ophthalmic ointments.
Burn wounds	Integumentary system	*Pseudomonas*	Gentamicin, amikacin, chloramphenicol	Dose regimen same as above. Additionally, necrotic tissue should be removed & lesions packed with an organic iodine ointment.
Mycotic dermatitis	Integumentary system	*Penicillium, Fusarium*	Tinactin®	Debride necrotic debris & apply topically.
		Trichoderma, Geotrichum	Chlorhexidine diacetate, aqueous povidone-iodine	Use as a soak; dilute 1:10 & soak 1 hr bid. In conjunction with drug therapy, the environmental temperature should be 27–30° C.
Amebiasis	Gastrointestinal system, liver	*Entamoeba invadens*	Metronidazole	275 mg/kg PO as a single dose repeated in 2 wk.
			Dimetridazole	100 mg/kg PO as a single dose repeated in 2 wk or 20 mg/kg sid for 10 days.

TABLE 4. COMMON ANTIMICROBIAL DOSAGES FOR LIZARDS AND SNAKES (Continued)

Primary Diagnosis	Location	Pathogen	Drug	Treatment
Trichomoniasis	Gastrointestinal system	*Tetratrichomonas, Monocercomonas*	Metronidazole, dimetridazole	Dosage regimens same as above.
Coccidiosis	Gastrointestinal, biliary system	*Eimeria*	Sulfadiazine, sulfamerazine, sulfamethazine	25 mg/kg sid for 1 wk.
Cestodiasis	Gastrointestinal system	*Bothridium, Bothriocephalus, Ophiotaenia*	Bunamidine	50 mg/kg as a single dose repeated in 2 wk.
			Niclosamide	150 mg/kg as a single dose repeated in 2 wk.
Nematodiasis	Lung/air sac	*Rhabditis*	Levamisole	10 mg/kg IP as a single dose repeated in 2 wk.
	Esophagus/stomach Stomach Large intestine Colon	*Ophidascaris* *Physaloptera* *Kalicephalus* *Oxyurids*	Thiabendazole	50 mg/kg PO as a single dose repeated in 2 wk.
			Mebendazole	20–25 mg/kg PO as a single dose repeated in 2 wk.
Ascariasis	Integument	*Ophionyssus natracis*	DDVP (Vapona Pest Strip)	Hang in cage for 3 days. Remove water bowl & ensure good ventilation.

TABLE 5. COMMON ANTIMICROBIALS FOR GUINEA PIGS*

Type of Infection	Primary Diagnosis	Common Pathogen	Reported Drug of Choice for Treatment
Bacterial infections	Upper respiratory disease &/or pneumonia	*Bordetella bronchiseptica, Streptococcus, Klebsiella pneumoniae, Pasteurella multocida, Pseudomonas*	Cephaloridine, chloramphenicol, tetracycline, gentamicin
	Enteritis	*Yersinia pseudotuberculosis, Salmonella*	Chloramphenicol, tetracycline
	Septicemia	*Bordetella bronchiseptica*	Cephaloridine
		Yersinia pseudotuberculosis, Salmonella, Streptococcus	Chloramphenicol, tetracycline, gentamicin
	Abscesses, torticollis	*Yersinia pseudotuberculosis, Streptobacillus moniliformis, Streptococcus zooepidemicus*	
Parasitic infestation	Coccidiosis Intestinal Renal	 *Eimeria caviae* *Klosiella cobayae*	Sulfaquinoxaline
	Nematodiasis	*Paraspidodera uncinata*	Piperazine citrate 2–5 mg/ml in drinking water for 1 wk, repeat in 1 wk
	Acariasis	*Chirodiscoides caviae, Trixacarus caviae*	Put 1/3 dichlorvos strip on the cage (not in it) for 24 hr, repeat in 1 wk; or dip weekly for 3 wk with lindane solution .025% or malathion solution 2%. For pediculosis, use above treatments of dust twice a week with carbaryl powder 5% or pyrethrin dust 0.05–0.1%.
	Pediculosis	*Gliricola porcelli, Gyropus ovalis*	

*See Table 9 for dosages not given.

COMMENTS

Guinea pigs are very susceptible to the changes in bacterial flora & subsequent toxin production associated with the use of antibiotics. The following drugs are reported toxic in guinea pigs: clindamycin, penicillin, lincomycin, erythromycin, bacitracin.

Broad-spectrum antibiotics generally provide greater margins of safety.

TABLE 5. COMMON ANTIMICROBIALS FOR GUINEA PIGS* (Continued)

Type of Infection	Primary Diagnosis	Common Pathogen	Reported Drug of Choice for Treatment
Fungal infections	Superficial	*Trichophyton mentagrophytes*	Griseofulvin 75 mg/kg PO sid for 4 wk. Tolnaftate 1% cream topically bid for 4 wk.

TABLE 6. COMMON ANTIMICROBIALS FOR HAMSTERS*†

Species	Type of Infection	Primary Diagnosis	Common Pathogen	Reported Drug of Choice for Treatment
Hamster (*Mesocricetus auratus*)	Bacterial	Upper respiratory disease &/or pneumonia	*Pasteurella pneumotropica*	Chloramphenicol, tetracyclines, cephaloridine
		Wet tail	Specific pathogens unknown	Tetracycline, neomycin
		Other enteritidies	*Bacillus piliformis, Salmonella*	Chloramphenicol
		Septicemia	*Bacillus piliformis, Salmonella*	Tetracycline, chloramphenicol
		Abscesses	*Pasteurella pneumotropica, Staphylococcus aureus*	Chloramphenicol, cephaloridine, tetracycline
	Parasitic infestations	Coccidiosis		
		Cestodiasis	*Hymenolepis nana*‡	Niclosamide 100 mg/kg PO, repeat in 7 days
		Nematodiasis	*Syphacia obvelata, Aspicularis tetraptera*	Piperazine citrate 10 mg/ml in drinking water for 1 wk, repeat in 1 wk
		Acariasis	*Demodex aurati, Demodex criceti*	1–5.5 mixture of ronnel & propylene glycol applied daily for 3–5 wk
	Fungal infections	Superficial	*Trichophyton*	Griseofulvin 25 mg/kg PO sid for 2–4 wk
Gerbil (*Meriones unguiculatus*)				Treat empirically as per hamsters
Ferret (*Mustela putorius*)				Treat empirically as per the domestic cat

*See Table 9 for dosages not given.
†Clindamycin is reportedly toxic in these animals. Their response to certain types of antibiotics is very similar to that of guinea pigs. Streptomycin 50 mg bid reportedly toxic.
‡Good sanitation is imperative in management of *H. nana*. Hymenolepids can infect humans.

TABLE 7. COMMON ANTIMICROBIALS FOR MICE AND RATS*†

Type of Infection	Primary Diagnosis	Common Pathogen	Reported Drug of Choice for Treatment
Bacterial infections	Upper respiratory disease &/or pneumonia	*Corynebacterium kutscheri, Pasteurella multocida, Pasteurella pneumotropica, Mycoplasma pulmonis, Klebsiella pneumoniae, Streptococcus pneumoniae, Bordetella bronchiseptica*	Chloramphenicol, tetracycline, cephaloridine, tylosin, sulfamerazine†

*See Table 9 for dosages not given.
†Hymenolepids can infect humans.

TABLE 7. COMMON ANTIMICROBIALS FOR MICE AND RATS*† (Continued)

Type of Infection	Primary Diagnosis	Common Pathogen	Reported Drug of Choice for Treatment
Bacterial infections (Continued)	Enteritis	*Salmonella enteritidis, Bacillus piliformis, Citrobacter freundii*	Chloramphenicol, tetracycline
	Septicemia, abscesses	*Pasteurella multocida, Salmonella enteritidis, Salmonella typhimurium, Bacillus piliformis, Pseudomonas aeruginosa, Corynebacterium kutscheri, Streptococcus*	Chloramphenicol, tetracycline, ampicillin, cephaloridine
	Skin infections	*Staphylococcus aureus*	Ampicillin, cephaloridine
	Torticollis, polyarthritis	*Mycoplasma pulmonis, Streptococcus, Streptobacillus moniliformis*	Chloramphenicol, tylosin
Parasitic infestations	Coccidiosis		
	Intestinal	*Eimeria falciformis*	Sulfaquinoxaline
	Hepatic	*Klossiella muris*	
	Cestodiasis	*Hymenolepis nana, Hymenolepis diminuta*†	Niclosamide 100 mg/kg PO, repeat in 7 days
	Larva form	*Taenia taeniaeformis*	
	Nematodiasis	*Syphacia obvelata, Aspicularis tetraptera*	Piperazine citrate in drinking water for 1 wk, repeat in 1 wk
	Pediculosis	*Polyplax serrata, Polyplax spinulosa*	Carbaryl powder or pyrethrin dust or place 1/3 dichlorvos-impregnated strip on cage (not in it) for 24 hr; repeat in 1 wk; or dip weekly in malathion solution 2% or lindane solution .025%
	Acariasis	*Myobia musculi, Radfordia affinis, Myocoptes musculinus, Psorergates simplex, Ornithonyssus bacoti*	Same as above
Fungal infections	Superficial	*Trichophyton mentagrophytes, Microsporum gypseum*	Griseofulvin 25 mg/kg sid PO for 4 wk

*See Table 9 for dosages not given.
†Hymenolepids can infect humans.

TABLE 8. COMMON ANTIMICROBIALS FOR RABBITS*

Type of Infection	Primary Diagnosis	Common Pathogen	Reported Drug of Choice for Treatment
Bacterial	Upper respiratory disease &/or pneumonia	*Pasteurella multocida, Bordetella bronchiseptica, Klebsiella pneumoniae, Pseudomonas aeruginosa, Streptococcus, Staphylococcus aureus*	Ampicillin, chloramphenicol, cephaloridine, tetracycline, gentamicin, furazolidone, sulfaquinoxaline
	Mucoid enteritis	Unknown	Tetracycline

*See Table 9 for dosages not given and for withdrawal times.

TABLE 8. COMMON ANTIMICROBIALS FOR RABBITS* (Continued)

Type of Infection	Primary Diagnosis	Common Pathogen	Reported Drug of Choice for Treatment
Bacterial (Continued)	Acute typhlitis	*Bacillus piliformis*	Sulfaquinoxaline, chloramphenicol, sulfamerazine
	Diarrhea	*Salmonella*	Furazolidone
	Vent disease	*Treponema cuniculi*	Penicillin
	Orchitis	*P. multocida*	Ampicillin
	Metritis	*P. multocida, Listeria monocytogenes*	Chloramphenicol, tetracycline
	Mastitis *(blue belly)*	*S. aureus, Streptococcus, Pseudomonas*	Gentamicin
	Septicemias	*Staphylococcus, Listeria, Salmonella, Pseudomonas*	Chloramphenicol, ampicillin, tetracycline, gentamicin
	Abscesses	*P. multocida*	Ampicillin
		Staphylococcus	Chloramphenicol
		Fusobacterium necrophorum	Penicillin
		Pseudomonas	Gentamicin
		Streptococcus	Tetracycline
	Skin infections	*Staphylococcus*	
	Torticollis	*P. multocida*	
	Conjunctivitis	*P. multocida, S. aureus*	Ophthalmic preparation bid
Parasitic infestations	Coccidiosis Hepatic	*Eimeria stiedae*	Sulfaquinoxaline
	Intestinal	*Eimeria magna, Eimeria media, Eimeria perforans, Eimeria irresidua*	Sulfaquinoxaline
	Cestodiasis larvae form	*Taenia pisiformis*	Niclosamide 100 mg/kg PO, repeat in 7 days
	Nematodiasis	*Passalurus*	Piperazine 200 mg/kg PO
		Trichuris	Thiabendazole 100–200 mg/kg PO
	Acariasis Ear mites	*Psoroptes cuniculi*	Mineral oil or commercial ear mite medication; retreat in 10–14 days
	Fur mites	*Cheyletiella parasitivorax, Listrophorus gibbus*	Rabon dust 3%, carbaryl powder 5%.
	Pediculosis	*Haemodipsus ventricosus*	Put 1/3 dichlorvos strip on cage (not in it) for 24 hr; repeat in 1 wk; or dip in lindane solution 0.25% or malathion solution 2%

*See Table 9 for dosages not given and for withdrawal times.

TABLE 8. COMMON ANTIMICROBIALS FOR RABBITS* (Continued)

Type of Infection	Primary Diagnosis	Common Pathogen	Reported Drug of Choice for Treatment
Fungal infections	Superficial	*Trichophyton mentagrophytes*	Griseofulvin 25 mg/kg PO for 2–4 wk
		Microsporum	Tolnaftate topically bid

TABLE 9. COMMON ANTIMICROBIALS FOR RODENTS AND RABBITS

Drug	Guinea Pigs	Hamsters	Rabbits	Rats/Mice	Comments
Ampicillin			10–25 mg/kg IM for 5–7 days		Wait 6 days before slaughter.
Cephaloridine	10–25 mg/kg IM or SQ tid for 5–7 days	10–25 mg/kg IM or SQ daily for 5–7 days	10–25 mg/kg SQ or IM sid for 5–7 days	10–25 mg/kg IM or SQ sid for 5–7 days	*Pseudomonas* often resistant to cephaloridine.
Chloramphenicol*	50 mg/kg PO tid for 5 days, or 30–50 mg/kg IM or IV for 5–7 days	50 mg/kg PO tid for 5–7 days, or 30–50 mg/kg IM, IV, or IP for 5–7 days	50 mg/kg PO tid for 5–7 days, or 30 mg/kg IV or IM tid for 5–7 days	50 mg/kg PO tid for 5 days, or 30 mg/kg IV or IM tid for 5 days	Not for use in food animals.
Furazolidone			.01% in drinking water for 2 wk, or 5 mg/kg sid PO for 2 wk		For prevention.
Gentamicin	5 mg/kg IM or SQ sid for 5 days	5 mg/kg IM or SQ sid for 5 days	5 mg/kg IM or SQ sid for 5 days	5 mg/kg IM or SQ sid for 5 days	Not for use in food animals.
Neomycin		100 mg/kg PO sid for 5 days & supportive care			
Penicillin	Contraindicated		20,000–60,000 IU/kg IM daily for 5–7 days, can add streptomycin at 20 mg/kg	Penicillin procaine & streptomycin reportedly toxic to small rodents	Wait 30 days before slaughter.
Sulfaquinoxaline	1% in drinking water for 2 wk		1% in drinking water for 2 wk (treatment), .025% in drinking water for 30 days (prevention)		For prevention. Do not slaughter for 2 wk posttreatment. Permitted by FDA as an additive to feed.
Sulfamerazine			.02% in drinking water for 7–10 days	1 mg/4 g feed, or .02% in drinking water for 7–10 days	
Sulfamethazine	1 g/L in drinking water		5–10 g/kg of feed; 1 g/L drinking water (prevention)		
Oxytetracycline	Soluble powder, 1 mg/ml in drinking water for 5–7 days	Soluble powder, 1 mg/ml in drinking water for 5–7 days	Oral suspension,* 50–100 mg/kg PO tid for 5 days; soluble powder, 1 mg/ml drinking water for 1 wk	Soluble powder, 3–5 mg/ml drinking water for 7 days	Wait 18 days before slaughter.* Prepare fresh every other day.
Tylosin				10 mg/kg IM sid for 5 days	

*Considerations in the use of chloramphenicol are as follows: Depression from acute overdose can be treated with 10% dextrose; chloramphenicol is antagonistic with penicillin & streptomycin; it prolongs pentobarbital anesthesia; it is not cleared for use in breeding animals; & it is possibly synergistic with tetracycline.

Ophthalmology of Exotic Pets

Michael G. Davidson, DVM
Department of Companion Animal
and Special Species Medicine
School of Veterinary Medicine
North Carolina State University
Raleigh, North Carolina

The recent increase in popularity of exotic pets has stimulated an interest in the ophthalmic disorders that affect these species. A wide variety of ophthalmic disorders, both primary (involving the eye) and secondary (causing systemic disease), affect exotic pets. Although most ocular disease problems in such animals can be managed by the same general principles applied to other species,[1,2] specific ocular characteristics of exotic animals affect the examination, manifestation, and treatment of their ophthalmic diseases. This article discusses the pertinent ocular anatomy and physiology and the specific ocular disorders afflicting the commonly encountered exotic animal species.

Exotic Mammalian Pets—Guinea Pigs, Gerbils, Hamsters, Ferrets, and Rabbits

Anatomy

The ocular structure of exotic mammalian pets is similar in most respects to that of other mammals. Being descended from nocturnal ancestors, most of their ocular development is directed toward seeing at night or in burrowing habitats. Characteristic features include a spherically shaped globe that is protected by an upper, a lower, and a third (nictitating membrane) eyelid. The upper eyelid typically is the most mobile; the action of the third eyelid is entirely passive, sweeping over the cornea as the globe is retracted into the orbit. There are two tear-producing glands: a lacrimal gland, situated in the temporal and dorsal aspect of the orbit, and a gland associated with the nictitating membrane. A venous sinus is located in the ventral orbit of rodents; its major clinical significance is to serve as a common site for collecting blood samples. The pupillary sphincter muscle is nonstriated, allowing pharmacologic blockage of its action by parasympatholytic agents, such as atropine. Rodents and rabbits have round pupils; ferrets have horizontally oval pupils that contract to small slits. Except in albinos, iris coloration is varying shades of brown. The accommodative ability of these species is limited by a relatively large, round lens and a small, rudimentary ciliary body.[2,3]

The most noticeable difference in ocular anatomy among exotic mammals is the pattern of the retinal vasculature system and the appearance of the ocular fundus. Gerbils and hamsters have a fundus typical of most rodents, with a holangiotic, or well-vascularized, retina. The optic disk is centrally located, with four to eight arterioles and venules radiating outward in a spokelike fashion. The fundus of ferrets also is holangiotic and is similar in appearance to that of dogs. The vessels emanate from a well-myelinated optic disk. The tapetum, a specialized reflective layer of cells in the choroid, is well developed in ferrets.

The guinea pig retina is paurangiotic, or poorly vascularized, with a few small arcades of vessels immediately surrounding the optic disk. In pigmented guinea pigs, the fundus is mottled red-brown; in albinotic guinea pigs, it is diffusely red. The fundus of rabbits is merangiotic, or partially vascularized (Figure 1). Retinal vessels, present only in a horizontal line along either side of the optic disk, overlie a band of heavily myelinated nerve fibers extending several disk diameters from the optic nerve. The optic disk, with its deep physiologic cup, is situated above the horizontal midline of the eye. The photoreceptors in the retina of these species are predominantly rods, which aid vision in diminished light.[2-5]

Examination

Ocular examination of most exotic mammalian pets is difficult because the globe is small. A focal light source or slit-lamp biomicroscope is used to examine the adnexa and the anterior segment. Because of the small size of the eye, mydriasis is especially important for visualization of the posterior segment. A solution of 1% tropicamide or 1% atropine effectively dilates the pupils of most exotic mammals.[1] The pupils of pigmented rodents occasionally are resistant to dilation because the melanin granules in the iris bind the mydriatic and thus inhibit its action. In such cases, 1% atropine solution mixed with equal parts of 10% phenylephrine solution and applied three to four times during a 15-minute period is an effective mydriatic.[1] Because of the small size of the eye, indirect ophthalmoscopy provides the best opportunity for fundus evaluation.

Diseases of the Eye

Pasteurellosis

Pasteurella multocida, the most common bacterial pathogen found in rabbits, is a frequent cause of rhinitis, pneumonia, otitis media, subcutaneous abscesses, and septicemia. *Pasteurella multocida* also can affect the eye, in association with these conditions or as an isolated ocular condition. Chronic conjunctivitis with resultant epiphora is the most common ocular manifestation of *Pasteurella multocida* infection. Anterior uveitis also occurs[6-8] (Figure 2). It is important to rule out other noninfectious causes of conjunctivitis and ocular discharge, such as entropion,[9] dust,[7] trauma,[6,7] and distichiasis,[9] in rabbits. *Pasteurella multocida* conjunctivitis is treated effectively with procaine penicillin G at 60,000 IU/kg intramuscularly once a day for 10 days, along with topical chloramphenicol ophthalmic solution or ointment applied four times a day.[6,8-10]

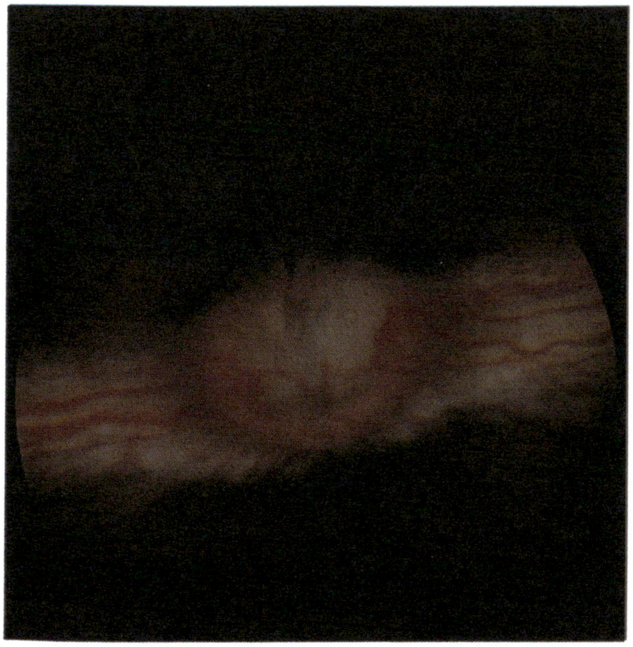

Figure 1—The fundus of a pigmented rabbit. Myelinated nerve fibers and vessels extend from the optic disk.

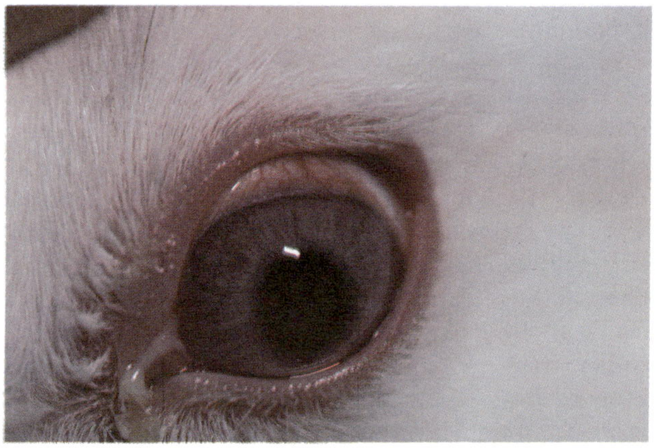

Figure 2—*Pasteurella* conjunctivitis in an albino rabbit.

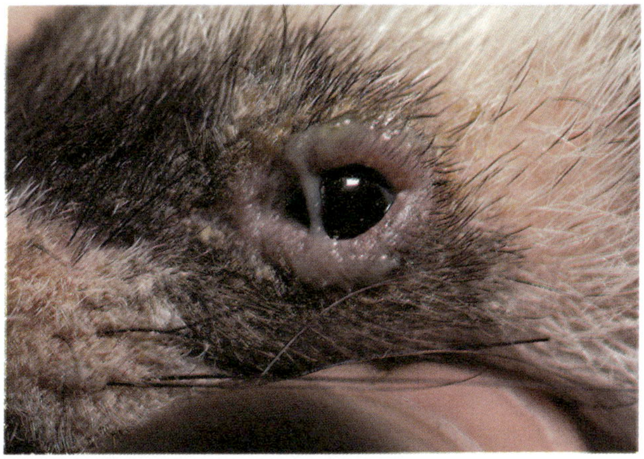

Figure 3—Canine distemper infection in a ferret. Note the severe blepharitis and mucoid ocular discharge.

Myxomatosis

Myxomatosis is a viral disease that is enzootic in wild rabbits along the West Coast of the United States. Transmitted by mosquitoes and fleas, the virus poses a constant threat to commercial and pet rabbits in that area. Blepharoconjunctivitis; swelling and closure of the eyelids; and a thick, mucoid ocular discharge are present in acute infections. When the disease is chronic, swelling of the face and the urogenital area can occur and subcutaneous tumors can develop.[10-12] Diagnosis is based on clinical signs and histologic examination of conjunctival biopsies for intracytoplasmic inclusion bodies in epithelial cells. Mortality in affected domestic rabbits ranges from 25% to 50%.[12] Infected animals should be culled and disposed of by burning to prevent further spread of the disease. Mosquito and flea control is helpful in epizootics.[10]

Canine Distemper Virus

Moderate to severe conjunctivitis accompanied by mucoid ocular and nasal discharge is a common finding in ferrets infected with canine distemper virus. The ocular discharge is an early clinical sign, occurring 7 to 10 days after exposure to the virus. Additional ocular findings can include severe blepharitis, keratoconjunctivitis sicca, and corneal ulceration (Figure 3). Several days after the conjunctivitis, an erythematous, pruritic skin rash consistently develops under the chin, in the inguinal region, and on the foot pads. The clinical course of distemper virus infection in ferrets is variable, largely depending on the strain of the causative virus. Animals infected with ferret-adapted strains die 12 to 16 days after exposure; those infected with canine strains succumb 21 to 35 days postexposure.[13-16] Clinical signs strongly suggest the disease; the diagnosis can be confirmed antemortem with serum antibody titers to distemper virus or with immunofluorescent antibody studies on conjunctival swabs or blood smears. Mortality in infected ferrets is virtually 100%, and euthanasia is a recommended alternative to supportive care.[14,15] To help prevent the disease, ferrets should be vaccinated with a distemper vaccine of chick embryo origin at 8 and 10 weeks of age and every 3 years thereafter.[14,15,17]

Guinea Pig Inclusion Conjunctivitis

Guinea pig inclusion conjunctivitis is a naturally occurring infection caused by a member of the *Chlamydia psittaci* group. Ocular changes include conjunctivitis with follicular formation, slight chemosis, and serous ocular discharge. Intracytoplasmic inclusion bodies are visible on cytologic examination of conjunctival scrapings taken during the acute stages of the disease. The disease is mild and self-limiting, and usually no treatment is necessary. Recovered animals are resistant to reinfection. The organism also infects the genital tract of guinea pigs, and offspring of infected animals can develop neonatal conjunctivitis. Guinea pig inclusion conjunctivitis is a proposed animal model for human ocular infection with *Chlamydia trachomatis*, a leading cause of blindness in Third World countries.[18,19]

Chromodacryorrhea

Secretion of pigmented tears is a normal physiologic process in many rodents, including gerbils. The pigment results from porphyrins synthesized in the harderian gland and excreted with the tear film. The red crusts that commonly accumulate on the medial canthus, the nose, and the paws of gerbils should not be misinterpreted as dried blood.[1,2,20,21]

Excessive pigment accumulation from epiphora is abnormal and signifies an underlying disease process. Overgrowth of the lower incisor teeth can obstruct the nasolacrimal duct in rodents and cause epiphora; corrective dentistry alleviates the condition.[1] Epiphora and excessive pigment accumulation in rodents also are attributed to stress, vitamin A or riboflavin deficiency,[20] and infection of the salivary and orbital tear glands with the sialodacryoadenitis virus.[22]

Lens Opacities

Cataracts are uncommon in small rodents; however, spontaneous opacification of the lens is observed in small mammals subjected to prolonged sedation or anesthesia. Such cataracts result from nonclosure of the eyelids, with subsequent evaporation of the aqueous humor and anterior lens opacification. Evaporation cataracts are reversible and usually resolve on recovery from anesthesia.[1,23]

Cataracts of juvenile onset occur in ferrets, possibly as a heritable trait.[15,24] Successful surgical removal of the lens is feasible despite the small size of the globe in ferrets.

Congenital and Hereditary Defects

Several congenital and/or hereditary anomalies that affect the eyes of rabbits have been described. These defects are significant primarily because of the widespread use of rabbits in comparative ophthalmic research. Colobomas—notchlike defects of the optic nerve, the retina, the sclera, and the choroid—occur in rabbits. Colobomas are believed to result from defective closure of the fetal ocular fissure during embryologic development. These defects occur frequently in rabbits with microphthalmic eyes and, less frequently, with eyes of normal size.[2,5] Congenital cataracts[25] and persistent hyperplastic vitreous with lens opacities[2,5] also have been reported in rabbits. In New Zealand white rabbits, inherited glaucoma is recognized by the development of buphthalmia, corneal edema, and conjunctival injection at three to four months of age.[2,5,7] Conjunctivitis and blepharospasm also have been reported in a litter of rabbits with congenital entropion of the upper eyelids. Surgical correction resulted in alleviation of the disorder.[9] Congenital ocular defects described in other species include corneal dermoids in ferrets[15] and microphthalmia in a hamster.[10]

Birds

Anatomy

The eyes of birds are interesting and highly developed. The globe is large relative to body size; a bird's eyes often outweigh its brain.[3] The large globe fits tightly in the bony orbit; eye movement is negligible or absent because extraocular muscles are small and rudimentary. The extreme neck mobility of most birds, especially raptors, compensates for the lack of ocular mobility.

Birds have a semitransparent third eyelid supplied with skeletal muscle. The nictitating membrane is positioned in the dorsomedial aspect of the globe and sweeps ventrolaterally across the cornea; in some species, it is believed to cover and protect the eye during flight. A lacrimal gland located ventrotemporally in the orbit and a harderian gland associated with the third eyelid supply the tear flow. Striated muscle is present in the iris, which forms a round pupil that responds poorly to light but is active during accommodation or excitement. Yellow, red, and brown are predominant iris colors. The ciliary muscle is composed of striated muscle fibers that allow voluntary control of accommodation. The large, pliable lens and the striated musculature of the ciliary muscle and the iris endow birds with excellent accommodative ability.[3,4,26-28]

The avian retina is devoid of blood vessels (anangiotic) and is characterized by the presence of a pecten, a structure unique to birds. The pecten is a pigmented, plicated structure arising from and obscuring the optic disk and extending into the vitreous body.[3,4,26-29] The function of the pecten has been debated for decades; although its purpose is still uncertain, it probably produces intraocular fluid.[30-32] The type, density, and number of photoreceptors vary with species; the retinas of nocturnal birds primarily contain rods, and those of diurnal birds primarily contain cones. The fovea, a specialized area in the retina responsible for visual acuity, is well developed in birds; some species are bifoveal.[3,4,26] The inner layers of the retina are absent in the fovea, allowing more light stimulus to reach the outer photoreceptor layer.

Examination

Although primary ocular disorders are encountered in birds, ocular involvement from periorbital or systemic disease processes is more common.[29-33] A thorough physical examination is required in birds presented with eye disease. The anterior segment and the adnexa can be evaluated with a focal light source. Hippus, a rapid, cyclic contraction and dilatation of the iris, is common in excited birds.[29] Consensual pupillary response is absent in birds and other submammalian species. Because of striated muscle fibers in the iris, mydriasis for examining the posterior segment requires a muscle-paralyzing agent. The pupils of most birds can be effectively dilated with 3 mg of tubocurare powder per ml of 0.025% benzalkonium chloride solution applied three to four times during a 20-minute period. The commercially available aqueous form of tubocurare (Tubocurarine chloride injection—Solvay Veterinary) is ineffective because of poor corneal penetration.[1,26,33]

Diseases of the Eye

Avian Pox

Periocular disease is common in patients affected with avian pox, a viral disease of many species of wild and pet birds. Avian pox occurs in two forms, which can exist singularly or in combination. In the wet (or diphtheric) form, fibrinous plaques develop in the oral cavity and in the upper respiratory tract. Ocular lesions include caseous plaques on the eyelids; swelling of the eyelids to the point of closure; and severe, exudative conjunctivitis (Figure 4). In the dry (or cutaneous) form, proliferative skin lesions develop around the eyes, the beak, the nares, and the feet. Scabs form on the eyelids 10 to 14 days after infection and often become secondarily infected with bacteria or fungi.

Diagnosis of avian pox is based on clinical appearance and histopathologic demonstration of characteristic intracytoplasmic inclusion bodies in pox lesions or conjunctival biopsies. Treatment should include systemic antibiotics (5 mg/kg of intramuscular gentamicin twice a day)[29] and high doses of vitamin A (30,000 IU/kg once every 10 days intramuscularly). A topical ophthalmic antibiotic (Gentocin® Ophthalmic Ointment—Schering) is applied two to three times a day if secondary bacterial conjunctivitis or blepharitis is present. Birds with extensive blepharal swelling have difficulty finding food and require tube feeding. Pox lesions can be treated with 1% to 3% merbromin (Mercurochrome®—Becton Dickinson) in a 70% alcohol solution

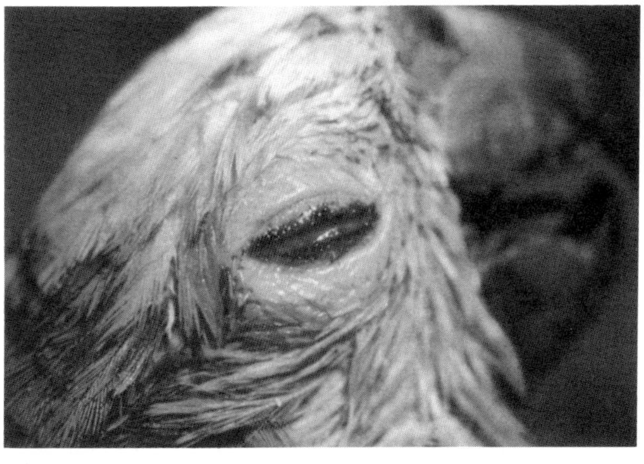

Figure 4—A blue-fronted Amazon parrot with the diphtheric form of avian pox. Severe blepharal swelling and secondary bacterial conjunctivitis are present.

twice a day. Scabs should be allowed to fall off; excessive damage to the lid margin can result if scabs are pulled off. Recovered animals can demonstrate scarring and depigmentation of the lids, lacrimal discharge, and chronic corneal ulceration. Mortality is variable, depending on the strain of the virus and the species affected. The canary, the lovebird, and the blue-fronted Amazon parrot are highly susceptible to the effects of the disease.[28,29,33-35]

Parasitic Diseases

Knemidokoptic (scaly-leg) mites commonly involve the beak, the cere, and the periorbital area of budgerigars. Long-term infestation results in hyperkeratosis with buildup of keratin and sebaceous material. Corneal irritation or ulceration can occur with extensive lesions. Diagnosis is based on direct observation and identifying the mites from a skin scraping. The mites usually are eliminated by a mild acaricide or plain mineral oil applied topically twice a week until the lesions resolve. A protective ophthalmic ointment is placed in the patient's eyes before treatment. Because topical therapy near the eyes can be irritating, an alternate effective treatment is a single intramuscular dose of ivermectin (Ivomec®—MSD AGVET) at 200 μg/kg.[28]

Oxyspirura mansoni

Oxyspirura mansoni is a small nematode that commonly infects the conjunctival sacs of cockatoos. When infestation is heavy, the eyelids swell and the patient might scratch its eyes. Treatment with ivermectin and washing the eye to remove dead worms are effective.[28]

Sinusitis and Rhinitis

Conjunctivitis and ocular discharge can occur concurrently with upper respiratory tract infection. Causes of sinusitis or rhinitis in birds include chlamydial, viral, mycoplasmal, and bacterial agents.[28] Abscessation of the infraorbital sinus or the periorbit is a possible sequela in chronic cases; this abscessation is evidenced by swelling and inflammation of the sinus and the surrounding structures above or below the orbit. Although many cases of sinusitis, rhinitis, or conjunctivitis respond to systemic antibiotics and vitamin A therapy, surgical curettage and flushing often is necessary in cases of sinus abscessation.[28,29,33] Ocular lesions usually resolve after treatment of the upper respiratory tract infection.[28]

Hypovitaminosis A

Hypovitaminosis A is an important nutritional problem encountered most frequently in psittacines fed an all-seed diet. Clinical signs associated with avian vitamin A deficiency include generalized unthriftiness and lethargy. Upper respiratory tract inflammation and secondary infection also occur and manifest as sneezing and nasal discharge. Ocular signs include keratoconjunctivitis sicca, blepharitis, and ocular discharge. Secondary bacterial or fungal infection of the eyelids can result from compromised epithelial integrity.[33,36] Therapy includes oral vitamin A (25 IU/g of body weight once a day for two to four weeks) and diet supplementation with foodstuffs high in vitamin A (leafy green or yellow vegetables, cod-liver oil, beef liver).[36]

Trauma

The large, protruding globes of birds predispose them to traumatic ocular injuries. This is evident especially in wild raptors in physical injury rehabilitation programs (Figure 5).[37] In one study, 18% of injured raptors had ocular lesions, the majority resulting from collisions or gunshots.[38] Superficial corneal wounds of raptors and caged birds are treated with frequent application of topical antibiotics. Cycloplegics, such as atropine, are useless in birds. Temporary tarsorrhaphy, using non-absorbable 3-0 or 4-0 suture material, is necessary for deeper corneal ulcers or descemetoceles. Third eyelid flaps are difficult to place and maintain in birds because of the skeletal muscle supply. Elizabethan collars can be used to prevent self-trauma. In the absence of corneal ulceration, traumatic uveitis or hyphema should be treated with topical corticosteroids.[26,28,33,37]

Enucleation of the Avian Eye

Enucleation might be necessary in birds with intraocular or orbital tumors, severe traumatic injury, abscesses of the globe or the orbit, or panophthalmitis.[39,40] The procedure is disfiguring and relatively difficult to perform because of the large size of the globe and its tight fit in the bony orbit. A subconjunctival approach is practicable in most pet birds (Figure 6). The orbital

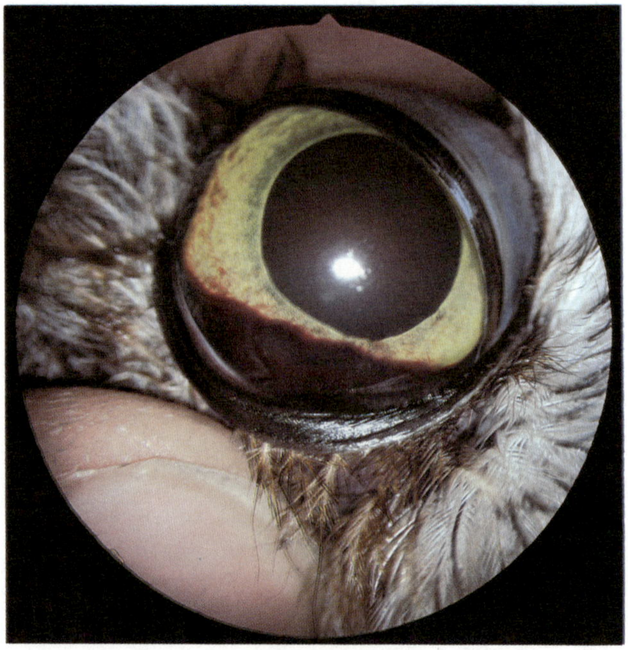

Figure 5—Ocular trauma causing hyphema in a screech owl.

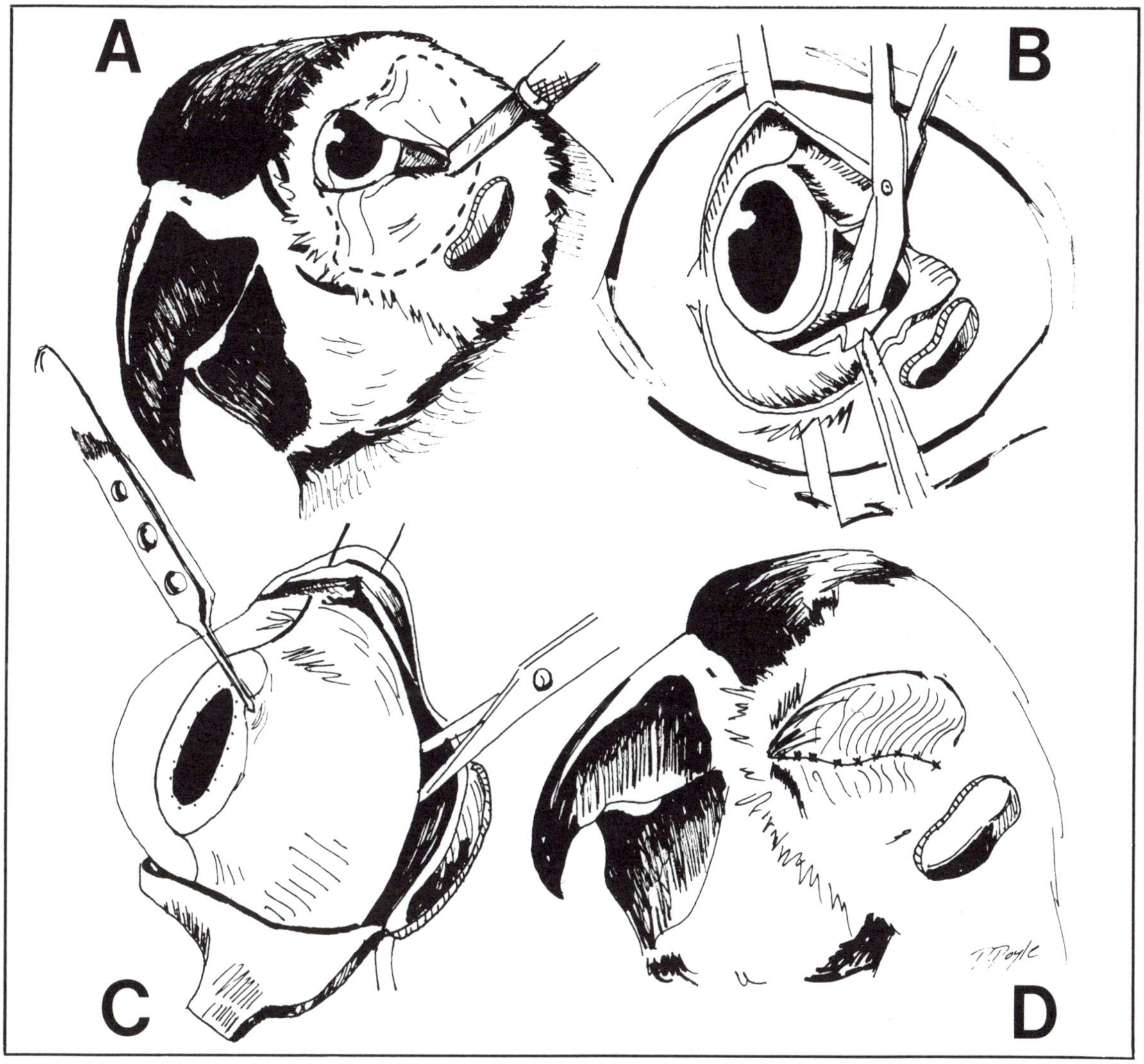

Figure 6—Enucleation in a caged bird. (*A*) Stay sutures are placed in the eyelids, and a lateral canthotomy is performed. The dotted line indicates extent of the globe in the bony orbit. (*B*) A circumferential incision is made in the conjunctiva and Tenon's capsule 1 to 2 mm from the limbus, followed by a 360° subconjunctival dissection. The extraocular muscles are severed at their attachment to the globe. Care is taken not to damage the orbital bones. (*C*) Tension is placed on the lateral limbus with fine forceps, and the globe is rotated medially. This allows access to the optic nerve and vessels, which are incised near the globe. The remaining conjunctiva and the third eyelid are removed. (*D*) A 1-mm strip is removed from each lid margin. The margins then are sutured with 5-0 nonabsorbable suture material. (From Murphy CJ, Brooks DE, Kern TE, et al: Enucleation in birds of prey. *JAVMA* 183(11):1234-1237, 1983. Modified with permission.)

bones are thin and fragile and easily damaged by excessive dissection. Care should be taken to avoid excessive tension on the optic nerve during the procedure—damage to the optic chiasm and the opposite optic nerve can result.

A globe-collapsing procedure also has been described, in which the sclera and the associated ossicles are severed to allow access to the optic nerve. The technique is suitable for removing the relatively large eyes of raptors, but it precludes complete histologic examination of the globe.[40]

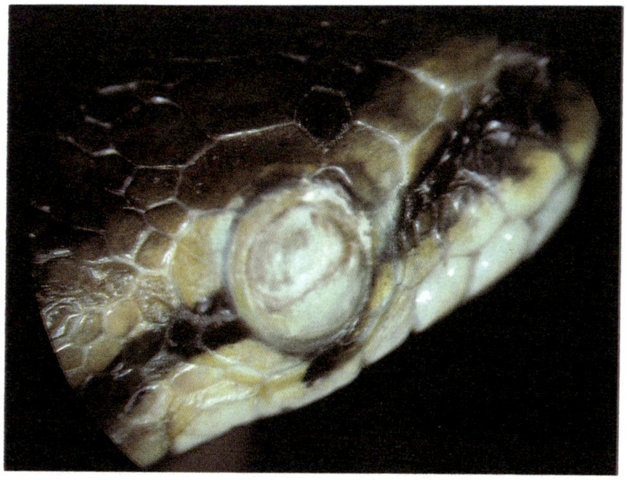

Figure 7—Retained corneal spectacle and secondary candidiasis in a ball python.

Cataracts

Cataracts have been reported in many avian species[2,26,28,29,41-43] and are a relatively common cause of blindness in older caged birds. Cataracts were noted in

0.4% of a group of birds from a zoologic collection.[44] Most cataracts in pet birds have no identifiable cause and are considered to be senile changes. Heritable, nuclear, and cortical cataracts have been identified in a group of related canaries.[43] Pet birds adapt comparatively well to blindness, provided items in their environments are not moved and they are fed on a routine schedule. Cage tops should be padded to prevent trauma to the thin cranial bones.[33] Surgical correction of cataracts, using lens extraction or phacoemulsification techniques, has been accomplished successfully.[45-47]

Neoplasia

Primary neoplasia of the eye and the adnexa is rare in birds.[33] Although budgerigars have the highest incidence of neoplasia of all animals, their eyes are not predisposed.[48] The few tumors reported include lipogranulomas of the eyelid,[33,49] gliomas of the optic nerve,[50] and orbital sarcomas.[51] Proptosis has been reported secondary to pituitary tumors in canaries.[52]

Reptiles

Anatomy

Reptilian pets generally are limited to three groups: the lacertilians (lizards), the chelonians (turtles), and the ophidians (snakes). The eyes of lizards and turtles closely resemble each other and are representative of most reptiles. The typical reptilian eye has a movable upper and lower eyelid and an active nictitating membrane. Similar to the avian eye, scleral ossicles surround the anterior globe and provide support. Striated muscle is present in the iris and the ciliary body. A harderian gland and a lacrimal gland provide tears, which flow directly into the oral cavity via the nasolacrimal duct; turtles lack this duct. The retina is avascular and is nourished by the choroidal vasculature. Most species possess a conus papillaris; this plicated structure overlies the optic disk and is analogous to the avian pecten.[3,4,53-55]

The ocular anatomy of snakes differs considerably from that of other reptiles. These differences are believed to result from an evolutionary period in which a burrowing, underground habitat resulted in rudimentary eyes that lost most specialized adaptations. When the snakes reemerged to their present habitat, their eyes redeveloped and underwent a phylogenesis separate from that of other reptilian species.[3,4,55] The globes lack scleral ossicles or other cartilaginous support. The eyelids are fused embryologically and form a transparent, protective spectacle. The space between the spectacle and the cornea communicates with the oral cavity via the nasolacrimal duct. The nictitating membrane is absent. Snakes lack a conus papillaris; instead the retina is covered by the membrana vasculosa, a fine network of capillaries overlying but not penetrating the surface of the retina.[3,53-55]

Examination

Examination of a reptile presented for ocular disease should include a thorough physical examination with special attention to the integument (especially periocular) and the oral cavity because diseases of these systems often accompany ocular diseases. The anterior segment is examined with a focal light source. In snakes, it is important to differentiate the subspecular space from the anterior chamber.[55] Visualization of the posterior segment and the fundus with the aid of mydriatics is impossible in reptiles because of the striated muscle in the iris and the ciliary body. In snakes, the relatively impervious spectacle further inhibits absorption of topical mydriatics. Reptilian mydriasis usually is best achieved under general anesthesia.[55]

Diseases of the Eye

Hypovitaminosis A

Vitamin A deficiency is frequently encountered in reptiles, especially turtles. Diets containing excessive quantities of skeletal muscle or poor-quality vegetables are likely to be vitamin A deficient. Hypovitaminosis A causes squamous metaplasia of the ducts and the parenchyma of the harderian and the lacrimal glands. Palpebral edema and conjunctivitis are clinically evident. Secondary bacterial or fungal blepharitis or keratoconjunctivitis also can occur. Treatment with a single intramuscular dose of vitamin A (5,000 to 10,000 IU) will reverse the clinical signs in early cases and halt progression of the disease in more advanced cases. Small amounts of cod-liver oil added to the diet will prevent hypovitaminosis A.[1,54-58]

Dysecdysis

Dysecdysis, or abnormal shedding of the skin, commonly occurs in snakes as the result of poor husbandry practices. A number of factors can lead to dyscedysis, including malnutrition, dehydration, low environmental relative humidity, systemic illness, thryoid dysfunction, or lack of proper cage substrate as an abrasive for initiating the shedding process. The normal shedding process begins with dulling of the skin and the spectacle. This cloudy appearance gradually fades in 7 to 10 days, just before the outer skin, including the spectacle, is shed. Dysecdysis often manifests clinically as retained, opaque corneal spectacles (Figure 7). Retained spectacles render a snake functionally blind and can impair seriously its ability to feed.[54,59,60]

A retained spectacle often can be removed with gentle traction using fine forceps. Care must be taken not to remove the underlying new spectacle because permanent corneal damage can result. Snakes with tightly adherent retained spectacles should be soaked in warm water (just enough to cover the snake) overnight. The spectacle is rubbed free gently with moistened cotton the next day. If the spectacle still is difficult to remove by this method, it is best left until the next shedding, thereby avoiding damage to the new spectacle. Systemic disorders or environmental conditions that might contribute to the problem should be corrected. Ideal relative humidity for snakes is 50% to 60%. Bricks or logs placed in the cage will aid the snake in removing the old skin.[53-55,60]

Distention of the Subspecular Space

Fluid distention and/or abscessation of the subspecular space in snakes can occur secondary to inflammatory conditions affecting the oral cavity, such as ulcerative stomatitis (Figure 8). The distention results from occlusion of the nasolacrimal duct at its oral opening. Bacterial or fungal infection of the mouth can ascend the duct and involve the subspecular space. To relieve the distention, a small wedge-shaped area in the ventral spectacle is removed using a #15 Bard-Parker scalpel blade. Removal is followed by flushing the subspecular space with a triple antibiotic ophthalmic solution. The stomatitis is treated concurrently with hydrogen peroxide mouthwashes and systemic antibiotics.[1,53-55]

Infectious Diseases

Abscessation involving the conjunctiva, the periorbit, or the retrobulbar area is common in reptiles.[53,55] Infectious keratoconjunctivitis also occurs, often as the result of poor hygiene. Local extension of these infectious conditions can produce panophthalmitis. Gram-negative organisms—*Proteus*, *Pseudomonas*, and *Aeromonas* spp.—are the predominant bacterial pathogens in reptiles. Opportunistic fungal infections also are commonly encountered.[54,61-65] Treatment of these infectious conditions follows basic ophthalmic principles, including drainage, topical and systemic antibiotics, topical antifungal agents, and enucleation in advanced cases. Topical treatment usually is ineffective in snakes because the keratinous spectacle is impermeable to topically applied medications. Infectious ocular diseases can indicate poor environmental conditions that should be corrected. To prevent trauma and infection to the eye, live prey should be killed routinely before feeding.[7]

Parasitic Diseases

Acariasis caused by *Ophionyssus* spp. is encountered frequently in snakes; mites are commonly found in the recess between the periocular space and the spectacle. A dichlorvos-impregnated strip (No Pest Strip®—Shell) placed in the cage effectively removes mites. The strip is left in the cage for three days, and the cage then is disinfected; the process is repeated in two weeks.[55]

Other Reptilian Conditions

A mucoid discharge appears in turtles after hibernation but requires no treatment.[55] Cataracts[54] and lenticular sclerosis[54,59] occur in snakes. Congenital microphthalmia, although uncommon, also has been reported in snakes.[55]

Summary

The eyes of exotic small mammals, birds, and reptiles have developed uniquely as dictated by the environments of their ancestors. Disease processes that involve the eyes of exotics often reflect these unique characteristics; however, the eye responds to insult in a limited number of ways. This limitation is no less true in exotic species than in common domestic animals. With this concept and a general understanding of the principles of veterinary ophthalmology, the clinician is equipped to manage ocular disorders of any species, including the exotics.

REFERENCES

1. Bellhorn RW: Ophthalmic disorders of exotic and laboratory animals. *Vet Clin North Am* 3(3):345-357, 1973.
2. Bellhorn RW: Laboratory animal ophthalmology, in Gellatt KN (ed): *Veterinary Ophthalmology*. Philadelphia, Lea & Febiger, 1981, pp 649-671.
3. Duke-Elder S: *Systems of Ophthalmology*, vol 1. St. Louis, The CV Mosby Co, 1958, pp 352-427.
4. Walls GI: *The Vertebrate Eye and Its Adaptive Radiation*. Bloomfield Hills, MI, Crenbrook Press, 1942, pp 607-675.
5. Rubin LF: *Atlas of Veterinary Ophthalmology*. Philadelphia, Lea & Febiger, 1974, pp 367-398.
6. Raphael BL: Pet rabbit medicine. *Compend Contin Educ Pract Vet* 3(1):60-65, 1981.
7. Fox JG, Cohen BJ, Loew FM: *Laboratory Animal Medicine*. Orlando, Academic Press, 1984, pp 149-204.
8. Harkness JE, Wagner JE: *The Biology and Medicine of Rabbits and Rodents*. Philadelphia, Lea & Febiger, 1983, pp 75-90.
9. Fox JG, Shalev M, Beaucage CM, et al: Congenital entropion in a litter of rabbits. *Lab Anim Sci* 29:509-511, 1979.
10. Hime JM, O'Donoghue PN: *Handbook of Diseases of Laboratory Animals*. London, Heinman Veterinary Books, 1979, pp 137-219.
11. Williams CSF: *Practical Guide to Laboratory Animals*. St. Louis, The CV Mosby Co, 1976, pp 148-170.
12. Patton NM, Holmes HT: Myxomatosis in domestic rabbits in Oregon. *JAVMA* 171(6):560-562, 1977.
13. Wallach JD, Beaver WJ: *Diseases of Exotic Animals*. Philadelphia, WB Saunders Co, 1983, pp 495-534.
14. Ryland LM, Gorham JR: The ferret and its diseases. *JAVMA* 173(9):1154-1158, 1978.
15. Ryland LM, Bernard SL, Gorham JR: A clinical guide to the pet ferret. *Compend Contin Educ Pract Vet* 5(1):25-32, 1982.
16. Dunkin GW, Lordlaw PP: Studies in dog distemper. I: Dog distemper in the ferret. *J Comp Pathol Therap* 39:201-212, 1927.
17. Rockbau G, Norby E, Lonnek N: Comparison between immunization efects in dogs and ferrets of living vaccines, attenuated in dog tissue cultures and embryonated eggs. *Res Vet Sci* 6:423-427, 1965.
18. Murray ES: Guinea pig inclusion conjunctivitis virus. I: Isolation and identification as a member of the psittacossi-lymphogranuloma-trachoma group. *J Infect Dis* 116:203-210, 1964.
19. Malaty R: Chlamydial conjunctivitis in the guinea pig, in Tabbara KF, Cello R (eds): *Animal Models of Ocular Disease*. Springfield, IL, Charles C Thomas, 1982, pp 79-86.
20. Harkness JE, Ridgeway MD: Chromodacryorrhea in laboratory rats (*Rattus norvegicus*): Etiologic considerations. *Lab Anim* 30:841-844, 1980.
21. Thiessen DD, Pendergrass M: Harderian gland involvement in fascial lesions in the Mongolian gerbil. *JAVMA* 181(11):1375-1377, 1982.
22. Weisbroth SH, Peress N: Ophthalmic lesions and dacryoadenitis: A naturally occurring aspect of sialodacryoadenitis virus infection of the laboratory rat. *Lab Anim Sci* 27:466-473, 1977.

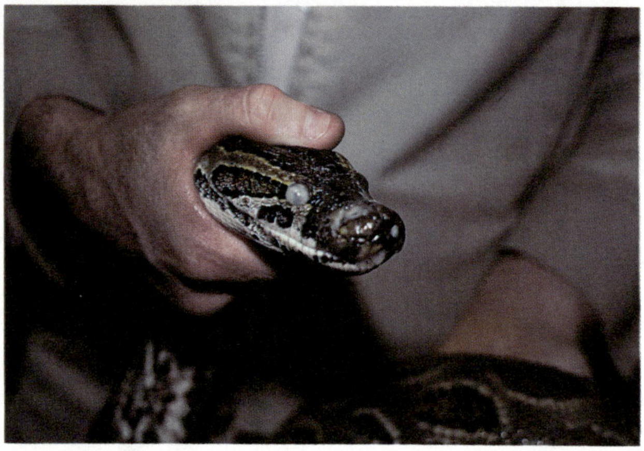

Figure 8—Distention of the subspecular space in a reticulated python. Note the discharge from the oral and nasal cavities. (Courtesy of Dr. Vicki Scheidt, North Carolina State University)

23. Frankfelder FT, Burns RP: Effect of lid closure in drug induced experimental cataracts. *Arch Ophthalmol* 76:559-564, 1966.
24. Utroska B, Austin WL: Bilateral cataracts in a ferret. *VM SAC* 74:1176-1179, 1979.
25. Gelatt KN: Congenital cataracts in a litter of rabbits. *JAVMA* 167(7):598-599, 1975.
26. Greenwood AG, Burnett KC: The investigation of visual defects in raptors, in Cooper JE (ed): *Recent Advances in the Study of Raptor Disease*. West Yorkshire, England, Cherion Publishing Co, 1981, pp 131-135.
27. Fox R, Lehmkukle SW, Broh RC: Stereopsis in the falcon. *Science* 197:79-81, 1977.
28. Karpinski C, Clubb S: Clinical aspects of ophthalmology in caged birds. *Annu Meet Assoc Avian Vet*: 216-227, 1983.
29. Zenoble RD: Selected diseases of the head and face in caged birds. *Compend Contin Educ Pract Vet* 4(12):995-1105, 1982.
30. Bellhorn RW, Bellhorn MS: The avian pecten. I: Fluorescein permeability. *Ophthalmic Res* 7:1-7, 1975.
31. Raviola E, Raviola G: A light and electron microscope study of the pecten of the pigeon eye. *Am J Anat* 120:427-435, 1967.
32. Seamson AR, Himelfarb TM: Correlated ultrafine structural changes of the avian pecten oculi and ciliary body of *Gallus domesticus*. *Am J Ophthalmol* 56:278-282, 1963.
33. Small E, Buke TJ: Diseases of organs of special senses, in Petrak ML (ed): *Diseases of Caged and Aviary Birds*. Philadelphia, Lea & Febiger, 1982, pp 491-495.
34. Arnall L, Keymer TF: *Bird Diseases*. Neptune City, NJ, T.F.H. Publishing Co, 1975, pp 95-100.
35. McDonald SE, Lowenstine LJ, Ardans AA: Avian pox in blue-fronted Amazons. *JAVMA* 179(11):1218-1222, 1981.
36. Pitts C: Hypovitaminosis A in psittacines, in Kirk RW (ed): *Current Veterinary Therapy VIII*. Philadelphia, WB Saunders Co, 1984, pp 622-626.
37. Murphy CJ, Kern TJ, Riis RC: Intraocular trauma in a red-tailed hawk. *JAVMA* 181(11):1340-1341, 1982.
38. Murphy CJ, Kern TJ, McKeever LLD, et al: Ocular lesions in free-living raptors. *JAVMA* 181(11):1302-1304, 1982.
39. Altman B: General principles of avian surgery. *Compend Contin Educ Pract Vet* 3(2):177-184, 1981.
40. Murphy CJ, Brook DE, Kern JE, et al: Enucleation in birds of prey. *JAVMA* 183(11):1234-1237, 1983.
41. Keymer IF: Cataracts in birds. *Avian Pathol* 6:335-341, 1977.
42. Tudor DC: Retinal atrophy in a parakeet. *VM SAC* 73:1456-1457, 1978.
43. Slatter DH, Bradley JS, Vale B, et al: Hereditary cataracts in canaries. *JAVMA* 183(8):872-874, 1983.
44. Schmidt RE, Toft JD: Ophthalmic lesions in animals from a zoological collection. *J Wildl Dis* 17(2):267-275, 1981.
45. Kern TJ, Murphy CJ, Riis RC: Lens extraction by phacoemulsification in two raptors. *JAVMA* 185(11):1403-1406, 1984.
46. Brooks DE, Murphy CJ, Quensenberry KE, et al: Surgical correction of a luxated cataractous lens in a barred owl. *JAVMA* 183(11):1298-1299, 1983.
47. Gandal CP, Amand WB: Anesthetic and surgical techniques, in Petrak ML (ed): *Diseases of Caged and Aviary Birds*. Philadelphia, Lea & Febiger, 1982, pp 304-325.
48. Ratdiff HC: Incidence and nature of tumors in captive wild mammals and birds. *Am J Cancer* 17:116-135, 1935.
49. Small E: Diseases of the organs of special senses, in Petrak ML (ed): *Diseases of Caged and Aviary Birds*. Philadelphia, Lea & Febiger, 1969, pp 351-355.
50. Arnall L: Anesthesia and surgery in caged and aviary birds. III: A systematic outline of surgical corrections. *Vet Rec* 73:188-192, 1961.
51. Arnall L: Anesthesia and surgery in caged and aviary birds. II: A regional outline of surgical considerations. *Vet Rec* 73:172-178, 1961.
52. Schalmberger HG: Neoplasia in parakeets, spontaneous chromophobe pituitary tumors. *Cancer Res* 14:237, 1954.
53. Marcus LC: *Veterinary Biology and Medicine of Captive Amphibians and Reptiles*. Philadelphia, Lea & Febiger, 1981, pp 42-46.
54. Frye FJ: *Biological and Surgical Aspects of Captive Reptile Husbandry*. Edwardsville, KS, Veterinary Medical Publishing Co, 1981, pp 228-240.
55. Millinchamp JT, Jacobson ER, Wolf DE: Diseases of the eye and adnexa in reptiles. *JAVMA* 183(11):1205-1212, 1983.
56. Wallach JD: Environmental and nutritional diseases of captive reptiles. *JAVMA* 159(11):1632-1643, 1971.
57. Elkon E, Zwart P: The ocular disease of young terrapins caused by vitamin A deficiency. *Pathol Vet* 4:201-222, 1967.
58. Wallach JD, Beaver WJ: *Diseases of Exotic Animals*. Philadelphia, WB Saunders Co, 1983, pp 979-1047.
59. Frye FJ: *Husbandry, Medicine, and Surgery in Captive Reptiles*. Bonner Springs, KS, Veterinary Medical Publishing Co, 1973, pp 70-75.
60. Jacobson ER: Histology, endocrinology, and husbandry of ecdysis in snakes (A review). *VM SAC* 72:275-280, 1977.
61. Marcus LC: Infectious diseases of reptiles. *JAVMA* 159(11):1626-1631, 1971.
62. Leonard JL, Shields RP: Acid fast granuloma in a turtle eye. *JAVMA* 157(5):612-613, 1970.
63. Collette BE, Curry OH: Mycotic keratitis in a reticulated python. *JAVMA* 173(9):1117-1118, 1978.
64. Barney CH, Hartfield DA, Schmidt RE: *Klebsiella* pneumonia infection with secondary hypopyon in Tokyo gecko lizards. *JAVMA* 173(9):1115-1116, 1978.
65. Townson FN, MacDonald SE, Wolf ED: Hypopyon in a tortoise. *JAVMA* 169(11):942, 1976.